Physician Assistant's Guide to Research and Medical Literature

SECOND EDITION

Physician Assistant's Guide to Research and Medical Literature

J. Dennis Blessing, PhD, PA-C
Professor and Chair
Department of Physician Assistant Studies
School of Allied Health Sciences
The University of Texas Health Science Center at San Antonio
San Antonio, Texas

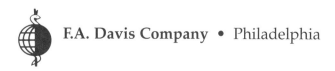
F.A. Davis Company • Philadelphia

F. A. Davis Company
1915 Arch Street
Philadelphia, PA 19103
www.fadavis.com

Printed in the United States of America

Last digit indicates print number: 10 9 8 7 6 5 4 3 2 1

Acquisitions Editor: Andy McPhee
Developmental Editor: Jennifer Pine
Art & Design Manager: Carolyn O'Brien

As new scientific information becomes available through basic and clinical research, recommended treatments and drug therapies undergo changes. The author(s) and publisher have done everything possible to make this book accurate, up to date, and in accord with accepted standards at the time of publication. The authors, editors, and publisher are not responsible for errors or omissions or for consequences from application of the book, and make no warranty, expressed or implied, in regard to the contents of the book. Any practice described in this book should be applied by the reader in accordance with professional standards of care used in regard to the unique circumstances that may apply in each situation. The reader is advised always to check product information (package inserts) for changes and new information regarding dose and contraindications before administering any drug. Caution is especially urged when using new or infrequently ordered drugs.

Library of Congress Cataloging-in-Publication Data

Physician assistant's guide to research and medical literature / [edited by] J. Dennis Blessing.—2nd ed.
   p. cm.
  Includes bibliographical references and index.
  ISBN 0–8036–1244–3
  1. Physicians' assistants. 2. Physicians' assistants-Research. 3. Medical literature. I. Blessing,
J. Dennis.
  R697.P45P488 2005
  610.73'72069-dc22   2005045473

This book is dedicated to my father, Oscar B. Blessing,
and to the memory of my mother, June J. Taylor.

I further dedicate this effort to my wife, Brenda G. Blessing,
and my sisters, Janice L. Blessing, Connie E. Blessing, and Sereta L. Summers.

I am pleased that the first edition of this book was received well enough to warrant a second edition. It is clear that research skills are becoming more and more important to physician assistants, physician assistant students, and physician assistant educators. There is so much that we don't know about ourselves as physician assistants and what we do. Today's ever changing world asks more of its health care providers than ever before. Resting on yesterday's knowledge will not solve today's problems or meet tomorrow's challenges. Research is the base for what we do as clinicians. Research brings us the medicines we use, provides better equipment and technology, informs us of what people think and feel, governs how we work, and helps us make decisions. Health care trends and today's medical environment make our understanding and use of research more important than ever. Whether you are a practicing physician assistant, student, or faculty member, research is important to you and a part of what you do now and will do every day.

One of the recurring comments from the people who reviewed and commented on the first edition of our book was that it was readable and easy to understand. One of my original intentions was to make the book a user-friendly guide. That commitment and understanding was shared and met by the first edition's contributors. While this book is greatly expanded, the basic commitment to readability remains.

You will find that this book contains much more content than its predecessor. We have expanded and added to the content of every chapter and added new chapters and sections. All the original contributors have returned and new contributors have joined us in this effort. Evaluations and comments from educators, researchers, students, and practicing physician assistants guided our decisions in what to include and change in this edition. We wanted to broaden the scope of the book and meet the needs of more people. From the very beginning we have intended that this book be a beginner's or introductory guide.

Every author has contributed to the literature on physician assistants. Every author is an experienced researcher and writer. The authors' skills and abilities represent a wide cross-section of the physician assistant and research worlds. All are committed to the advancement of physician assistants and research.

This guide is especially appropriate as a textbook to accompany medical research courses in PA programs. It will cover research as it applies to practice, education, and social aspects related to the PA profession. Of particular interest are the chapters on interpreting the medical literature and the chapter on grant writing. The chapter on presenting research results has been expanded to include oral and poster presentations. The data analysis chapter has been expanded and includes decision trees for choosing statistical tests. A chapter on human subjects and dealing with Institutional Review Boards is added. Introductions to clinical investigations, evidence-based medicine, clinical reviews, surveys, and needs assessments are now presented.

Currently there are over 60,000 practicing PAs in the United States, and they are involved in every type of medical practice, setting, and specialty. There are a number of clinical, legal, social, and ethical aspects of practice that warrant investigation, using precise, formal research techniques. In addition, there are 134 PA educational programs with approximately 10,000 students enrolled. Accreditation requires all programs to educate students on research and how to interpret medical literature. Approximately 70% of PA programs are offered the master's level, and students are required to complete a major paper, project, or thesis. In addition, research and scholarly activity are integral components of the expectations for PA educators, especially those in tenure track positions. This book can act as a resource, reference, and text for all PAs, whether they are practicing clinicians, educators, or students. This book should be a starting point and one of many tools as you seek the answers that are so important to the care of people and the advancement of the physician assistant profession.

J. Dennis Blessing

No textbook is entirely the result of a single individual's effort, and this one is no different. So many people have contributed in so many ways that it is impossible to thank them all. For all those I fail to name in this acknowledgment, please forgive me. Everyone I know has contributed in some way.

The contributors to the text deserve much praise for their work. Their efforts have resulted in a body of work that is truly greater than the sum of its parts. All of these individuals believe in the value of research for the physician assistant profession. Any one of them could have undertaken the production of this book and succeeded. They are a truly dedicated group of people and we are fortunate to be able to share in their expertise.

I know that each of our authors would agree that we must thank the students who inspire us to work harder and our clinical colleagues who put our work to the test. For many of us, it is the curiosity and quest for knowledge of our students that drive us in our research efforts. The dedication and quality care of our practicing colleagues inspire us to equal their efforts. The physician assistant profession is a pool of challenges and questions that need answers. It is our hope that this book will help our students and colleagues develop the skills they need to provide answers to the many challenges of medicine and society.

Equal thanks must go to the people who work "behind-the-scenes" at F.A. Davis. I know working with editors and authors is like herding cats, but the folks at F.A. Davis are special people with high levels of tolerance and patience. Without the efforts of Carl Holm, Jennifer Pine, Margaret Biblis, Kimberly Harris, Andy McPhee, and all the other folks at F.A. Davis, you would not be reading and using this second edition. Their guidance has been invaluable. While he was not involved with this edition, I want to thank Sandy Reinhardt for his help in getting all this started.

I also want to express special thanks to my boss, Dr. Marilyn S. Harrington, Dean of the School of Allied Health Sciences, The University of Texas Health Science Center at San Antonio for her support of scholarly activity and research across the health sciences. She is a model for us all. Dr. Douglas Murphy, Associate Dean, Mr. Terry Duffey, Assistant to the Dean, and Ms. Denice Trevino, Administrative Assistant, have all contributed to my efforts along the way.

Next (and certainly not least), my colleagues in the Department of Physician Assistant Studies, The University of Texas Health Science Center at San Antonio have been unrelenting in their support of my writing efforts. These people are the faculty and staff who carry out the day-to-day activities of an educational unit that frees me to undertake my writing. They put up with my idiosyncrasies, offer advice, make suggestions, and, sometimes, yell back. They may not always know it, but they are keys to any success that I have and that this book may achieve. Very special thanks to Judith E. Colver, J. Glenn Forister, Lisa N. Reyna, Miguel Ramirez-Colon, Daniel W. Wood, Estela Sifuentes, and Kathy Mercado-Vasquez. They are a remarkable group.

Special thanks go to Dr. Cindy Olney and Dr. Douglas Murphy, both at The University of Texas Health Science Center at San Antonio, for making suggestions and critiquing chapters in their areas of expertise.

Lastly, I must make a special note of thank you to my mentor. We all need role models and people who guide us as we grow and develop as professionals. Most of us can identify a number of people who help us along the way, but there is always one person who seems to contribute or inspire a little more. For me, that person is Dr. Richard R. Rahr. Long before I ever wrote a single word or became a chairperson, I recognized that Dr. Rahr was a model for physician assistant educators. We have had a long relationship as colleagues, and the 11 years that I worked for him were a truly formative period for me as teacher, administrator, and physician assistant. I have never met anyone as unselfish as Dr. Rahr. I still call on him for advice and help. I hope that everyone who reads this book can find a mentor like him.

Salah Ayachi, PhD, PA-C
Associate Professor
Department of Physician Assistant Studies
School of Allied Health Sciences
The University of Texas Medical Branch at Galveston
Galveston, Texas

Debra L. Benfield, MEd, RD, LDN
Master Project Director
Physician Assistant Program
Wake Forest University Health Sciences
Wake Forest University School of Medicine
Winston-Salem, North Carolina

Christopher E. Bork, PhD
Dean, School of Allied Health
Director, Center for Creative Instruction
Professor of Physical Therapy
Professor of Orthopedic Surgery
Medical College of Ohio at Toledo
Toledo, Ohio

James F. Cawley, MPH, PA-C
Professor and Director, Physician Assistant Master of Public Health Program
Department of Prevention and Community Health
School of Public Health and Health Services
Professor of Health Care Sciences
School of Medicine and Health Sciences
The George Washington University
Washington, D.C.

Meredith A. Davison, PhD
Professor and Director
Physician Assistant Program
Midwestern University
Downers Grove, Illinois

Richard W. Dehn, MPA, PA-C
Clinical Professor and Associate Director
Physician Assistant Program
University of Iowa
Iowa City, Iowa

Anita Duhl Glicken, MSW
Professor of Pediatrics
Child Heath Associate/Physician Assistant Program
University of Colorado Health Sciences Center
Aurora, Colorado

Constance Goldgar, MS, PA-C
Director of Graduate Studies
Physician Assistant Program
University of Utah
Salt Lake City, Utah

William D. Hendricson, MA, MS
Director, Division of Educational Research and Development
The University of Texas Health Science Center at San Antonio
San Antonio, Texas

Roderick S. Hooker, PhD, PA
Professor
University of Texas Southwestern Medical Center
Medical Staff, The Department of Veterans Affairs, Medical Service
Dallas, Texas

Robert W. Jarski, PhD, PA-C
Professor and Director, Complementary Medicine and Wellness Program
School of Health Sciences
Oakland University
Rochester, Michigan

P. Eugene Jones, PhD, PA-C
Professor and Chairman
Department of Physician Assistant Studies
The University of Texas Southwestern Medical
Center at Dallas
Dallas, Texas

Marvis J. Lary, PhD, PA-C
Dean, The Herbert H. and Grace A. Dow
College of Health Professions
Central Michigan University
Mt. Pleasant, Michigan

Raylene Lawrence, PA
Physician Assistant Student
The University of Washington Medex
Program
Teaching Intern
The University of Texas Medical Branch
at Galveston
Galveston, Texas

Anthony A. Miller, MEd, PA-C
Associate Professor and Director
Physician Assistant Program
Shenandoah University
Winchester, Virginia

Bruce R. Niebuhr, PhD
Associate Professor
Department of Physician Assistant Studies
Department of Preventive Medicine and
Community Health
The University of Texas Medical Branch
at Galveston
Galveston, Texas

Suzanne M. Peloquin, PhD, OTR, FAOTA
Professor
Department of Occupational Therapy
School of Allied Health Sciences
The University of Texas Medical Branch at
Galveston
Galveston, Texas

Richard R. Rahr, EdD, PA-C
Professor and Chair
Department of Physician Assistant Studies
School of Allied Health Sciences
The University of Texas Medical Branch at
Galveston
Galveston, Texas

Virginia A. Rahr, RN-C, EdD
Associate Professor
School of Nursing
The University of Texas Medical Branch
at Galveston
Galveston, Texas

Scott D. Rhodes, PhD, MPH, CHES
Assistant Professor
Section on Social Sciences and Health Policy
Department of Public Health Sciences
Wake Forest University Health Sciences
Winston-Salem, North Carolina

Albert F. Simon, DHSC, PA-C
Chair
Department of Physician Assistant Sciences
St. Francis University
Loretto, Pennsylvania

Bonnie, A. Dadig, EdD, PA-C
Professor
Physician Assistant Department
Medical College of Georgia
Augusta, Georgia

Catherine Gillespie. DHSc, PA-C
Assistant Professor
Physician Assistant Department
Gannon University
Erie, Pennsylvania

Dawn Morton-Rias, PD, PA-C
Dean, Collge of Health Related Professions
State University of New York
Downstate Medical Center
Brooklyn, New York

Martha Petersen, MPH, CHES, PA-C
Assistant Professor
Physician Assistant Program
Rangos School of Health Sciences
DuQuesne University
Pittsburgh, Pennsylvania

Sara H. Reffett, MSA, PA-C
Professor
Physician Assistant Department
Medical College of Georgia
Augusta, Georgia

Robert J. Spears, MPAS, PA-C
Assistant Professor
Physician Assistant Program
University of Findlay
Findlay, Ohio

Gary R. Uremovich, MS, MPAS, PA-C
Assistant Professor
Department of Allied Health
Kettering College of Medical Arts
Springfield, Ohio

SECTION I

Contemplating Research

chapter 1

Research: A Powerful Tool

J. Dennis Blessing, PhD, PA-C

The beginning of research is curiosity, its essence is discernment, and its goal truth and justice.
Isaac H. Satanov

If we knew what it was we were doing, it would not be called research, would it?
Albert Einstein

There is no doubt that the physician assistant (PA) profession has had a significant impact on American medicine and American health. The PA concept initially was developed in response to the specific health-care needs of rural America and the loss of physicians from general practice, but it was nurtured by the social changes of the 1960s and 1970s and influenced by the availability of experienced medics and corpsmen from the war in Viet Nam.[1] The profession has been greatly affected by external factors that had little relationship to the field itself, but that generated expansion and contraction of federal support and the opening and closing of educational programs, particularly in the 1980s. The 1990s were a boom decade for PAs. Demand for PAs was fueled by attempts on the part of government and big business to control costs and by expanded practice privileges for PAs, acceptance by physicians and other health-care professionals, and acceptance and recognition by the public. In 1992, 57 PA programs were educating and training approximately 3,500 students, with about half graduating each year. In 2004, 133 PA programs were educating and training 9,800 students.[2] The American Academy of Physician Assistants estimated that in December 2002 57,879 individuals were eligible to practice as PAs.[3] This is remarkable growth and, yet, there is much that we do not know about the practice of PAs and their short-term and long-term effects on the health of our country's population.

A major issue for our profession is that we have not developed a cadre of PA researchers. This is understandable because the profession has concentrated on creating practitioners, and clinical practice has been the reason that individuals choose to become PAs. This author believes that clinical practice and service should continue to be the major driving force for PAs. However, it is time for our professional organizations and educational institutions to support and develop a core of researchers who will take the lead in developing an understanding of the social and medical impact of PAs. The changing climate of medical practice in light of developing evidence-based medicine, new technology, population demographics, and the challenges of new and changing disease patterns places a research burden on all practitioners, including PAs.

More and more PAs are involved with clinical investigations and other types of research today, and this will continue to an even greater extent in the future. As students develop research skills as part of their education and training, they will carry those skills to practice. Even within those practices that do not participate in organized or structured research activities, research skills and understanding will be important. Practices that survive and thrive in the difficult medical environment of both the present and the future will have to examine how they do business, conduct practice, and make decisions about what works for their patients and what does not. This takes research skills.

In our practice lives, we have always needed the skills to interpret the medical literature, as we do today. Beyond that, in the past, research was what someone else did. If it affected PAs, then perhaps we were interested. In the future, research will be part of every PA's work and usual activity, either in the search for new knowledge or for everyday improvement of service to those in need.

Research and Physician Assistants

Saying the word "research" may conjure up images of egghead nerds hidden away in labs doing work few can understand—Dr. Frankenstein at his creation, or perhaps just the bored faces of students as they attempt to make sense of information garnered from research. Certainly many may imagine that the pursuit of research information has little, if any, application in the real world, and you, as a PA, may not believe research is relevant to clinical practice.

For many people, the research process is difficult to understand. It requires manipulations of impossible-to-learn formulations that end up in language that only other researchers can understand. Research sometimes produces results that contradict each other, leaving the rest of us wondering what is going on. Research intimidates clinicians and keeps PA educators from taking tenure-track positions. The process of conducting research can cause wholesale panic in many students, or it may be regarded as boring, regimented work that may have little to do with the "real world."

However anxiety-producing the concept of research is for students, faculty, and practitioners, it is the basis for what we do. Research is the key to our present and future, regardless of our position and function in the profession. The practice of medicine is based in scientific research that PAs apply in the care of every patient. The only way health care can advance is by research, developing evidence of what works, and applying the results. Even if we are not actively involved in research, we must possess a basic understanding of the process to allow us to interpret what the results mean, differentiate between conflicting results, and discern what is useful to us. As evidence-based medicine becomes more and more the basis for what we do, understanding and conducting research also become more important. More and more practicing PAs will find that research or some aspect of research will be part of their day-to-day job.

Research Equals Curiosity

Whether we have realized it or not, we have all done research in some manner. If you have ever sought the answer to a question, you have done research. Your mom's admonition to "Look it up!" sent you off on a research effort to find the meaning of a word in the dictionary. Curiosity and the need for information create the drive to find answers in medicine and in everyday life. Finding those answers is research. Needing to know, and seeking answers to our questions, motivate us to do research. Certainly, much of our "research" is informal and without the systematic constraints required in formal research, but we all have done it. If you are a practicing PA, you do research every day as you investigate the medical literature for solutions to your patients' problems. If you are a student, you do research as part of your education and preparation to enter the profession. The very act of study is investigation in some ways, regardless of what we call it. Preparation for an examination by a student or for the recertification exam by an experienced PA is a form of research. If you are a faculty member, one of your major roles and responsibilities as an academician should be scholarly activity and the advancement of knowledge. Research is the way that is done.

Research occurs in the laboratory, classroom, office, practice, and society at large. The results can be applied directly to a problem or make up a small piece of larger solutions. Research is a tool that can help us prepare for what will happen and understand what has happened. Our personal needs and desires direct how we use research and the part it plays in our careers and lives in general. Learning to use this tool helps relieve our anxieties and increases our ability to appreciate and to even enjoy the process.

Research that involves our interests or needs for discovery is most important, as we may dislike doing something in which we have no interest. In some ways, research may be more important to the practitioner than to the student or academician. Similarly, what interests us may be mundane, but necessary to our profession or livelihood. For example, the practicing PA may have little interest in the differences in practice census flows by disease type, but that information may have a great impact on patient scheduling and provider assignments.

Research may provide answers that allow for the most efficient use of PA time and expertise in a practice. Many questions about one's practice can be answered by research. It may or may not require enormous statistical analysis, but it requires the systematic gathering, analysis, and interpretation of information.

Another example of research application in practice is patient outcomes. What is the difference in outcomes in a practice if we treat a disease with drug A versus drug B? There may be a wealth of information in texts and the literature, but what about your specific practice? Your personal research provides the answer. The clinician can do the research formally or informally. The value to the practice may be equal, but a formal investigation could lead to dissemination beyond the practice if significance is discovered.

For the Student

For the student, research is part of the task of discovery and learning, providing the information needed to build a fund of knowledge that will determine what we do as health-care providers. Every student must learn to interpret the medical literature and be an informed consumer of research literature. At a minimum, learning what research means and how to interpret research findings teaches a process that we can use for the rest of our lives to provide information, learn new skills, and deliver an acceptable level of care to our patients. In many ways, the research process is comparable to medical reasoning and critical thinking. Much of the discipline needed to develop and conduct research is the same as that needed to systematically assess and manage disease processes.

PA education is consistent with adult learning theory. We must all be lifelong learners, and the PA who stops building his or her knowledge base will soon be lost. Experience is part of that knowledge base, but continuing to understand and interpret research will be the foundation for maintaining, redefining, and increasing that base. Research can help us change to meet the challenges of the future. It can be as simple as studying for the next test or finding the answer to a question asked by a patient. It is a tool that allows us to "learn how to learn."

For the Physician Assistant

For PAs who are expected to conduct research as part of their jobs, good research skills can serve as a tool for advancement. It also can provide the opportunity to contribute to the profession and to the practice of medicine. Research can provide information applicable to a particular setting or to the profession and society. For many

PA faculty members, mastering research skills and performing research or scholarly activities are major job expectations. The process involves discovery, synthesis, and presentation of ideas and concepts that can benefit many people. Research and scholarly activity are one of the three basic components of the faculty roles. It is incumbent on faculty members to master research skills and contribute to medicine and society's fund of knowledge and to our understandings of the PA profession.

Another consideration in developing research skills for the practicing PA is that clinical investigations are an expanding enterprise. The development of new drugs, procedures, and medical equipment and devices give practices an opportunity to be a part of cutting edge developments offering advancements to their patients, as well as additional sources of income for the practice. Practice income should be a minor consideration for participating in clinical investigations, however. Every practice that is involved with clinical investigations needs an on-site coordinator for the study. This certainly could be part of a PA's job and an activity that PAs can find engaging and important. A PA involved in clinical investigations must understand the elements of the scientific process, informed consent, and methodology. Working as a research coordinator in a clinical practice offers challenges and opportunities that can be a very satisfying component of a PA's work.

Fear of the Unknown

The unknowns and seemingly complex methods of systematic research and its processes frighten many people. So, too, the unknowns of analysis, statistics, and interpretation can be daunting. Research may be held in high regard by many but in low regard (almost thought of as a "dirty word"?) by others. This is particularly true for many PAs because we entered the profession with a service orientation and commitment to clinical practice. Research had been left to others. But as we have become more involved in and invested with the practice of medicine and have taken on roles that extend beyond those of a dependent provider, we must meet society's expectations and take on additional responsibilities. We must be more involved in the science of discovery, which includes the advancement of medical science, including the science of application and delivery. We must be involved with the investigation of PAs and medical care in every aspect, whether it involves the provider and patient; social, behavioral, delivery, and political components; or concepts and philosophy. Research is necessary to discover who, what, and where we are. Despite the tremendous growth in our numbers and practice privileges, we must continue to justify our role in medicine and society. The more we know, the more we realize we need to know. Research is the tool that will allow us to go where we want to go in the future and define what we need to do to meet the medical needs of humankind.

Research Takes Many Forms

The research you may do can take different forms (Table 1–1). Research can be categorized in several ways, including pure, experimental, clinical, applied, descriptive, laboratory,[5] and outcomes research. The types of research an individual does depends on many factors. PAs are in a position to participate in and conduct any category of research.

The design of a research study is an important factor that confuses many beginning investigators.[4] Some research can be done without any special knowledge or skills, such as counting how many patients have a particular diagnosis. Some research requires specialized skills and must follow an exact methodology, such as clinical drug trials. Research also has a language of its own that must be learned and understood. The recording and writing of research procedures and results have special requirements that must be learned, practiced, and perfected. For most of us, research is about phenomena (something that can be perceived) that affect what we do and what we want to know. It is about observation and interpretation of what we learn in order to answer our questions.

Research can be challenging and difficult. It also can be enjoyable and rewarding. At every level and in every format and design, it should add to our knowledge. It is unlikely that any of our research will make headlines, but we can be content to answer our questions and to make small contributions to the body of knowledge. We have questions that need answering. Medicine has questions that need answering. Society has questions that need answering. If we accept the challenge of answering those questions, then we need at least a basic understanding of research and how to apply it to our situation or practice. Learning the process of research gives us the greatest likelihood of finding the answers. You do not have to be a genius to do research. You do not have to be mathematically gifted. You only have to have the interest. The PA can use research and its results in the classroom, laboratory, or clinic. It is a process to be learned and used to help yourself and others (see Fig. 1–1).

Table 1–1
Types of Research*

Type	Description
Pure	Abstract and general, concerned with generating new theory and gaining new knowledge for the knowledge's sake. Example: theory development.
Experimental	Manipulation of one variable to see its effect on another variable, while controlling for as many other variables as possible and randomly assigning subjects to groups. Examples: double-blind random assignment control groups, response to an intervention.
Clinical	Performed in the clinical setting where control over variables is quite difficult. Examples: drug trials, therapeutic outcomes.
Applied	Designed to answer a practical question, to help people do their jobs better. Examples: time use studies, evaluation of different types of interventions with the same purpose.
Descriptive	Describing a group, a situation, or an individual to gain knowledge that may be applied to further groups or situations, as in case studies or trend analyses. Examples: surveys, qualitative research, measurement of characteristics, response to phenomena.
Laboratory	Performed in laboratory surroundings that are tightly controlled. Example: basic science research.

*Adapted from Bailey,[4] p. xxii.

Our Goal

The goal of this book is to provide you with an introduction to research. It is directed to PAs, PA students, beginning PA researchers, and PA faculty. This book was written by experienced educators, practitioners, and researchers. Certainly, there are many ways to approach research beyond what is in this book. We hope this book helps you begin your research efforts and advance your skills and abilities. Each small piece that we can add to the whole results in improvement for the profession and for the physical, mental, and social health of those for whom care is provided.

This book is just one piece of what you need. Use this book as an introductory tool, a starting point, and add to it from other resources. Learning the process of research is as important as understanding the research results. You will need to add other resources to your research library and references. Use many books and resources in your work.

Developing a Research Agenda

Developing a personal research agenda is dependent on many factors. Some introspection is required and it must include a personal assessment of your attributes,

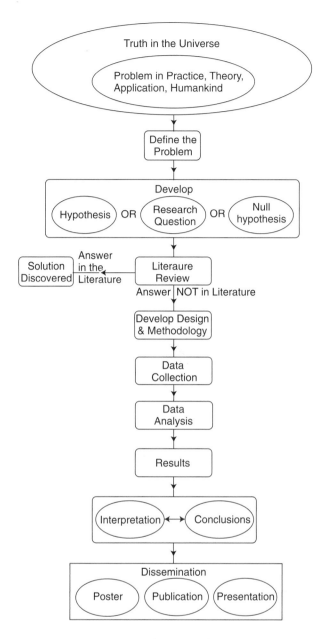

FIG. 1–1. Outline of the scientific process.

their help. Find the people who are doing what you want to do. Explore the possibilities of collaborating with someone on his or her research as a learning activity. The other key element to a successful research effort is to allow adequate time for your investigations. For PA faculty, students, and clinicians the research agenda must include a timeline and adequate time must be set aside and protected for your efforts. So as you plan your research, mark specific research time that can be disrupted only by extenuating circumstances. Then, stick with that scheduled time and use it for your research.

When you are ready to embark on this journey, this author believes the first step is to brainstorm and be as expansive as possible. Sit down with pencil and paper or at the computer keyboard and make a list of everything that interests you in any way. When you have recorded everything you can think of, walk away for a period of time, whether for a few minutes or a few days. The key is to NOT think about your agenda for a while (a short while). Then come back and refine your list. Add new items and subtract those that do not seem important to you. You may want to repeat this process more than once before you get down to defining your agenda. Once you have a list of possibilities, start the defining process:

1. Make a list of everything that interests you or questions for which you would like to learn the answer.

2. Prioritize your list in the order of your interests.

3. Make a second ordered list (from the first) of the things that you have the capability to do.

4. Make a third ordered list (from the first) of the things that are important to your job.

5. Make a fourth ordered list (from the first) of the things that are important to society or medicine or the profession.

6. Compare your lists. Items that appear at the top of all four lists should then be prioritized and merged into a single list.

7. Make the decision about what you can do and cannot do. Mark off the things that you cannot do. This includes financing your work. Financial support is just as important as time and expertise to the success of a project.

8. This is your research agenda. It contains a list of challenges that need to be researched: challenges that you have the capability to research; challenges that are important to your job, the profession, society, and medicine; and challenges you have an interest in investigating. What could be better?

9. Choose the investigation that is number one, develop a timeline for the study, set aside your research time, and plan your step-by-step process. Then

interests, resources, and your expectations and the expectations in your situation (Jones PE, personal communication, 2004). Part of this personal assessment must consider your strengths as a researcher and abilities to accomplish your agenda. You cannot do quantum physics if you do not have the required background, no matter how strong your interest. You must also be able to concentrate your research effort so that you develop or use the expertise you have to the maximum. It is better to be an expert in one small, specific area than somewhat of an expert in several. As a beginning researcher, you need mentors and collaborators. Find people who have skills in the area you are interested in and seek

10. GET STARTED. A respected PA educator has said, "Time goes by regardless of what you do. When it does, make sure you are not still waiting for the best time to begin" (Rahr RR, personal communication, 2004).

11. Revise, adjust, and renew periodically as necessary, particularly after completing a project.

12. Think about what you have done, your research agenda, and start your next project.

Summary

Whether you love it, dislike it, or would rather not think about it, research is a part of your professional life as a student or clinician. Research provides the basis for all that we do as health-care providers. Although most researchers will not make world shaking discoveries, each small piece that we are able to add that improves our understanding of the world around us is important. Remember, research isn't a dirty word. It is a powerful tool we must all learn to master in order to care for others.

References

1. Hooker RS, Cawley JF. Physician Assistants in American Medicine, 2nd ed. Philadelphia: Churchill Livingstone, 2003, pp. 5–7, 15–16.
2. Association of Physician Assistant Programs. Eighteenth Annual Report on Physician Assistant Educational Programs in the United States, 2001–2002. Association of Physician Assistant Programs, Alexandria, VA, 2002.
3. American Academy of Physician Assistants. AAPA 2003 Physician Assistant Census Report, at *http://www.aapa.org/research/03census-intro. html*
4. Bailey DM. Research for the Health Professional: A Practical Guide, 2nd ed. Philadelphia: FA Davis, 1997, p. xxii.
5. Campbell DT, Stanley JC. Experimental and Quasi-Experimental Designs for Research. Boston: Houghton Mifflin, 1963, p. 1.

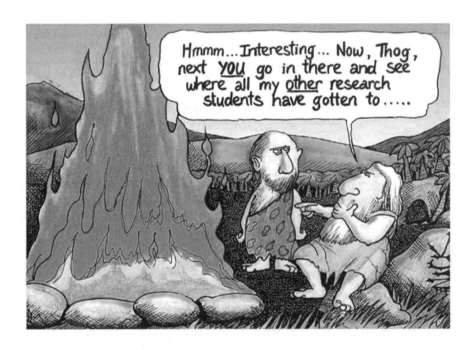

Proto-Professor Algarth Zag, pioneer in fire research.

Reprinted by permission of Nick D. Kim.

chapter 2

Interpreting the Medical Literature

Roderick S. Hooker, PhD, PA and J. Dennis Blessing, PhD, PA-C

In no affairs of more prejudice, pro or con, do we deduce inferences with entire certainty, even from the most simple data.

The Narrative of A. Gordon Pym, by E. A. Poe

Questioning: The beginning of genius without which no progress would flow
Anonymous

Chapter Overview

More than two million biomedical articles are published in medical, health, and professional journals each year.[1] For most clinicians, wading through even a small number of journals or articles can be daunting. The challenge is to not only stay abreast of current changes in medical practice but also to make the educated health care consumer aware of the information the articles are presenting. Never has so much information been available to so many people. Patients appear in the medical office with information from sources such as news releases, newspaper and television reports, and Internet sites; sometimes new advances are reported to the public before they are described in the medical literature. In a profit-driven system, frequently the information that is delivered focuses on the benefits without the downside of new advances.

Like all medical clinicians, the practicing physician assistant (PA) must be able to interpret the scientific and medical literature quickly and completely in order to meet the challenge of applying new information and meeting the needs of eager patients. For centuries, textbooks were a reliable source of information in the practice of medicine. By the mid-twentieth century, their slow revisions and lag time from completion to distribution meant they were never completely up to date. Today the role of textbooks is to provide a good foundation, but current medical literature is the key to modern practice. Reading journals remains a source of current information for many clinicians. Even in print journals, however, there is some delay in the source to provider pipeline. In the new century, the speed and access capabilities of the Internet provide resources unavailable to previous generations of health-care providers. Information is posted quickly, efficiently, and is accessible to all.

Ultimately, an important question for every clinician is, "What is important to my patients and my practice?" Answering that question is the key to providing the most current and effective care, and it requires developing skills to critically examine the medical literature and determining what is applicable to your practice and what benefits your patients. This chapter is designed to provide some guidelines in the process of interpreting the medical literature. Professional growth and experience are aided by the ability to interpret the medical literature.

Introduction

Interpreting the medical literature is defined as integrating, synthesizing, and summarizing information obtained from different medical and scientific studies into a recommendation for some sort of guidance. The intent is to apply the best knowledge available to make the best choice for the circumstance before you. This summarizing of information, known as integrative literature, comes in many forms. It can be composed of systematic reviews, overviews, meta-analyses, practice guidelines, decision analyses, and cost-effectiveness analyses. The concept of evidence-based medicine is expanding and the extraction of evidence from the literature into practice, while logical, presents some challenges. Busy clinicians must develop skills that allow them to become critical consumers of select literature and decide what applies to their practice and patients. It is "The application of the best available evidence to patient care."[2] As you develop your skills in interpreting the medical literature, remember that "patient care" is at the heart of what you do. Being patient-centered allows the correct patient care decisions to be made when interpreting and applying medical knowledge.

The goal of this chapter is to introduce the concept that integrating the literature is one of the keystones to understanding research. It is a skill that must be learned, practiced, and applied. Those who are reading this book in preparation for a research project or course will recognize that research results, especially those that deal with health and medicine, can sometimes be confusing, conflicting, and confounding. Add to all this the recent advent of evidence-based medicine, systematic reviews, meta-analysis, and outcome data, and it is no wonder that we sometimes come away from readings and searches more uncertain and unclear than when we began. Because it is necessary to anchor our work in previous works of a similar vein, we must develop skills in how

to interpret the medical literature and then add new data to our fund of knowledge.

As you become more immersed in your research efforts and more experienced as a researcher, your abilities to synthesize and use the literature will improve. The same is true for the clinician seeking to interpret the literature on a medical problem. To become an expert in interpreting the medical literature takes years of experience and a broad understanding of process, statistical design, and analysis. There must be a starting point, and you are taking the first steps now.

To undertake a research project and to obtain the maximum benefit and usefulness from your literature search, you must understand and have the ability to interpret what the research problem is and what has occurred in this area of interest. For example, students may wonder if they are entering a profession that will be the right career for them. The problem is they do not know much about this subject and may not be sure where to go for the answers. At the heart of this question is one of satisfaction. Is the PA profession a satisfying one? If someone is entering a profession in which job satisfaction is low and attrition is high then patients are not well served. For example, historically nursing home aides were poorly paid, worked hard, kept long hours, and had a high turnover. With the development of better management and organization, that industry has begun to change and the incidence of nursing home malpractice has dropped.

The literature search is often a quest for theory building and discovering what research has been done and how it could be done better or differently. The scholar's research should say something new, or validate existing work, while connecting with research that already has been reported. Rather than serving as an attempt to develop a unique idea, using the literature allows a foundation to be laid that is conducive to discussion and debate. How the literature is interpreted will influence your research process and your interpretation of the results. Interpreting the literature may develop a knowledge base and make the case for the investigation. The research project or scientific investigation literature search is presented in Chapter 4.

Interpretation of the literature takes on greater importance when it involves the care of others; misinterpretations can lead to significant errors in health-care and medical applications. This chapter is based on several resources and the authors' experience to provide a general guide on how to interpret the medical literature.

Interpreting the Literature: First Things First

To understand an article in the proper context, some baseline knowledge is important. If the information is new to individuals, they will probably be reading a basic version or at least one that leads the reader to understand the background of the subject. For example, persons who are knowledgeable in rheumatology will be selecting journals that assume the reader knows about prostaglandins and interleukins. Their skill and knowledge base in reading this literature will surpass those of people outside of the disciplines of rheumatology and immunology.

Most medical readers have developed some literature interpretation skills by reading or studying various medical literature resources. A rudimentary step in literature interpretation is to understand certain terms used in research (e.g., percentages, means, validity, limitations, probability, subjects, and population). Most of these terms can be found in the glossary of this book or in other chapters. Recognizing the meaning and significance of research terms or incorporating research terms in the context of your work will come with time and experience as your interpretation of the literature progresses. One suggestion is to *never* let a term go undefined as you review the literature, particularly if the material is important to your own efforts or in your practice and care giving. Look up terms as you progress through the literature material. Another suggestion is to develop a bibliography of useful references. Historically many researchers tore articles out of journals or made copies of important articles and kept them in file cabinets. Because so many articles are retrievable, a simple Word document may be all you need to keep a record of useful material. Many journals and articles are now online and can be accessed quickly.

The Scientific Method

Understanding the medical literature can be a challenge for most because it is so dynamic and fueled by new technology. To convey medical and other pertinent information requires being factual and informative and employing some rigor in the process of obtaining accurate and applicable information. When information is communicated in a real-world situation, certain principles that everyone can trust and rely on must be in place. The way to ensure this is to use the scientific method. Its principles are integral to the literature process (searching and interpreting) because they stress the acquisition of knowledge through the rigorous process of systematic observation, analysis, and reasoning. Schematically it is the scientific method corridor through which all concepts must pass. This process adds value and becomes part of our fund of knowledge. Our literature search must include and incorporate scientific observation and data collection. The formal process of acquiring scientific knowledge, whether

through reviewing the literature or recording observations, is done in a logical and reproducible manner. In essence, this means that any competent clinician could replicate the literature search and reach the same conclusions. A research project incorporates the scientific method into the literature by defining each step in the process as follows:

1. Problem: a precise statement of what knowledge was sought and why it was sought.
2. Question: a single sentence that asks a question related to the problem.
3. Method: the plan of how the research was done and how the knowledge was gained.
4. Results: unequivocal statements of the knowledge that was gained.
5. Interpretation: application of the knowledge gained.

How you interpret the results of this process is key to understanding how you will apply the results to the better care of your patients. Recognizing the steps of sound scientific investigation and application of scientific concepts will help you interpret the results and outcomes in a meaningful manner.

Questions to Ask (and to Answer)

Whether reading and interpreting the medical literature for application in practice or gathering data for a research project, part of your task and challenge is to assess what is published on the topic of interest. Box 2–1 outlines a set of questions to be asked and answered before making any assumption about the piece of literature.

Ultimately, this line of literature questioning or evaluation will become second nature to you. Writing out your answers to these questions as you evaluate an article or series of articles will help to reinforce the steps in being a critical evaluator of literature. As you move through this process, new questions of your own will emerge.

Although many of these questions are self-explanatory, commentary and clarification are needed to ensure that the thought processes are consistent and clear to you. As you move among various sources for information, new suggestions on evaluating the medical literature will emerge allowing you to develop your own style and process. Only through scrutiny, analysis, and replication can answers to questions be found, and the scientific process and the information that results from the process be validated. This scrutiny, analysis, and replication occur when consumers of the medical literature ask the right questions and challenge the answers.

BOX 2-1

Questions to Ask and Answer

1. What is the source (journal) of the article?
2. Was the publication peer reviewed?
3. Who are the authors and what are their affiliations?
4. What is the main subject of the study?
5. What was the problem(s) investigated?
6. What is the purpose or rationale for the study?
7. Who or what constituted the sample or population?
8. What was the design of the study?
9. What are the statistical analyses used?
10. What are the results?
11. Are the results clear?
12. Did the results answer the identified questions?
13. Do the results seem valid?
14. Are the interpretations (conclusions) of the results consistent with design and analysis?
15. Are the results consistent with findings from similar studies?
16. What do the results mean to medicine and health care and you and your patients?
17. Can the results be applied to your research or clinical practice?

The Questions

1. *What is the source (journal) of the article?*

The reputation of a source can be important as a citation. Journals that tend to have the highest subscription rate tend to hold a high degree of prestige. Generally those journals in a discipline within the top 10th percentile are the most often cited. For clinical articles, these include *The Journal of the American Medical Association (JAMA), The New England Journal of Medicine, Lancet,* and so forth. Although not everything they publish is beyond reproach or question, they tend to use a rigorous peer-review approach to ensure that their reputation remains where it is. This is not to say that other journals do not produce high-quality work. Lower ranked journals do publish sound scientific findings and good journals have on occasion published bad science (Wooley FR, personal communication, 2004). The rigor of submitting a paper for publication can be assessed by looking at its guidelines for authors.

2. *Was the publication peer reviewed?*

Peer review is a process of manuscript critiquing by someone familiar with the same body of literature that the author is submitting. Since the 1950s the majority of scientific manuscripts submitted for publication have been undergoing a peer-review process. This type of review is intended to critically evaluate a manuscript so the reader is offered some confidence that the resulting publication has been scrutinized for soundness, the results are valid, and the conclusions are consistent with the findings. Journals are ranked on the basis of their scientific merit and readership. Readership often rests on the journal's ability to bring new and important information that can be confidently accepted. However, not every article in a "peer-reviewed" journal is necessarily subjected to the peer review process. Many journals have "departments" or "special sections" or "features" that undergo a different manner of review or oversight, even in a "peer-reviewed" journal.

3. *Who are the authors and what are their affiliations?*

The reputation of the author(s) can be important, particularly if the findings are controversial. Experts in a particular field may know many of the contributors to their body of literature but the person just entering a field of study may need a period of time to become familiar with the major subjects and the important names. To help feel confident about the literature you are reviewing, you may have to do some homework on the reporting media and the authors, particularly if the literature concerns important discoveries or contributions. You may recognize the work of some authors and the reputation they bring to the literature. On the other hand, a note of caution is needed before accepting every finding.

The authors' affiliations (who they work for or where) can have some influence in the consideration of a reported study. Certain institutions and universities tend to be centers of excellence in particular areas of science and learning and tend to attract a body of scientists and writers expanding work in this area. Knowing this information will help you understand where the authors are coming from or what may influence their work environment. It will also help you understand why they are studying these problems to begin with.

4. *What was the problem(s) investigated?*

The answer to this question should be self-evident from the text. The research problem is the issue or topic of focus. For example, we know little about the career patterns of female PAs. The problem is the difficulty in predicting how long various types of PAs will remain in the workforce. Health economists and labor experts need these questions addressed for education or health policies to be implemented. The research question is always a narrower portion of the research problem. A hypothesis is the method of addressing a research question. If the problem to be solved is a test of theory, a test of applications, replication or proof of prior work, or any combination of these, then the problem should be elucidated early in the report. Research questions and the hypotheses tested should be stated clearly and linked to the problems being investigated. You should also look for any assumptions made by the investigators. Assumptions can confound and influence the study and report.

5. *What (or who) is the main subject of the study?*

The answer to this question may be similar to or the same as the problem investigated, but depending on the type of investigation could be different in some way from the problem. For example, in a study of student performance on test taking, the subjects of the study are the students. However, the problem investigated could be how the students study for tests, how they act during tests, and what they remember after the tests. In medicine, the subject of a research study could be cholesterol, but the problem investigated may be the response of cholesterol to some intervention.

6. *What is the purpose or rationale for the study?*

This question is the "why" of the study. Why was it done? What purpose did it serve? Was it an important problem? There is no dearth of questions one can ask, but for research literature to be valid, it should serve a useful purpose with sound rationale for its undertaking.

7. *Who or what constituted the sample or population?*

Sample size is often critical for population research. One needs to ask who or what was studied and how many were in the sample or subsamples studied. It is important to understand this aspect of the study if the results are to apply to your work or patients. The number of subjects studied can affect outcomes: too small a number may not be representative or may miss a pertinent factor; too large a number may minimize some important or key findings. To extrapolate data and apply it outside a study, the characteristics of the sample must be evident and comparable to the population from which the sample is selected. Caution needs to be kept in mind that what may be true for one group of individuals may not be true for another.

8. *What was the design of the study?*

Oftentimes the design of the study can be critical to the outcome. The methods should be described in enough detail to allow you to draw conclusions about the results and applications. Each type of study design has its limitations, threats to validity, threats to statistical analysis, and threats to conclusions. Even the fundamentally sound "random assignment, double-blind" studies have limitations. You should become familiar with the limitations of the various types of studies and look for biases in the design since these flaws may affect conclusions and your effort to interpret the results.

9. *What are the statistical analyses used?*

Are the data analyses performed appropriate for the data type and study design? A statistics book is a very useful resource to have if you are unfamiliar with data analysis. It may also be good to consult a statistician to help you. Statistics confuse many of us, and even experienced researchers make mistakes. So, look closely at how the data were analyzed. Do the data and statistical analyses make sense? Sometimes reviewing the statistics may be helpful in understanding the results and conclusions.

10. *What are the results?*

The results should be reported as unambiguously as possible. Two researchers undertaking the same study should report their findings in much the same way without any subjective interpretation. Determine if the results of the study seem consistent with the study design and the analyses used. Do the data make sense and are the results consistent with my understanding? Results that indicate extremes in analysis should be examined closely.

11. *Are the results clear?*

Do the results have meaning to the intent of the study? Are they understandable? Are they consistent with the methods and analyses proposed? When results are not clear then either the study was done in an obfuscating manner or you are not familiar with the statistical methods used.

12. *Did the results answer the identified questions?*

Although results may not be what you expected, that does not mean that they are wrong. If the methodological process was undertaken correctly, the results should stand on their own and most people would draw similar conclusions. Results should answer the questions posed earlier in the study. Although the answers often lead to more questions, the research questions should be addressed in the Results section.

13. *Do the results seem valid?*

Validity is at the heart of most studies and is defined as something that makes common sense, is persuasive, and seems right to the reader. Face validity simply means the validity at face value. As a check on face validity, test/survey items are sent to teachers to obtain suggestions for modification. Because of the vagueness and subjectivity of face validity, psychometricians have abandoned this concept for a long time. However, outside the measurement arena, face validity has come back in another form. The validity of a theory refers to results that have the appearance of truth or reality.

14. *Are the interpretations (conclusions) of the results consistent with design and analysis?*

It is here that the article's writers make the correct conclusion about the data, although this area can be open to personal bias and misinterpretation. In your own evaluation, therefore, it is important to decide if the conclusions are consistent with the type of information that the study design and analysis can yield and the results presented.

15. *Are the results consistent with findings from similar studies?*

Before reading a research article, you should have a sense of the problem from past similar studies either from previous literature reviews or from your own clinical practice. This will give you some sense of the results of the study in question. Studies that deviate greatly from what is already known should be examined more closely. This does not mean they are wrong; earth-shaking discoveries do occur from time to time. Most research, however, adds only a small piece to our fund of knowledge. This is especially true in medical research and literature.

16. *What do the results mean to medicine and health care in general and to you and your patients?*

This question may be the most important one the clinician can ask. What does it mean to your practice and to the people for whom you provide care? For medicine and health care, it is important to examine the validity of an intervention and make sure it is applicable to your patient population. You should be able to understand the risks and benefits of an intervention study and what the results mean

to the overall well-being of your patients' social, mental, and physical health.

17. *Can the results be applied to your research or clinical practice?*

This question is probably the ultimate one to ask, and only you can answer it. If you have examined the literature carefully and analytically, it is hoped that you will have the answers for your research or practice.

Evidence-Based Medicine: A New Way of Looking at the Medical Literature

There is a general assumption that if something claims to be "evidence based" it is the guiding light for medical practice. However, remember that the key is the applicability to "patient care." "Evidence-based" does not replace clinical experience/expertise. Evidence-based research should be a way to bridge the gap between rigorous research and clinical investigations for the clinician and ultimately to your patient's benefit. Evidence-based outcomes can come from research studies (the more rigorous, the better) or from the synthesis of existing data and outcomes (e.g., meta-analysis). Regardless, you must still interpret or evaluate the study in relationship to your needs or your patients' needs.

Friedland et al.[3] have developed a very straightforward approach to evaluation, evidence-based medicine (EBM). His five-step approach is presented in Table 2–1. While this is a nice concise approach, it does not eliminate the need to ask and answer the previous questions presented by the authors. The table outlines a process that is a part of the larger overall evaluation and interpretation of the medical literature.

Table 2–1
A Five-Step Study Guide for EMB*

Step 1	Do I want to evaluate the study?	Is it interesting, novel, relevant?
Step 2	What are the research question, study design, study findings?	What is the population studied, variables, study design, results/outcomes/findings/conclusions?
Step 3	Are the findings believable?	Do the subjects and variables represent the research question? Are the findings attributable to chance, biases, or confounding variables? Are the findings believable in the context of existing knowledge?
Step 4	What are the important findings?	Are the findings clinically relevant?
Step 5	Will the study help my patients?	Are the subjects similar to my patients? Are the interventions applicable to my patients? Will the findings/outcomes result in an overall benefit for my patients?

*Adapted from Friedland.[3]

Table 2–2
Levels of Evidence

Level	Description
A	High-quality evidence that considers all important outcomes. Randomized controlled trials (RCT), well done systematic reviews of randomized controlled trials, meta-analysis systematic reviews using comprehensive search strategies.
B	Well designed, nonrandomized clinical trials. Systematic reviews of studies other than RCTs with appropriate search strategies and well-substantiated conclusions, lower quality RCTs, cohort studies, case-control studies with nonbiased subject selection and consistent findings, quality retrospective studies, certain uncontrolled studies, well-design epidemiological studies with compelling findings.
C	Consensus or expert opinion

From American Family Physician.[4]

Table 2–3
Level of Evidence Modifiers

Modifier	Description
1	Nonrandomized clinical trial
2	Systematic review of nonrandomized clinical trial
3	Lower quality of randomized clinical trial
4	Clinical cohort study
5	Case control study
6	Retrospective study
7	Uncontrolled study
8	Epidemiological study

From American Family Physician.[4]

The last consideration in the interpretation of evidence-based literature is the level of evidence. When a study or groups of studies are analyzed for best evidence, a rating system is used. This rating of the evidence can be a guide for clinicians about the strength of the evidence and its source (Table 2–2). In addition to the rating of the level of evidence, qualifiers are used to describe the source of the evidence (Table 2–3).

Another presentation format for evidence-based medicine is the POEM™ or Patient Oriented Evidence that Matters. The POEM is a commercially available format in which the EBM literature is reviewed and summarized.[5] The intent of the POEM is usual evidence-based results in a concise and easily readable format that have application in clinical practice. A number of medical journals have a POEM section or as a feature. These types of summaries are very helpful, but for those interventions or outcomes that affect your patients, go to the original work.

A General Approach to Reading the Literature

Asking all the right questions, going through all these steps, and reading as much as you can are still very time consuming. There are large numbers of resources out there and all types of services that can be used or accessed. Still, the amount of information is overwhelming. With more than 2.5 million biomedical publications a year, it becomes important that you develop an approach to the medical literature. No single approach will work for every PA in every situation. You must tailor your approach to your situation, need, and environment. A general approach follows, but it can be modified in many ways.

1. Identify the journals that are pertinent to your specialty.
2. Develop a strategy for reviewing those journals.
3. Set aside a specific time period each week when you can review your journals. (Allow yourself uninterrupted time for the reading and review.)
4. Identify those articles of interest by their title or by reading the abstract.
5. Make a quick review of the tables and figures.
6. Make a decision to read the article.
7. Apply the techniques for interpreting the article.
8. Apply the results to your practice.

A key to a successful strategy for accomplishing your goals is "protected" time for browsing, reading, and interpreting the literature important to your practice and patients. You must establish that time.

Summary

Interpreting the literature is the synthesizing of information obtained from different medical and scientific studies and integrating pertinent outcomes into practice and patient care. A PA must develop a sound process for review and evaluation of the medical literature. Skilled interpretation of the medical literature will lead to up-to-date practice and patient benefit. The PA who fails to stay abreast of the medical literature is not going to be a competent practitioner. As evidence-based analyses increase, so will the pressure for practice trends to follow that evidence. However, evidence must be balanced with clinical experience and expertise for the best likelihood of improved patient outcomes. The literature must be a part of everyday PA activity and pursued with a critical eye.

References

1. Lee KP, Schotland M, Bacchetti P, Bero LA. Association of journal quality indicators with methodological quality of clinical research articles. JAMA 2002;287:2805–2808 at *http://jama.ama-assn.org/cgi/content/full/287/21/2805* Accessed May 5, 2005.

2. Sackett DL, Richardson WS, Rosenberg W, Haynes RB. Evidence-Based Medicine: How to Practice and Teach EBM. New York: Churchill Livingstone, 1997.

3. Friedland DB, Go AS, Davoren JB, Sblipak MG, Bent SW, Subak LL, Mendelson T. Evidence-Based Medicine: A Framework for Clinical Practice. New York: Lange Medical Books/McGraw-Hill, 1998, pp. 145–246.

4. American Family Physician. Levels of evidence in AFP. At *http://www.findarticles.com/cf_0/m3225/4_66/90607847* Accessed May 5, 2005.

5. InfoPOEMs at *http://www.infopoems.com* Accessed May 5, 2005.

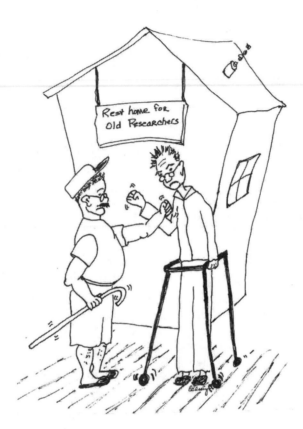

Blessing and Hooker continue to disagree about their own research. No one else cares.

Reprinted by permission of Brenda G. Blessing.

chapter 3

The Research Problem

Salah Ayachi, PhD, PA-C

Chapter Overview

This chapter discusses the development and refinement of a research problem. Developing a research question, hypothesis, or null hypothesis is not automatic and can be difficult. Identification of the research problem and defining it in terms that can be investigated, studied, and researched are critical steps in the research and scientific process. Sound methodology can be developed only when the research problem is well defined in a format that can be investigated. Defining the research problem and developing your research question, hypothesis, or null hypothesis requires time and effort. For many of us, refinement of our research interests and quests is a challenge.

Introduction

Research provides a systematic process for uncovering answers to clinical and other questions. It also expands on current knowledge that can then be applied to education, clinical practice, and the benefit of society. Although some problems may be evident, others are not as easily recognized or defined. Refining and defining our problems is a must for successful research.

The first step in a research project is to identify the problem that needs investigation. To the novice this may constitute the most difficult step.[1] So, how does one go about identifying the problem to research? The process involves more than just asking or writing down a question; it calls for moving stepwise from general to more specific questions, thereby focusing on and defining the question as specifically as possible so that it can be studied. Like any other ability, this skill needs to be learned, developed, and honed.

Why go through the mental exercise and invest time on the front end? The reason is that it helps define the problem effectively and accurately (i.e., clarifies it) and sets the tone for the entire exploratory process and your subsequent work. Generally, you, the physician assistant (PA), or any other health-care professional will investigate a problem that interests you or has an impact on what you do. Any question in your practice, specialty, or interest is therefore worth researching.

Identifying the research problem is not always a simple task. Often, the difficulty stems from confounding factors that keep one from focusing on what needs to be studied. This challenge is particularly true for those who are new to research. For many of us and for those who are not familiar with the research process, getting to the exact problem that needs to be studied is like looking through foggy glasses or a smudged windshield. This is not only confusing but also frustrating, time consuming, and wasteful. In fact, failure to develop a clear and concise research problem can lead to unsuccessful research. Think of the research problem as your guiding light that points you in the right direction. Until the fog has dissipated or the windshield has been cleaned, the view remains unclear. And, until the researcher develops an exact, defined problem(s), the picture may remain blurred and the path uncertain.

Developing the Research Question: The Process

How do you select topics? Generally, the topic of interest comes from your environment, work, or interest in a particular subject or problem. Sometimes what you read in journals may create a topic for you; often research articles end up generating more questions than they answer, giving you a chance to take a study one step further or to answer some of the questions raised by the article. For example, a study on PAs that concludes that PAs spend relatively more time with patients may raise the question of what component of care allows or causes PAs to take more time. Anyone interested in the subject would realize that a research problem has been identified for further investigation.

Study replication can be an exciting adventure and may lead to confirmation of findings or perhaps new findings. You may find a study of a problem and want to investigate a similar problem in a group or area not covered by the first study. Or perhaps you believe the methodology was flawed or the author's conclusions were wrong, in which case you could replicate the study. Regardless of the problem or type of study, choose something that interests you.

In general, familiarity with the specific research field being used is necessary to discern what has been achieved and what needs to be done. One must be sufficiently knowledgeable about what has been accomplished, where current knowledge stands, and where to go from there. A literature review and search is conducted to provide you with current information and to help further define your problem or research question. Otherwise, if you remain uncertain about the nature of the issue or problem, it will remain unclear. Your research problem needs to be defined by both your literature search and what you already know (Box 3–1).

What Constitutes a Research Problem?

A research problem may be viewed as a situation that begs resolution or needs improvement, modification, or an answer. In other words, it is a situation that warrants examination and study, whether for the purpose of

---

BOX 3–1

Topics come from:

- Work environment (clinical observations, problems, or challenges)
- Personal interest (medical condition of self, family member or acquaintance)
- Prior studies (journal articles or reports in medical and lay literature)
- Mentor or preceptor interest (in the case of PA students)
- Literature review
- Others' studies
- Graduation requirements (students)

---

doing things more effectively and efficiently; to validate observations made in the classroom, clinic, or other setting; or to provide an answer to a question. The research problem could be just something you are curious about or that interests you.

An example of a research problem that PAs and others have studied and continue to study is identifying factors that determine patient satisfaction with care provided by PAs in general or within a specific practice (e.g., within your practice). A related problem of interest has been to contrast patient satisfaction with care provided by PAs versus that provided by other midlevel providers or physicians. Another example of a research problem is to identify the factors that affect patient adherence with medication regimens and to determine the influence of religious beliefs, cultural and ethnic standards, or socioeconomic and other issues on compliance. These are examples of problems that should interest not only PAs and the PA profession, but also others—both within and outside the health-care system—because of the significant impact, not only on the patient's welfare and health care in general, but also on the economic welfare of the country. Still another example of a research problem that should interest the PA profession is the question of a difference in patient care between that provided by PAs who graduate from master's programs and that provided by graduates of bachelor's or associate degree programs. This is a sensitive topic with political overtones that has been broached in editorials, but not addressed in a scientific way using an analytical approach. For the researcher the results are the results, and the politicians should be left to deal with the fallout. Many other problems come to mind as well.

Getting Started

You are encouraged to take a few moments and list five problems/questions for which you would like to know

---

Exercise 3–1

List five research problems that interest you (see Table 3–1) and rate your degree of interest in each (Most interesting = 5; Least interesting = 1)

	Problem	Rating
1.	_____	_____
2.	_____	_____
3.	_____	_____
4.	_____	_____
5.	_____	_____

---

the answers. Use the box above to prioritize them. Keep in mind that substantive research is not accomplished overnight. Research, especially substantive research, is a lengthy process with the potential of becoming tedious and frustrating. You sometimes have to work to maintain your enthusiasm for your research, but without continued enthusiasm, you are likely to stop short of reaching your goals.

Identifying a Research Problem

Identifying the research problem is the first step in conducting research. You begin by asking yourself, "What is the question that I want to answer?" It is a good idea to write down your questions and begin the record keeping for your study. You must be able to manage the problems because having a large number of problems (as research questions or null hypotheses or hypotheses) in one study is probably not going to be beneficial. Remember the acronym "KIS!" ("Keep it simple!"). It is best to identify a problem in its basic form and do a thorough investigation rather than tackle a large number of problems. This is analogous to the predator that succeeds only after it has learned to identify and focus on the appropriate prey. As a predator, you have to chase one prey, not the whole herd. Otherwise, the outcome of the chase is a foregone conclusion and, as a predator, you will be left hungry. The same is true for identifying your research problem. One well identified problem is much better than a number of ill-defined or general problems. It is also worth keeping in mind that it is unlikely that any of us will make an earth-shattering discovery, but each of us can add a small piece to what we know.

As a PA determined to investigate a problem, you must be able to focus on what needs to be done to resolve the problem (situation) at hand. To identify the problem, you may pose several questions including the following:

1. Given a situation, what can be done, or what approach should be taken to improve it?

2. What is known (what does the literature say) about it?

3. What is not known about the situation?

4. What information or data are needed to improve the situation?

Based on answers to these and other questions, the PA should be able to better define the problem(s).

Consider the following as examples of a process for development of a problem and study:

Scenario 1: A clinical PA, who is keeping a log of ideas and observations, notes an unusual number of postoperative infections in a particular patient population. The PA discusses this observation with the supervising physician. After perusing several patient charts, the two concur that the problem is real and decide that "someone should look into it" to determine the reason for these infections (purpose of the study) to ultimately minimize the number of cases of postsurgical infections (goal of the study). Other reasons for carrying out the study would include reducing morbidity and mortality, reducing the costs of care, and other equally important goals.

The PA and supervising physician then devote time to deciding what to do (brainstorming) and formulate questions to narrow the focus, determine the importance of the study, and decide the degree to which it can be researched. They consider, among others, the following questions:

1. What information to gather

2. Where to access the information

3. Whether to rely solely on medical records or to include survey data from patients, nursing staff, or others

4. What, if any, consents to obtain

5. Whether or not to recruit a consultant to help design the study or analyze the data after it is gathered

6. Whether the results should be published and in which medium (i.e., how the information should be disseminated)

7. Whether there are any ethical issues, and how to address them

8. Where to find financial support to carry out the study

Figure 3–1 is a schematic of the process of developing a hypothesis from an observation based on scenario 1.

Some examples of possible research questions for this scenario may include the following:

1. Are there procedural differences between infected patients and noninfected patients?

2. Are there demographic differences between infected and noninfected patients?

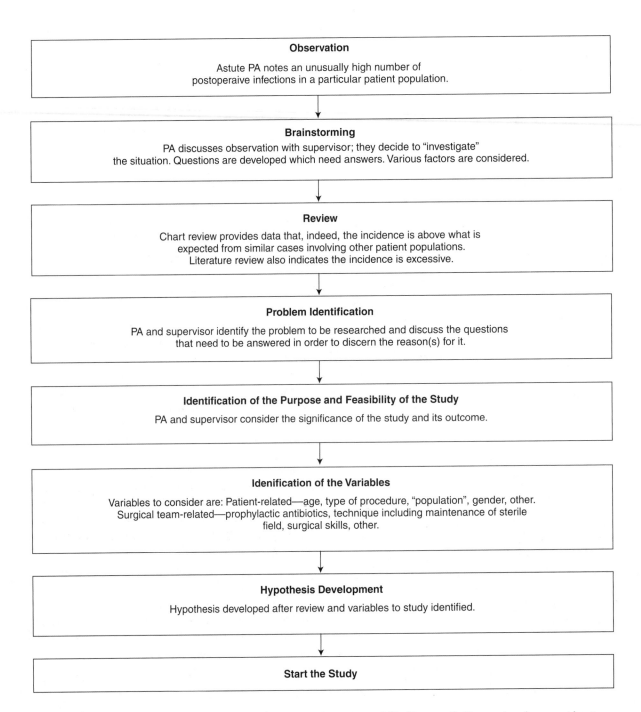

Observation

Astute PA notes an unusually high number of postoperaive infections in a particular patient population.

Brainstorming

PA discusses observation with supervisor; they decide to "investigate" the situation. Questions are developed which need answers. Various factors are considered.

Review

Chart review provides data that, indeed, the incidence is above what is expected from similar cases involving other patient populations. Literature review also indicates the incidence is excessive.

Problem Identification

PA and supervisor identify the problem to be researched and discuss the questions that need to be answered in order to discern the reason(s) for it.

Identification of the Purpose and Feasibility of the Study

PA and supervisor consider the significance of the study and its outcome.

Idenification of the Variables

Variables to consider are: Patient-related—age, type of procedure, "population", gender, other. Surgical team-related—prophylactic antibiotics, technique including maintenance of sterile field, surgical skills, other.

Hypothesis Development

Hypothesis developed after review and variables to study identified.

Start the Study

FIG. 3–1. Developing a hypothesis from an observation.[2] (Adapted from Mateo MA, Newton C. Progressing from an idea to a research question. In Kirchhoff KT, Mateo MA [eds]: Using and Conducting Nursing Research in the Clinical Setting, 2nd ed. Philadelphia: WB Saunders, 1999, p. 198.)

3. Are there care differences between infected and non-infected patients?

Using the null hypothesis format, you would answer these questions with the following statements:

1. There are no procedural differences between infected and noninfected patients.
2. There are no demographic differences between infected and noninfected patients.
3. There are no care differences between infected and noninfected patients.

Using the hypothesis format, you would address these problems with the following statements:

1. There are procedural differences between infected and noninfected patients.
2. There are demographic differences between infected and noninfected patients.
3. There are care differences between infected and non-infected patients.

You would then proceed to identify your variables and design your study. Statistical analyses will determine the answers to your research questions or indicate whether you should retain or reject your null hypotheses, answer your research questions, or prove your hypotheses.

Scenario 2: A group of three PA students, required to identify a research problem and conduct a project as part of the curriculum, develop interest in studying the effectiveness of a new surgical method for managing low back pain in patients with herniated disks. They discuss the idea with their mentor and decide it is a worthwhile endeavor to determine whether the "new" method is "better" than the older methods. They discuss the following (suggested answers in parentheses):

1. What information to gather (patient satisfaction)
2. Where to access the information (surgical practice)
3. Whether to rely solely on subjective data (reported pain score) or to include objective data (type to be determined)
4. What, if any, consents to obtain (patient and physician consent)
5. Whether or not to recruit a consultant to help design the study or analyze the data after it is collected (perhaps a faculty member who is savvy in statistical methods)
6. Whether the results should be published and in which medium (i.e., how the information should be disseminated)
7. Whether there are any ethical issues, and how to address them (patient consent, confidentiality, etc.)

8. Where to find financial support to carry out the study (could this be accomplished without incurring financial expenses?)

Example research questions related to Scenario 2 include

1. How safe is the method?
2. How much more costly is the procedure?
3. What are the morbidity and mortality rates associated with this method (as compared to older methods)?
4. What is the degree of patient satisfaction with this method?
5. How many workdays are saved using this method (as compared to established methods)?

As an exercise, use the null hypotheses below to develop the appropriate hypotheses.

1. There are no differences in patient satisfaction between new and older methods.
2. There are no differences in morbidity and mortality between patients undergoing the new versus older methods of patient management.
3. There are no outcome differences.

Stating the Research Question

A good research question is one that can be answered using observable data and includes the relationship between two or more variables, and is logical.[3] According to Sutherland et al.,[4] the three most frequently identified indices of the merit of a research question are potential impact, justification, and feasibility. Consider these terms as you develop your research questions. Put the questions in straightforward sentences, hypotheses, or null hypotheses format. Deal with only one variable per research question, if possible. Develop enough questions, hypotheses, or null hypotheses to fully explore the problem that you are investigating. Remember that one question answered well with sound methodology is better than many questions not answered well.

Narrowing the Focus of the Question

In order to achieve the kind of focus necessary, you would do well to be systematic in your approach to honing and defining your problems and questions. Generally, you need to start broad and become more specific[5] (Box 3–2). Here is an example of one approach.

Problem statement

There is no information on how many PAs do not practice clinically following successful completion of PA curricula.

Going from Broad to Specific

- Problem statement
- Question (problem converted into question that can be answered)
- Aim/purpose
- Objective/s (what the researcher/s will do to answer the question

Question (Problem converted into a question that can be answered):

How many PAs do not practice clinically following successful completion of PA curricula?

Aim (or purpose) of the research project:

To determine how many PAs do not practice clinically following successful completion of PA curricula

Objective/s (more specific than the aim):

What the researcher is going to do to answer the question:

1. Collect information on the number of PA graduates who do not practice clinically.
2. Determine how many are men and how many are women.
3. Determine the age distribution of these graduates.

4. Determine how many practiced initially then stopped and how many never practiced.
5. Identify the reasons provided for not practicing clinically.
6. Determine whether the type of practice has any impact on the decisions to not practice.
7. Determine the impact of personal, marital, financial, or other considerations on the decision.

Here is a second (reverse) approach using a different problem. Say you are interested in the subject of hyaline membrane disease, but are not quite sure what to study/research. Moving from the more general to the more specific, you could take the following approach:

1. Incidence of hyaline membrane disease ("Too broad! What about it?")
2. Incidence of hyaline membrane disease in African American neonates (Getting warmer!)
3. Incidence of hyaline membrane disease in female African American neonates.
4. Incidence of hyaline membrane disease in female African American neonates born to teen mothers. (Getting more specific!)
5. Incidence of hyaline membrane disease in female African American neonates born to teen mothers between 1998 and 2004. (Even more specific.)

Exercise 3-2

Consider your top choice problem (from Exercise 3–1). Work from general to specific in the manner outlined above.

Problem statement: _____

_____

Question: _____

Aim/purpose: _____

_____

Objective/s

a. _____

b. _____

c. _____

d. _____

e. _____

f. _____

g. _____

6. Incidence of hyaline membrane disease in female African American neonates born to teen mothers between 1998 and 2004 in Colin County.

You have now carved out a research project aimed at determining the incidence of hyaline membrane disease in a specific population. Is such a project feasible? The answer is "theoretically, yes!" However, other factors, including costs and available resources, have to be considered before the study can be successfully carried out.

Sources of Ideas for Research Problems

Some topics that are certainly in the realm of possibility for PAs or PA students that can be explored for research studies include the following:

1. PA role in health promotion
2. Learning styles of PA students (for academic PAs)
3. Patient attitudes toward PAs and other midlevel providers
4. Cost-effectiveness of PAs and cost-effective for whom
5. PA attitudes toward specific patient populations (e.g., people with HIV/AIDS, minorities, gays, and lesbians)
6. Impact of PAs and other midlevel providers on health care in medically underserved areas
7. Any type of clinical investigation
8. Relationship between master's degrees and quality of patient care
9. Research training in the curriculum – Is there a lasting effect?
10. The PA profession niche in research
11. PA applicant selection—predictive value of the Graduate Record Exam (GRE), grade point average (GPA), and other parameters
12. PA program graduate success rates with the Physician Assistant National Certification Examination and curriculum differences
13. Differences in PA practice by specialty
14. Economic impact of a PA on a community
15. PA malpractice and liability

PAs, especially those new to research, may glean research ideas from various sources. These sources may include clinical practice (as in the scenario described earlier), literature review, interaction with students in didactic and clinical settings, interactions with colleagues at meetings (such as the American Academy of Physician Assistants or the Association of Physician Assistant Programs meetings or state and local meetings), interaction with supervisors, or research papers in which authors point out "further" aspects that need exploring. Ideas can also be obtained from government and from private and public organizations (e.g., requests for proposals, also known as RFPs) that seek information and data on or about a particular subject or point of interest. These types of requests are distributed by government agencies or private foundations and often are formulated by experts and specialty groups.[5]

Determining Need for the Study

As alluded to previously, the need for studying a particular problem is determined by many factors such as the following:

1. Significance in medical, legal, and socioeconomic terms
2. Whether or not the issue has already been addressed (i.e., its novelty)
3. Acuity or seriousness
4. Human, time, and financial costs or economic burden
5. Contribution to knowledge

A survey of nurse researchers[6] indicated that focus on "real-world concerns" and soundness of methodology are criteria of greatest significance in research projects, and focus on timely or current concerns was less important. On the other hand, personal interest in a particular problem may be the most important driving force. This may be true for many PAs and PA students as well. This question could be another research project for you.

Must a Study Be Original?

Although some researchers view replication studies as less scholarly and less valuable than original studies (an attitude that is more pervasive in some disciplines than in others), the fact remains that there are many instances in which replication may be both indicated and valuable. Some of the reasons studies are replicated include extending the generalizations of the findings, establishing credibility, reducing errors (types I and II), and providing support for developing theories.[7] For novice researchers who might find identifying research topics and problems confusing and overwhelming, replication studies may actually be "just what the PA ordered."

Summary

The first step in your research effort is to identify the problem(s). Each problem is then put into a research question or null hypothesis form. Your statements should be concise and deal with only one variable or subject each. Each statement must be in a form that allows investigation. In developing your questions, try to deal with a manageable number of questions or variables. Small steps are best. It is better to do a complete job with research that adds a small piece to our knowledge base than to do an incomplete job with multiple problems. Keep in mind certain key tips when developing your research question (Box 3–3).

Box 3–3

Pearls

1. Carry a pocket notebook or piece of paper and write down research ideas as you think of them.

2. Define your research problem to its simplest format.

3. Learn what is known or has been done about the problem or related issues.

4. Be able to define your goals, objectives, and purposes.

5. Be able to describe the significance of your research and why it can be the solution or part of the solution of the problem.

6. Be able to answer the questions of why your project is important to society, medicine, and profession.

References

1. Bailey DM. Research for the Health Professional—A Practical Guide, 2nd ed. Philadelphia: FA Davis, 1997, p. 2.
2. Mateo MA, Newton C. Progressing from an idea to a research question. In Kirchhoff KT, Mateo MA (eds): Using and Conducting Nursing Research in the Clinical Setting, 2nd ed. Philadelphia: WB Saunders, 1999, p. 198.
3. Lindeman CA, Schantz D. The research question. Journal of Nursing Administration 1982;12(1):6.
4. Sutherland HJ, Meslin EM, Cunha DA, Till JE. Judging clinical research questions: What criteria are used? Social Science and Medicine 1993;37(12):1427.
5. Jenkins S, Price CJ, Straker L. The Researching Therapist—A Practical Guide to Planning, Performing and Communicating Research. Philadelphia: Churchill Livingstone, 1998, p. 24
6. Moody L, Vera H, Blanks C, Visscher M. Developing questions of substance for nursing science. Western Journal of Nursing Research 1989;11(4):393.
7. Beck CT. Replication studies for nursing research. Image–the Journal of Nursing Scholarship 1994;26(3):191.

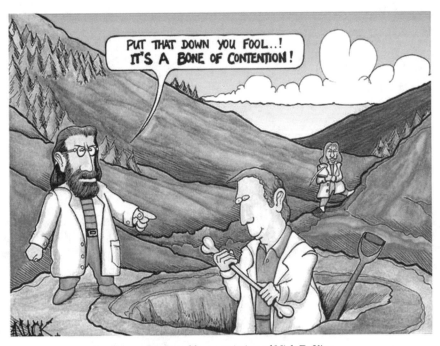

Reprinted by permission of Nick D. Kim.

SECTION II

Your Research

chapter 4

Review of the Literature

Marvis J. Lary, PhD, PA-C

Science has discovered that it is the lower part of the face that gives away one's thoughts, not the eyes. This is especially true when one opens the lower part of the face.

Elbert Hubbard

Chapter Overview

This chapter is a "how to" resource designed to provide basic mechanics for doing a literature review. It defines some of the common terminology associated with the process of searching the literature and provides helpful hints in locating selected information most effectively and efficiently. The review of the literature (some may call it a "review of the pertinent literature") is where the background for your investigation and what is known about your subject is reviewed and presented to the reader. The review of literature is typically a large section (many times the largest) of your thesis, dissertation, or manuscript and well referenced. When a reader finishes reading the Review of Literature, he or she should have a good basis for evaluating and understanding your investigation and its significance. A good Review of the Literature will also allow the reader to contrast your results and conclusions to what is known about the problem(s) being investigated.

Introduction

What is a Review of the Literature? A literature review identifies and discusses published information in a particular subject area. The format of a review of the literature will vary from assignment to assignment and by the type of manuscript to be produced. A Review of the Literature can be a self-contained unit—an end in itself (you may find the answer to your question when you do your literature search)—or it can be a preface to and rationale for engaging in primary research. A literature review can be just a simple summary of what has been published on a topic, but more commonly, it combines both summary and synthesis of the subject and points of interest. Although a literature review evaluates methods and results, the main emphasis is on knitting together theories and results from a number of studies to describe the "big picture" in a field of research. One way to think about the Review of Literature is that it is the history of what is known about your problem.

In writing the literature review, your purpose is to convey to your reader what knowledge and ideas have been established on a topic, and what the strengths and weaknesses of those ideas are. Besides enlarging your knowledge about the topic and providing a background for readers, writing a literature review lets you gain and demonstrate skills in two areas:

- Seeking information: ability to scan the literature efficiently, using manual or computerized methods in order to identify useful publications and information
- Critical analysis: ability to identify and analyze unbiased and valid studies and determine if further research is indicated

A thorough review of the literature involves the systematic identification, location, and analysis of documents containing information related to the research problem or question. Documents include a variety of publications and unpublished resources, such as dissertations, speeches, and even personal communications.

For your research purposes, a successful literature review will do the following:

1. Provide an overview of scholarly work related to and organized around the research question you are developing.
2. Allow you to synthesize results into a summary of what is and is not known.
3. Identify areas of controversy in the literature.
4. Formulate questions (form the basis for your investigation) that need further research.
5. Provide tools, such as instruments that have already been validated, studies that can be replicated, and data that can be used for both correlation and research design ideas.

What Is the Purpose of Literature Reviews?

Published literature reviews provide a handy guide to a particular topic. If you have limited time to conduct research, literature reviews can give you an overview or act as a stepping stone. For professionals, they are useful reports that keep them up to date with what is current in the field. For scholars, the depth and breadth of the literature review emphasize the credibility of the writer in his or her field. Literature reviews also provide a solid background for a research paper's investigation. Comprehensive knowledge of the literature of the field or subject is essential to most research papers.

Where Do I Begin?

Determine the purpose of your literature review. What do you need to know? For a research project, define the research problem/question. Try stating the problem in the form of a question. You might start with a broad question such as, "Are physician assistants (PAs) satisfied with their profession?" Then try making your question more specific, such as, "What are primary-care PAs most and least satisfied with in their career choice?" Specificity will focus the search.

Gather background information from various resources to define terms, identify previous research areas, and identify key researchers and studies. Never before have there been so many excellent resources for finding information. Although libraries still present the best resources for your search, you can find many at your fingertips on your own computer. Resources for gathering this literature type of background information include the following:

1. Dictionaries in specialty areas that give definitions of terms and phrases used within the specific field of interest.
2. Bibliographic databases prepared by authorities in your specialty field that list previous research (often with annotations). These bibliographies may come in various forms, including the following:
   - Books
   - Journal articles (to review articles on a particular topic)
   - Published proceedings from professional meetings
   - Publications on the World Wide Web

An excellent resource for bibliographies published in books or journals is the Bibliographic Index, 2004. This index is published by the H.W. Wilson Company and can be found in the reference collection of many libraries and accessed online. Directories may also assist in identifying related agencies or associations in your field. An excellent resource for this is the Encyclopedia of Associations, which lists 135,000 nonprofit organizations also found in libraries and online. There are variations in the titles found in libraries, so it may be helpful to work with a reference librarian to identify the most useful background information sources for your research area.

Prepare for the Search

Identifying key words and concepts is vital to a successful literature search. Break your research statement down into its key concepts. For example, the research question, "What are primary care physician assistants most and least satisfied with in their career choice?" could include key concepts such as "primary care," "physician assistants," and "career satisfaction." These key concepts (and key words) can then be used as you progress in your literature search.

Once you have determined the key concepts for your search, you should consider all terms that may be synonymous with or similar to these terms. It is important to have synonyms, narrower terms, and broader terms to narrow or expand the search. Examples of similar terms for the same subject are as follows:

1. Primary care: general internal medicine, pediatrics, family medicine
2. Physician assistant: physician extender, practitioner, midlevel practitioner, health-care provider, clinician, and the outdated but still used physician's assistant
3. Career satisfaction: career choice, professional satisfaction, job satisfaction, career change

Depending on the keywords and concepts associated with your research topic, you may find a vast amount of information or very little. For example, if the keywords "physician assistant" were used, volumes of information would be available. If the words "physician assistant referrals" were used, fewer specific resources would be found.

Where to Search

The subject of your research topic will provide direction as you begin your search. You don't want to limit yourself, however, and overlook a valuable resource—that's why it's called a search. You want to be confident that you have explored all resources. This thoroughness strengthens the quality of your work and increases your expertise on your research subject. A lack of rigor in your search and subsequent literature review will put your whole effort into question.

Countless resources are available for literature reviews. Become familiar with all of them, including library and computer resources. Research literature resources can be found in local medical centers, higher education institutions, medical societies, public libraries, and other places. For computer resources, it is important to keep in mind that even though publications can often be identified on the Web, the full document may be available only from a library.

Books

Each library's catalog contains the record of all cataloged materials owned by that library, including books.

Some libraries also have mega-databases that list the shared holdings of many other libraries. These databases are useful if your local library does not have an adequate collection in the area of your search; most libraries participate in interlibrary loan systems to greatly expand the resources available to you. Remember, there is a lag time between the point when information in a book is submitted and the time the book is published. In general, books are very useful for background work in theory and history, but may not be the most up-to-date resource for a particular subject.

Magazine and Journal Articles

Periodical indexes contain indexing for thousands of journals or magazines. Electronic versions cover spans of years, but may cover only the recent years of publications in detail. For historic research in journal literature, it may be necessary to go to a library with a back file of paper indexes. Always check the dates covered when searching an index. It is important to know the different types of indexes available, including the following:

1. Multisubject periodical indexes are useful when searching for magazines or journals on a subject with multidisciplinary aspects.
2. Subject-specific periodical indexes are available if you want to do an in-depth search in a specific journal, field, or subject.

Government Documents

The U.S. government is uploading more information to the Internet; statistics, reports, and a myriad of other types of publications are available. In some cases, standard publications are no longer being produced in paper form, but are available only via the Internet. Search indexes are available in various formats to identify these resources. One online resource example is the Center for Disease Control's (CDC) *Morbidity and Mortality Weekly Report (MMWR)*. Government information is public property and usually does not require a fee for access. This information can also be reproduced and used without direct permission, but you should reference the source appropriately.

Dissertations

Doctoral dissertations, and to some extent master's theses, are often available in the library of the institution at which the degree was granted. They can also be accessed through electronic indexes for dissertations.

Information on the Internet

Almost anything can be found on the Internet these days. Using your keywords or concepts along with one of many search engines, you can find a vast amount of information on almost any subject. The great amount of available information can, however, require significant time and ability to sort through and interpret. This is where using more specific keywords and concepts becomes necessary to narrow and focus the search. Be careful when using Internet sources. Make sure they have the scientific rigor you need. Almost anyone can put almost anything on the Internet.

At Last—Launching the Search

Remember that more is not necessarily better. In all likelihood, you will not use all the resources you find. The real skill lies in your ability to determine the most relevant, pertinent, and important literature to cite. Once you begin writing your research manuscript, you will need an organized method of making that determination.

Get organized from the very outset of your literature search! You need a method of keeping track of resources. Developing a working bibliography can be done in various ways ranging from a simple index card file to a more complex computerized database utilizing one of the many software packages available for indexing. Each working bibliography entry should contain the following information (with some variations) for books, periodicals, and government documents:

  Author's name

  Title of work

  Publication information

  Library call number

  The URL for Internet sources

  (optional) A personal note about the contents of the source

A file for actual copies of documents, journal articles, abstracts, and so forth will also be needed so that you can refer to them as you are writing. A file of index cards is a simple way of keeping track of resources as you find them (Figure 4–1).

Which Database Should Be Used?

There are hundreds of databases; some are subject specific and some are multidisciplinary. Two examples of subject-specific databases are Medscape, which is specific to medicine, and ERIC, which is specific to education. Both can be accessed on the Internet. Academic

TITLE	Job Satisfaction Among Rural Physician Assistants
AUTHOR	Phillip T. Strange
PUBLICATION	Journal of Rural Medicine
DATE	September, 2004, vol. 6, No. 5, pp 122-123
SOURCE	Internet: www.ruralfamilymedicine.org/joRMMEno/winter99.htm
COMMENTS	Survey of 250 primary care PAs in Midwest rural communities. Results reflect high degree of satisfaction with PA role in the rural setting (76%). Specific areas of dissatisfaction were not identified. Recommendation for further study to identify reasons for dissatisfaction in one quarter of the respondents.

FIG. 4–1. Example of an index card for keeping records of resources.

Index is an example of a multidisciplinary index to more than 1,500 general magazines and scholarly journals, and can be found in libraries.

Your research topic will dictate which databases to access for your search. It is important, however, to remember to not overly limit your search. You want to learn as much as possible, even if you don't include everything in your final document. Your keywords andconcepts may dictate using many databases to accomplish a comprehensive search pertaining to your content area.

Most databases limit the search by indicating the field in which a word or words should appear. For instance, there are likely to be ways to search in one or more specific fields, such as the following:

1. Author field (by author's name)
2. Title field
3. Publication date
4. Subject field

Most databases are searched using keywords. This means that the words that appear anywhere withinthe search field of a record may be found by entering a keyword search. For instance, in the example givenearlier, the terms "primary care," "physician assistant," or "practice satisfaction" would produce documents using one of those keywords. If desired, using a combination of two or more of the keywords or concepts could narrow the field of information. This approach can be used until the information sought is specific enough to identify resources directly related to your research topic.

Boolean Operators

The Internet is a vast computer database; therefore, its contents must be searched according to the rules of computer database searching. Much of database searching is based on the principles of Boolean logic. To expand your search for keywords and concepts, Boolean "operators" can be used to expand your search for keywords and concepts. The Boolean operators "AND," "OR," and "NOT" are connecting words (usually in all uppercase letters, but not always) that allow you to combine two or more keywords or concepts. For example:

1. If you are doing a search on PA practice satisfaction, you would type in the words "Physician Assistants AND Practice Satisfaction." The search will include the terms on either side of the Boolean connector and retrieve articles that discuss physician assistant practice satisfaction (Figure 4–2).

2. If Physician Assistants OR Practice Satisfaction is used, articles with either term will be retrieved (Figure 4–3).

3. If Physician Assistant NOT Practice Satisfaction is used, only records with the term Physician Assistant will be retrieved. No record with practice satisfaction will be retrieved even if Physician Assistant is in the article (Figure 4–4).

Internet Savvy

The convenience of doing a complete literature search from your own personal computer, along with the fact that almost any subject can be found on the Internet today, makes it the most popular way of searching databases. When using the Internet for your search, be cognizant of the fact that anyone can put information on the Web; accuracy or quality is not a prerequisite. When searching the Internet, the following criteria should be considered:

1. Why has this site been created? Is someone trying to sell you something? Inform you? Persuade you?

2. Where did this site originate? Was it from a sponsoring entity or individual? The resulting content ranges from definitive to false. Only some of the sites located will be relevant to a given topic.

3. What is the content? Check for accuracy: Websites are rarely refereed or reviewed; the source of information should be clearly stated. Check for comprehensiveness: Does content cover a specific time period or aspect of the topic? Check for currency: Has the site been updated recently and is the information current? Check for hyperlinks to connecting sites that should relate to the same topic: Are they relevant and appropriate? Look elsewhere for additional sites.

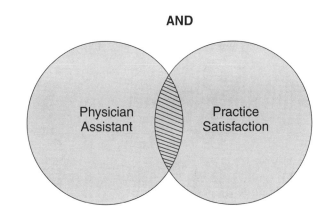

FIG. 4–2. In this search, you will retrieve only records in which BOTH of the search terms are present.

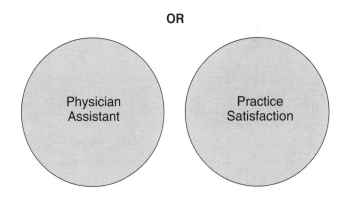

FIG. 4–3. In this search, you will retrieve records with ONE or BOTH of the search terms present.

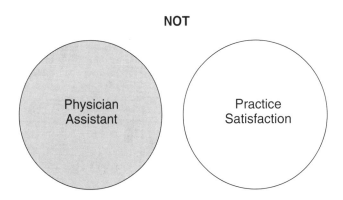

FIG. 4–4. In this search, you will retrieve only records in which the term Physician Assistant is present. No record with the term Practice Satisfaction will be retrieved even if the term Physician Assistant is present.

4. Style and functionality: Good Internet sites enhance the information offered. The site should be well organized and easy to navigate.

Results of the Search

Methods for interpreting the literature are found in great detail elsewhere in this book (Chapter 2), but you should consider some preliminary criteria as you perform the search. Questions to address about specific subjects include the following:

1. Author: Who is the author? Can you find any identifying information?
2. Type of publication: Is it a scholarly journal? Academic book? Popular magazine? Website?
3. Date of publication: Is it current? Does the date matter?
4. Relevance: How relevant is the content of the material to your research topic?
5. Publisher: Is the publisher a professional association or organization? Academic press? Government? Commercial press?
6. Citations or reviews: Are other authors citing this material? If the source is a book, is it listed in the Book Review Index?

All of this information can be recorded using the system that you have chosen to organize your search. As you begin analyzing and interpreting the information that has resulted from your search, you will have at your fingertips all the information needed to draw conclusions and write your research document.

Writing the Literature Review

After gathering all that information and copying all those articles and book chapters, you are at last to write about your literature review. Here are some suggestions for organizing your paper. You should also see Appendix A and Chapter 13.

Title:	Title of your project
Introduction:	The Introduction prepares the reader with a framework for what is to follow.
	Explain the focus of the literature review and the questions you wanted to answer. Summarize the main issues.
Body:	Describe studies and do a comparison and evaluation of findings. Discuss controversies, implications, and questions remaining to be answered.
Conclusion:	Summarize your findings and provide recommendations for future research on the subject.
References:	List according to adopted format

Once you begin writing your literature review, be sure to reference key points, quoted information, and controversial stances. Remember you want your reader to understand the driving points of your research and what has gone before is just that. The review should allow the reader to understand your problem and why answering that problem is important. A good review of the pertinent literature should almost be a stand-alone document. Once you have that: You are off and running. Congratulations!

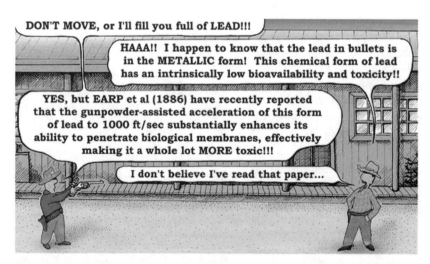

ENVIRONMENTAL SCIENTISTS IN THE WILD WEST

Reprinted by permission of Nick D. Kim.

chapter 5

Methodology

Christopher E. Bork, PhD and Robert W. Jarski, PhD, PA-C

Overview

This chapter covers research design and methodology, which becomes the "Methods" section of your research project. Choosing the right design adds validity, reliability, and strength to your findings and results. The best-intentioned and most meaningful of projects can be derailed by errors in design and weakened by failure to choose the best design. Challenges to validity and reliability must be considered when developing the methods for your investigation. You cannot make a decision about the correct statistical analysis for your study until you have made your design decisions. This is another area in which you should seek the help and consultation of an expert or someone with experience in research design. This chapter gives you a starting point.

Introduction

Once the topic and specific research questions or hypotheses have been identified (and the literature review completed and digested), the investigator must choose a method suitable for achieving the project's objective. This objective is specified as a hypothesis, purpose statement, or a clear and specific research question. In addition, your objective should be evaluated primarily by the following criterion:

Is it important to medicine, the profession, or society?

That is, will it be a significant contribution to our fund of knowledge? Some journals refer to this as the "so what?" section. In many cases, authors are required to respond in writing to this question when submitting a manuscript for publication. Think about how you would answer this question, even if you were never asked. At least for your sake, answering this question will help give some value or meaning to your study. This question should be a guiding principle for research.

Your research project's methods should be driven by the objective. When choosing a method, two mistakes may distract beginning investigators. The first is selecting a method that is familiar or novel without first defining the research objective (e.g., "I want to use a video recorder."). The second common mistake is planning to use already available data. Although convenient, this backward approach almost always leads to trivial information that is unlikely to contribute significantly to our knowledge base. "When all you have is a hammer, the world looks like a nail." The methods should generate data that achieve worthwhile objectives.

The Methods Section

The Methods section describes what was actually done in carrying out the study. It should be sufficiently clear and detailed so that others may duplicate the study. The Methods section includes descriptions of the following:

- Subjects
- Instrumentation used (including questionnaires, when used)
- Procedures carried out
- Analytic procedures used for evaluating and summarizing the data

Data analysis must be suited to the particulars of the study: the number of subject groups (e.g., two, an intervention and control group), the number of subjects within each group, and the procedures used for data collection (e.g., single or repeated measures). One might automatically assume that the analysis would involve a statistical method. Although this is often the case for many research efforts, you may want to consider whether a specific question might be best answered using a qualitative approach.

A Methods Scheme

Each study plan poses its own challenges. Beginning researchers will find it useful to refer to a system such as the one presented in Table 5–1 for identifying some available study options. First, the researcher must decide whether the approach will be analytic or descriptive by answering the question, "Is there a comparison between groups?"

Understanding Research Design

Controlling Bias

The design of research considers several factors and is best described as an attempt by the researcher or investigator to limit or control factors and biases that potentially can contaminate an experiment or study. As mentioned in previous chapters, all research starts with an idea or a problem. The research hypothesis is the investigator's expectation for the outcome or the solution to the problem; it is, however, only a hunch.

Table 5–1
Selected Research Designs

Name	Design	Statistical Test
One-shot case study	X O	None
One group pre-test–post-test	O X O	Dependent or paired t test Wilcoxson matched-pairs, signed ranks
Static group comparison	X O ‒‒‒‒‒‒‒‒‒ O	Independent t test Chi-square Mann-Whitney U
Post-test-only control group	R X O R O	Independent t test or ANOVA Mann-Whitney U Kruskal-Wallis ANOVA
Nonequivalent control group	O X O ‒‒‒‒‒‒‒‒‒ O O	ANCOVA or ANOVA
Pre-test–post-test control group	R O X O R O O	ANCOVA or ANOVA
Solomon four group	R O X O R O O R X O R O	ANCOVA or ANOVA
Counterbalanced	X_1 O X_2 O X_3 O X_2 O X_3 O X_1 O X_3 O X_1 O X_2 O	ANOVA
Time series	O O O O X O O O O	ANOVA, trend analysis

X indicates experimental treatment or intervention; O, observation, measurement, or evaluation; R, randomization of a large number of subjects; ‒‒‒‒‒‒‒‒, nonequivalent group; ANOVA, analysis of variance; and ANCOVA, analysis of covariance.

Selection of a research design is a method that takes into account the researcher's expectation (the research hypothesis) and creates a means of controlling biases that may result from the expectation. In other words, if an informed observer knows what the investigator's expectations were, the research design is contrived as a means to eliminate bias and allow the results of the study to truly represent the effect of the independent variable. The observer could conclude that the researcher's bias did not influence the result.

Other reasons for an understanding of research design include recognizing and minimizing the effect of threats to validity, both internal and external. In this chapter, the learner becomes familiar with the concepts of error, reliability, forms of validity, and a method of identifying and diagramming typical research designs.

Error

All research involves measurement and all measurements involve error. The common formula for a given measurement is:

Observed measurement = true measurement + error

The astute reader immediately deduces that as error decreases, the observed measurement begins to approximate the true measurement. In everyday life one commonly contends with errors in measurement. Consider an all-too-common example. If you have ever tried to cut a shelf to put inside a closet, you may be painfully aware of the formula for an observed measurement. In this example, if the observed measurement includes too large an error, then the shelf will not fit in the closet. The shelf may be either too large or too small because the error term can be either positive or negative.

Types of Error

Error can be categorized into two forms, random and systematic. Random error consists of those errors that occur strictly because of chance and may be thought of as "noise in the system." Small sample sizes tend to be more vulnerable to random error. For example, if one takes five measurements versus one measurement, the average of the five measurements is less likely to be incorrect or have a large error term. The carpenter's proverb of "measure twice, cut once" recognizes the role of random errors.

Systematic error can be thought of as a series of consistent biases affecting a measurement. Typical researcher errors include poor technique such as sloppiness, inappropriate protocols or research designs, inappropriate measures, and incorrect statistical applications. For example, if a researcher is using heart rate (beats per minute) as an indicator and calculates heart rate using 10-second readings sometimes and 15-second readings at other times, then the error risk increases. (Sloppiness has been introduced by not using a consistent reading time.)

Similarly, if a researcher is using a survey to assess a clinical outcome, error may be introduced by several factors, including the subjects' differences in verbal fluency or even the conditions under which the survey is completed. Consider the differences in response to a telephone survey about practitioner satisfaction from an individual who has just experienced a 2-hour traffic jam and from one who has just exercised and feels wonderful. Differences in their levels of stress may affect their responses.

By choosing appropriate measures, using a reliable technique, and employing valid instruments to obtain measurements, a researcher can eliminate a substantial number of errors. Of fundamental importance to obtaining appropriate and useful data are the concepts of reliability and validity.

Reliability

Reliability focuses on the consistency with which a measurement is taken. If a measurement lacks reliability, then the data obtained may be useless because of error. In other words, if substantial error exists in the measurements, then the researcher cannot know whether observed changes in the dependent variable are caused by manipulation of the independent variable or variability in measurement. Reliability is also of paramount importance to the physician assistant (PA) in clinical practice. If a clinician does not gather reliable data, then there is no way of knowing whether apparent changes in the patient are the result of actual physiological changes or poor technique. In other words, the clinician will not know if progress is taking place as a result of treatment.

Forms of Reliability

There are three common forms of reliability: instrument reliability, intra-rater reliability, and inter-rater reliability. Instrument reliability focuses on the consistency of measurement by a particular instrument. For example, if a weighing scale has a worn spring, it may measure light weights accurately but heavy weights inaccurately. The method to improve instrument reliability is to consistently calibrate the instrument.

Intra-rater reliability focuses on the consistency with which an individual takes measurements. For example, does the PA measure blood pressure in the same way each and every time? If not, there is a strong possibility that the measurements will differ because of technique rather than actual differences in the patient. One method to improve intra-rater reliability is to consistently follow an established protocol and to routinely check for consistency.

Inter-rater reliability focuses on the consistency in measurements between or among more than one individual taking the measurements. If more than one individual is taking a measurement, there must be adequate assurances that results are caused by changes in the true measurement rather than fluctuations in the error. The concept of inter-rater reliability is often ignored and has important ramifications for clinical practice as well as research. Besides being poor practice, inattention to inter-rater reliability may obscure differences in a patient's progress. If individuals who are seeing the patient do not collect data in the same way, they will not be able to ascertain if differences are caused by differences in the patient or differences in the way the measurement was performed (error). In other words, if data are not gathered in a consistent or reliable manner, their accuracy is questionable, and therefore the data may be useless.

The "two P rule"—protocol and practice—is prudent when two or more individuals are taking measurements. The individuals should take measurements using a standard protocol that they have practiced. They should also compare their measurements periodically, and they may wish to ascertain their consistency by using one of the tests that assess inter-rater reliability.* When reading or reviewing any article that involves measurements, one should look for an assessment or other assurance that the data were gathered reliably.

Validity

Another concept that must be considered regarding data and measurement in an investigation is validity, which asks questions about the usefulness or appropriateness of the data being gathered. In a practical sense, reliability and validity are related concepts. Reliability focuses on consistency of measurement, whereas validity focuses on the appropriateness of a given measurement. A simple illustration may help. In a game of darts, reliability can be thought of as the consistency of the pattern or spread of the darts; validity can be thought of as ensuring that the darts are aimed at a dartboard. There are two principal types of validity: measurement or test validity and design or experimental validity.

---

*A discussion of the measures of reliability is beyond the scope of this text. Interested readers are advised to read the classic articles by Shrout and Fleiss and Bartko and Carpenter listed in the readings for this chapter found in Appendix B.

Measurement or Test Validity

Measurement or test validity asks the question: "Does the test or measure actually do what it is intended to do?" For this to occur, a given measurement should have a defined purpose and relate to a given phenomenon. (For example, a clinician routinely takes a temperature because this vital sign can be an indication of an inflammatory process.) For the purposes of this chapter, we focus on some common forms of test validity.

The first form is face validity, which addresses the question, "Does the particular measurement or method appear to be appropriate?" This form of validity often relies on the opinion of experts. Most authorities consider face validity the weakest of the forms of test and measurement validity. Construct validity asks whether the measurement is based on theory. In the example of taking a temperature, the construct that an inflammation involves heat provides modest construct validity. Content validity, on the other hand, asks whether the test is broad enough to address the scope of the content. For example, if one wanted to test PA students' knowledge of anatomy but tested them only on the anatomy of the upper extremity, then that particular test would lack content validity. Criterion validity asks how well the test performs and if it is useful when judged against a standard.

There are generally two subcategories of criterion validity: predictive validity and concurrent validity. Predictive validity assesses whether and how well a test predicts a specific phenomenon or outcome. For example, how well does a positive Ober test (a straight leg raise) accurately predict a lumbar disc protrusion? Concurrent validity asks whether the test performs as well as an accepted test. Generally, this category is used to validate a short or noninvasive version of a test. For example, concurrent validity would be used to establish the validity of a urine test as opposed to a serum glucose test to monitor diabetes mellitus.

Design or Experimental Validity

There are two forms of design or experimental validity: internal and external. Internal validity is concerned with limiting or controlling factors and events other than the independent variable, which may cause changes in the outcome or dependent variable. These factors or events are termed threats to internal validity. External validity, on the other hand, is concerned with factors that may affect the generalization of the conclusions drawn from the study. These factors are referred to as threats to external validity. The next sections examine these two concepts.

Threats to Internal Validity

As mentioned, threats and concerns related to internal validity are unintended factors and conditions that can affect the results. For example, if one were assessing the effects of two dietary regimens and did not take into account the subjects' levels of activity, then the internal validity of the study would be threatened.

There are two broad categories of threats to internal validity: temporal or time-based effects and measurement effects. Temporal or time-based effects consist of history, maturation, or attrition. History refers to effects on the dependent variable that are a result of the passage of time. For example, suppose an investigator is interested in a new topical ointment for the common cold sore, caused by the herpes simplex virus. The researcher treats one group of patients with a new drug or topical ointment for 7 days and obtains excellent results. The fact is, however, that cold sores from the herpes simplex virus are thought to be self-limiting anyway, with symptoms that generally resolve in 7 days. Thus, the passage of time has obscured the effect or noneffect of the topical ointment.

The next temporal effect or threat to internal validity is maturation. Maturation can be thought of as those threats that happen by changes resulting from development. Suppose an individual is suggesting that a particular type of rehabilitative therapy improves the development of infants' motor skills. In this example, the individual contends that the therapy helps infants walk sooner. The effects of that therapy and potential changes in the infants' motor skills may be the result not of the type of therapy involved but rather of the developmental process. Thus, the experiment may be flawed by threats to internal validity, specifically maturation.

The third temporal effect or threat to internal validity results from attrition. Stated quite simply, when subjects leave a study, the results may be distorted. Consider the consequences of a study of a hypothetical new drug for migraine headache sufferers. In this hypothetical study, one group of subjects receives the new drug, and their results are compared with those of another group of subjects who receive a placebo. The subjects will be seen every 3 weeks for a period of 6 months. Consider what occurs if subjects taking the new drug no longer have migraine headaches, so they no longer come to their appointments. The only individuals left in the study will be those for whom the drug did not work. Thus, at the end of 6 months, when it comes time to compare the placebo to the experimental drug, there will appear to be no difference because the majority of people who continue to have migraine headaches will remain in the study. The people who were helped by the drug dropped out of the study, and their attrition affected— and may distort—the results.

Measurement effects are those threats to internal validity that result from an investigator trying to measure a phenomenon. The first threat is testing, especially when the test is repeated several times. Sometimes the act of testing a patient affects the results of the study. Consider an investigation in which the researcher is interested in the effect of a particular type of setting on function in a group of individuals who have suffered a cerebral vascular accident. One of the measurements may be a functional test (e.g., how well the individual is able to dress without help from others). In this hypothetical study, the investigator decides to administer a pre-test to determine the baseline time needed for an individual in the study to self-dress. In this case, having the patient get dressed may help the patient discover new and better strategies for getting dressed, thus contaminating the results.

A second example would be an investigator who wishes to compare two forms of drug therapy on patients with cardiac problems. In this study, the investigator chooses to use a step test, having the subjects step up and down repeatedly, recording the number of times they can do so until the heart rate reaches a predetermined percentage of maximum. In this study, the patient's performance may be affected by the motor learning that takes place. In other words, the patient may improve just by virtue of a pre-test using the step test.

The next threat to internal validity is instrumentation. Quite simply, the type of instrumentation used may affect the results. Consider a study in which the investigator is interested in whether youngsters with handwriting problems press their pencils harder on the paper. To measure the point pressure of the writing implement, the youngsters are asked to use a pencil-type instrument containing a force transducer and a wire that leads to a recording device. The fact that the instrument represents an unnatural pencil may affect the results. Thus the instrument itself is a threat to internal validity.

Another threat to internal validity is sampling. Sampling effects include the confounding effect of the selection of subjects for a study according to some bias, whether recognized or not. If selected by virtue of a bias, the subjects are not representative of the population. For example, if subjects were surveyed in a study via a mail questionnaire that was sent only to residents in an affluent suburb, then the conclusions drawn from the results may be affected by the sample that was surveyed.

The final measurement effect that is a threat to internal validity is termed statistical regression to the mean. Simply stated, this is the tendency for a group of outliers to move toward the mean (the average), not necessarily because of any difference in the subjects' characteristics, but rather because of the laws of probability. A classic example of statistical regression to the mean can be illustrated by what happened when students with developmental and learning challenges were mainstreamed into a classroom with so-called "normal" students. After a period they were tested, and their scores on a developmental and learning inventory improved. Buoyed by success, these researchers decided that if scores improved by putting challenged students in a "normal" class, then perhaps putting "normal" students in a class with gifted students would bring the "normal" students' scores up. When this was tried and all the students in the class were retested, the exceptional students appeared to do more poorly on the test. Did the exposure to "normal" students somehow contaminate these learners? No. What was happening was simply statistical regression to the mean. In both cases, the group that was being tested (the developmentally challenged and the gifted students) came from the ends of the distribution of test scores—the highest and lowest scores. On the retest, their scores tended to migrate toward the mean, toward that typical score within a population. The message here is that investigations using subjects who may be considered outliers (physically challenged individuals or elite athletes, for example) may be affected by statistical regression to the mean.

Threats to External Validity

As mentioned earlier, threats to external validity include factors and conditions that affect the ability to generalize the results of a study. Threats to external validity can be placed into two categories: threats related to the populations used and those related to the environment in which the study takes place (that is, environmental threats).

The first population-related threat to external validity concerns the subjects' accessibility to the study. When one performs a study, one usually studies a portion of a given population—a sample. If the sample used in an experiment or investigation is substantially different from the population, then the ability to generalize the results to the population may be compromised. This threat may be of particular interest in clinical studies because in the typical clinical study subjects generally has access to medical care and the wherewithal to seek medical care and continue with treatment. Thus, in some clinical studies, the subjects may not represent the entire population, which may include individuals who have compromised access to medical care and treatment.

The second threat to external validity in the population category is termed subject–treatment interaction. This threat can be thought of as the confounding effects of attributes of subjects on the dependent variable. Because of genetic makeup, lifestyle, or some other confounding variable, certain subjects react differently, either more positively or more negatively, to any given treatment. For example, you may know people who are blessed with a metabolism that allows them to eat whatever they wish without gaining any weight. On the other hand, if placed on the very same diet, other people gain appreciable and potentially copious amounts of weight.

The first of the environmental or experiment-related threats to external validity is the description of the variables. If the variables used in a study are not described precisely and in sufficient detail, then it may be difficult, if not impossible, for subsequent investigators to replicate the study or for clinical practitioners to obtain the same results. For example, consider a study of a new antihypertensive drug in which the control subjects receive "conventional therapy," but this is not specified in detail. A clinician may not be able to determine whether the new drug is preferable to current therapy that the practitioner already uses because there is not enough detail to ascertain how similar the current therapy is to the control therapy.

A second environmental threat takes place when there are multiple treatments and can involve test order. In some cases, when two treatments or two drugs are given, one may potentiate the effects or otherwise affect the actions of the other. Failure to recognize the effect of treatment order or multiple treatments may affect the ability to apply the results of the study.

The Hawthorne effect is a threat to external validity named after a classic experiment by Elton Mayo, who was looking at worker productivity at a plant located in Cicero, IL. Mayo was interested in the effect of lighting on worker productivity. He explained to the workers that they would be in an experiment on productivity. Mayo then proceeded to increase the ambient lighting in the factory. As expected, productivity went up. In the next phase of his study, Mayo then dimmed the ambient lighting. Worker productivity went up again. Finally, Mayo raised the ambient lighting to the previous high-intensity level, and yet again the productivity went up. Mayo concluded that the ambient lighting was unrelated to the workers' productivity, but the fact that they knew they were being studied affected their performance. Thus, the Hawthorne effect is an effect on results caused by the subjects knowing that they are participating in an experiment. Typically, subjects in clinical experiments have better compliance with treatment regimens than patients who are not participating in an experiment.

The Rosenthal effect refers to measurement errors caused by the involvement of the investigator in a study. In other words, the personal attributes, charisma, and abilities of the researcher affect the results. For example, if an investigator is a charismatic practitioner, then patients may improve partially because of their belief in the clinician treating them. Other practitioners who attempt to obtain similar results are likely to be unsuccessful.

In summary, in every study the investigator must consider and try to control factors, conditions, and the effects of circumstances that threaten internal or external validity. Similarly, professionals critically reading the literature must be aware of these threats to validity to determine the credibility of the conclusions and the applicability of the work to their practice. In many cases, the choice of research design affects the investigation's susceptibility to threats to validity.

Types of Studies

Descriptive Studies

Descriptive studies generate data that are either non-numerical or numerical. Non-numerical information may be presented as verbal commentaries about subjects' clinical characteristics and behaviors, histologic slides, radiologic images, and so forth. For these data, descriptive methods from the subdiscipline of qualitative research would be appropriate. For ethical and legal reasons, when qualitative findings are presented, a subject's identity must be impossible for readers to track.

Similarly, numerical data on individual subjects are almost never presented in a research report. Numerical information is usually presented as statistical summaries such as averages and measures of variability (see following sections). The mean, median, and mode are averages; when unspecified, "average" refers to the mean. The measure of variability most frequently used in medical literature is standard deviation. Occasionally, a range or standard error (SE, also called standard error of the mean, SEM) is used. When confidential information is not disclosed, numerical reports may be supported by exemplar, anecdotal, or model information that conveys valuable research or teaching lessons.

Analytic Studies

Analytic studies test for the following:

- Between-group differences (e.g., a group of patients receiving a drug compared to those receiving a placebo)
- Relationships among variables (e.g., the correlation between cholesterol levels and coronary artery occlusion)
- Both differences and relationships

The specific statistical test and which data are analyzed by the test are included and described in Chapter 9. Although the term is used loosely in medical literature describing analytic studies, the "true experiment" is a prospective design in which the researcher controls as many subject, treatment, and environmental variables as possible.

A cross-sectional study is a data-based "snapshot" of subjects at one period. For example, childhood bone maturation may be studied by describing bone densities in a group of children ages 1, 3, 6, and 9 years old. A longitudinal approach would follow a group of 25 one-year-old children over the next 8 years. If the researcher could control all or most variables over time, then a longitudinal study could also be experimental. It would be difficult to ascertain that intervening variables have not crept into the design, however, so long-term experiments involving human subjects are rare.

When there is substantial risk to human subjects, it is not always possible to conduct a true experiment ethically. The risk may be caused by inducing the disease or condition being studied, or by testing an experimental intervention or treatment. As an alternative, it may be possible to study a disease (e.g., cervical cancer) by identifying those who already have it and those who do not, and then comparing the two groups for factors that might have been responsible for the disease (e.g., human papillomavirus exposure). This is the case-control study design.

Another experimental approach is to identify people who have and do not have a particular risk factor (e.g., human papillomavirus exposure) and then examine the two groups over time to identify those who later develop the disease or condition (e.g., cervical cancer). This is called the cohort study design. Whether a cohort or case-control study design is used, a control or reference group is necessary. For example, if a newscast reports that all subjects in a group of heroin addicts have used marijuana, can we conclude that marijuana use leads to heroin addiction? If the heroin addicts were found to have consumed whole milk, can we conclude that whole milk leads to heroin addiction? A control or reference group composed of people who do not use heroin is likely to show that many have used marijuana and whole milk.

Prospective versus Retrospective Designs

Data collection for prospective studies is planned in advance. Prospective designs include true experiments and concurrent cohort studies. The concurrent cohort design involves subjects who do not have the disease in question, but do have a suspected risk factor, and are tested at a later time to determine if the disease developed in them. In many cases, the prospective approach is the only way to obtain information about a new or recently discovered phenomenon such as a previously unrecognized disorder or a newly developed technique.

True experiments attempt to gain strict control over the conditions of the study, including subject selection, instrument calibration, and the experimental environment. Compared to retrospective designs, prospective designs are credited with having better control of variables and a greater possibility of having valid and reliable standardized measurement methods. Disadvantages include cost (which may limit subject numbers) and the difficulty of extrapolating the results of strictly controlled methods to the clinical setting, where a similar level of control is not possible.

Retrospective studies examine already existing data, including chart reviews and case-control studies. A retrospective approach may be the only ethical way to study the mechanisms of certain interventions. For example, thalidomide was widely prescribed outside the United States for nausea and vomiting during pregnancy, and later was found to cause developmental defects. Because the researcher often cannot know exactly how and under what circumstances data were collected, it may be difficult to verify that retrospective data were collected properly. This is not always the case for retrospective data, however. For example, the electrocardiogram tracings collected decades ago, with their standardization curves, are known to be reliable and valid. Retrospectively collected data are usually inexpensive and readily available in large quantities, and a large N value (the total number of participants in a study) may be used to compensate for variability. For these reasons, the value and usefulness of a study should not be based solely on whether its data were collected prospectively or retrospectively. The particular method of data collection should be evaluated on its own merit.

Uses of Statistics

Many skilled clinicians are skeptical or even fearful of statistics. They contend that "anything can be proved or disproved," and that readers are easily fooled. This is not true for those who have knowledge about research methods and the basic statistical principles presented here. Statistical information is commonplace in medicine. A few easy-to-learn concepts will enable you as a clinician to become an astute and informed consumer of medical information. This ability is invaluable for interpreting study results in journal articles, conference presentations, and drug advertisements. Clinicians do not need to become statisticians, but because we rely on scientific information throughout our professional lifetimes for understanding new information, the astute clinician should be familiar with clinical research methods and basic statistical terminology.

In medicine, statistics are used primarily in three ways. First, they are used to describe and summarize group information. Second, they allow us to infer or generalize sample results to the larger population, which is essential because it is impossible or impractical to measure each and every individual. Instead, samples are used, and a reader needs to know the degree to which a study sample represents a particular patient population. Third, statistics test for significant relationships or differences between groups of subjects. "Subjects" is a technical term referring to samples of individuals who have been selected (often randomly) to represent the population from which they came. Many clinicians resist using the word "subjects" when referring to patients. This term does not imply lack of concern or empathy, however; it is a technical term that refers to individuals admitted to a study from which data will be collected.

Types of Data

A datum (singular of data) is a unit of information about a subject. An example would be the total cholesterol value of 178 mg/dL on Ms. M., who is one subject in a study on the lipid profile of women. Data may be non-numerical (nominal or ordinal, also referred to as nonparametric because of the statistical tests that can be legitimately performed on these types of data), or numerical (interval or ratio, also called parametric).

Nominal data are characteristic names that have no numerical value. Examples would be male or female, black or white, osteoarthritis or rheumatoid arthritis, smoker or nonsmoker. Ordinal data have characteristics that are comparative and can be rank ordered. Examples are shorter or taller, less painful or more painful, darker or lighter, an increased size of a palpable mass. Interval data have numerical values between units but no actual zero point. Examples include degrees centigrade and blood glucose (a patient could not have a body temperature or blood glucose value of zero). Ratio data have numerical values between units, and a zero value is possible. Examples include milligrams of alcohol per deciliter, basophils per cubic millimeter, and number of pack-years smoking history.

Like clinical data, numerical research data are preferred to non-numerical data. For instance, in a study on smokers, knowing the number of pack-years (numerical data) provides better information than knowing only that a patient smokes (non-numerical). The more powerful parametric statistical tests can be applied to numerical data.

Although it is not always possible to quantify data, they can nevertheless be valuable in their descriptive, qualitative form. For example, a narrative about a radiograph of a hairline fracture with a detailed description of its important characteristics, landmarks, and possible origin may be more informative than just a report of a "hairline fracture: present or not present" on 100 films.

When it is not possible to use numerical data, nonparametric statistical tests (such as the Spearman's correlation or Chi-square) must be used. It is an error to apply parametric tests (such as Pearson's correlation or the *t*-test) to nonparametric data because a falsely low P value (probability value) is likely to be fabricated (referred to as an alpha or type I error). A falsely high P value is likely to result when nonparametric tests are used for analyzing numerical (parametric) data. In this case, it is unlikely that a false hypothesis will be accepted, but consequentially a true one may be overlooked (referred to as a beta or type II error). This may occur especially when the calculated P value is close to the desired alpha level.

These classifications of numerical data are commonly used in most scientific articles; however, qualitative research methods also serve invaluable roles in some medical studies and are used as extensively in clinical research as they are in clinical problem solving.

Experimental Designs

An investigator must decide whether a qualitative or quantitative approach will more effectively address the research objective. A second question is whether the study will involve retrospective data (such as clinical records) or prospective data (information that will be newly generated as part of the project). The implications of these questions have been discussed earlier in this chapter.

If the investigator decides to use an experiment to answer the research question, then choosing the appropriate experimental design is imperative. In a project proposal, the investigator describes the methods to be used for analyzing the study's data. Many proposal guidelines suggest creating mock data that are likely to resemble the study's actual data. This often adds a sobering dose of reality in terms of the magnitude and required timeline for the project. This process also helps the investigator plan for both computer needs and possibly consultation with a statistician or methodologist.

The selected research designs presented in Table 5–1 are likely to accommodate the needs of most investiga-

tors. Although experimental and epidemiological studies share some methodological similarities, epidemiologists have developed specialized techniques for the needs of their discipline. Although infrequent, some PA investigators may need to use advanced epidemiological techniques for their studies. In these cases, consulting an epidemiology textbook or an epidemiologist is appropriate. The statistical principles presented here apply to most experimental and epidemiological studies, whether prospective or retrospective. Familiarity with these principles should enable the clinician to converse knowledgeably with most clinical research methodologists and consultants.

Pre-experimental, Experimental, and Quasi-experimental Designs for Research

The purpose of this section is to provide the reader with a shorthand way of recognizing typical research designs and the associated threats to validity inherent in those designs. Much of the work done in this area can be attributed to Campbell and Stanley, who wrote theclassic text *Pre-Experimental, Experimental and Quasi-Experimental Designs for Research*. In this text they develop a shorthand method for diagramming research designs similar to the way that English grammar has been classically taught: by diagramming sentences, students learned to understand proper grammar and sentence construction. Similarly, individuals can more easily recognize a research design by diagramming it.

Campbell and Stanley and others have used certain conventions. For the purposes of this section, the following symbols are used:

1. An R represents randomization and indicates that a particular group was randomly selected or assigned.
2. An M indicates that the groups were matched.
3. An X (with or without a subscript) indicates a treatment.
4. An X_0 indicates no treatment or, in some cases, the control condition.
5. An O indicates a measurement. If multiple measurements are taken, then subscripts, such as O_1, O_2, O_3, and so forth, may be used.
6. A dashed line, _____, indicates nonequivalency and denotes that the groups may be substantially different.

Pre-experimental Designs

The pre-experimental designs are the weakest of the research designs and are subject to many threats to internal and external validity. They are characterized by the lack of a control group, sensitivity to temporal threats to internal validity, and poor generalizability.

One-Shot Case Study

The first pre-experimental design, the one-shot case study, is diagrammed as follows:

X O

In this design, a treatment is given and a measurement is made. This particular design is typical of survey research. A group of respondents are identified based on one or more preexisting criteria and then are administered a questionnaire, which is measured. Another example of the one-shot case study is to use the typical high school or college classroom. The instructor assumes that the students have a certain level of baseline knowledge when they enter the class, but this baseline is not measured. The treatment consists of the exposure in the class, and the measurement is the student's performance in the class. If the students do well, then the instructor may conclude that it's because the students learned so much in the class; however, the instructor cannot justifiably arrive at that conclusion because the students' baseline level of knowledge in the subject upon entering the class is unknown. This demonstrates how the one-shot case study is a weak design because of its vulnerability to threat to both internal and external validity.

Even with its limitations, the one-shot case study is useful for certain types of research such as descriptive studies wherein the investigator wishes to describe what currently exists. Most surveys can be characterized as one-shot case studies. Often the data they yield are very useful to clinicians and therefore published in the medical literature. For example, Levine was interested in the clinical practice of lung transplantation and wanted to ascertain if there were wide differences among transplantation programs.[1] In order to describe the state of clinical practice he surveyed 65 active lung transplantation programs. By asking for information on a number of key areas of practice, such as lung preservation and post-transplantation care, he was able to conclude that there was substantial consensus as well as a few areas of variance among transplantation centers. The results cannot be generalized to centers that did not respond nor do they have a long "shelf life" because a survey is most often a snapshot of a phenomenon or a sample at a specific time. Nonetheless staff members of lung transplantation centers are able to determine if the practices at their center are consistent with those at other centers.

One Group Pre-Test–Post-Test

Slightly more robust is the one group pre-test–post-test design. In this particular design, subjects receive a pre-test, the treatment, and a post-test or retest:

O X O

This design is characteristic of clinical practice in which a patient (or a group of patients) is evaluated and diagnosed, a treatment is administered, and the patient (or a group) is then subsequently reevaluated.

Another example includes providing a group of high school students with education about alcohol abuse. The pre-test and post-test may be a questionnaire on alcohol use. This design is particularly vulnerable to the temporal threats to internal validity, and therefore the investigator theoretically cannot conclude that the outcome was the result of treatment because the illness may have been self-limiting or the subject may simply have outgrown the problem as a result of development. In the case of high school students, changes in alcohol use may be related to the time of year and lack of parties where alcohol is served rather than to a result of alcohol abuse education.

Without being able to compare the group to a reference or control group, one cannot evaluate the effects of temporal threats to internal validity. Similarly, one cannot generalize from the results because it is not known whether the patient or group is representative. Nonetheless studies utilizing a one-group, pre-test–post-test design may be found in the medical literature.

In a study of the effects of a five-day immersion leadership development experience on current and aspiring nursing leaders, Tourangeau et al. assessed and compared self-appraisals by participants and assessments by colleagues before and 3 months after the experience.[2] Although they concluded that "a concentrated leadership experience is effective in strengthening leadership behaviors" critical readers may point out several issues that challenge their conclusions. Because participants' colleagues assessed leadership behaviors before the experience and knew they would be completing another assessment later on, they may have become more sensitive to observing leadership behaviors. In other words, some of the observed differences may be due to changes in the raters rather than the participants. If there is skepticism in the reader's mind just think about and compare the differences in your powers of observation before entering PA school and now. The study could have addressed the concern about differences in the raters by having them also rate individuals who did not undergo the leadership program. Ideally, the raters would have been blind to the subjects' participation, or in other words, they would not know if a person they were rating had or had not participated in the leadership development program. If changes in leadership were observed for individuals who had not participated in the program then at least some of the observed change could possibly be attributed to the changes in the raters. This concern about the raters is further supported by the fact that the participants' self report on leadership behaviors was not significantly different after the program. Finally, because the subjects were volunteers those who felt they would benefit from the program may have self-selected to participate. Hence the subjects may not have been representative of aspiring nurse leaders.

Static Group Comparison

The third pre-experimental research design is entitled the static group comparison. In this design, a group that has received a treatment or been exposed to a condition is compared to a group that did not receive the treatment or was not exposed to the condition:

$$\begin{array}{c} X\ O \\ \hline O \end{array}$$

Remember that the dashed line indicates that these groups are nonequivalent. This design, which attempts some form of control with the group that was not treated or exposed, is better than the previous designs, but because the groups were not randomly assigned, one cannot conclude that they are equivalent.

This design is typically used in epidemiological studies, particularly in environmental or occupational epidemiology. For example, one may be interested in a group of people who are living in an area that may be contaminated with an agent that is a suspected carcinogen. The investigator may hypothesize that living in this area may result in a greater incidence of certain types of cancers. People who live in the contaminated area are compared with similar people who live in an uncontaminated area. Should there be a greater and statistically significant difference in the number of people with cancer for the contaminated area, then the researcher could conclude that the suspected carcinogen might be related. Please note that one cannot conclude causality from this type of design.

The usefulness of the static group comparison is that it allows studies of variables that generally cannot be manipulated by the investigator. Legally and ethically, an investigator cannot require people to live in an area that is suspected to cause a disease or disability or even participate in an optional learning experience. On the other hand, if individuals choose to live in that area or participate in an experience, then one can measure and analyze the effects and compare them to a similar group of individuals who live in a different "control" area or did not participate in an experience.

An example of a static group comparison from the medical literature is a study by Lynch et al. that compared residency choices by medical students who did or did not participate in an optional rural health awareness program.[3] One group of medical students participated in an enrichment initiative entitled the Rural Health Scholars Program (RHSP), which included both didactic and experiential learning focusing on practice in underserved and rural areas. The proportion of participants that chose residencies in primary care, family medicine, community hospitals, and known underserved areas were compared to their classmates who did not participate in the RHSP. While the results demonstrated that significantly more students who participated in the RHSP choose residencies in family medicine and community hospitals the authors could not conclude that the RHSP was the "cause." Because the groups were nonequivalent, the possibility that medical students self-selected participation in the RHSP because of an interest in primary care in a rural setting could not be ruled out.

In summary, one of the major problems with a static group comparison occurs because the groups are nonequivalent. Therefore, there is always the possibility that some factor other than the treatment is causing the results. For example, students who came from a rural area or those who had a spouse from a rural area may have already made the decision to practice in a rural area before they participated in the experience.

Experimental Designs

The next series of research designs are the true experimental designs. These studies are characterized by randomization of the subjects and a control group. The reader should remember that randomization does not mean that the groups are identical, but rather that they are equivalent. Randomization works on the law of probability, which suggests that when a group is selected or subjects are assigned randomly, the traits, characteristics, and conditions that may affect the outcome (confounding variables) are distributed roughly equally among the groups, thus canceling out their effect.

Pre-test, Post-test, Control Group Design

The first experimental design is the pre-test, post-test, control group design. In this design, subjects are randomly assigned to a group, pre-tested, given a treatment or no treatment, and then tested after exposure to the treatment or no treatment:

$$R \; O_1 \; X_0 \; O_2$$

$$R \; O_1 \; X_1 \; O_2$$

In the diagram above, two groups are compared on a single variable with two conditions (X_0 and X_1), but more than two groups or conditions can be analyzed using this design. In addition, it is possible to examine more than one variable.

The pre-test, post-test, control group design effectively rules out most threats to internal and external validity. Because it is the most rigorous design, the pre-test, post-test, control group design is commonly accepted as the "gold standard" and is typically used in randomized clinical trials. It should be noted that in clinical trials and other research involving human subjects, it is unethical and often illegal to withhold treatment. Thus the control group may be the group that receives the conventional treatment while the experimental group receives the new treatment. In other words, the conventional treatment is used as a control or the baseline.

Patients will often ask a PA for advice about claims made about various health-care products, including food and nutritional supplements. Many foods make the claim that they are enriched or fortified with vitamins, inferring that they are better than their nonenriched competitors. Thankfully, the medical literature includes some robust studies that shed light on the subject.

In a study to examine if fortified cereals actually increased subjects' blood levels of selected B vitamins, Tucker et al. compared a fortified cereal to a cereal that was not fortified in a sample of older adults.[4] Their approach was to measure blood levels of homocysteine (an amino acid), folic acid, and vitamins B_6 and B_{12} in subjects on two occasions to obtain baselines. According to the authors: "High homocysteine and low vitamin B concentrations have been linked to the risk of vascular disease, stroke and dementia" (p. 805). After baselines were obtained, the subjects were randomly assigned to a group that ate a cup of a fortified cereal daily or a cup of cereal that was not fortified. At 12 and 14 weeks the blood levels of homocysteine, folic acid, and vitamins B_6 and B_{12} were measured.[†] Neither the subjects nor the investigators performing the tests knew whether a subject was consuming fortified cereal or not. When the group membership is unknown to the subject and the investigator (until the tests are concluded) the study is termed a double-blind study because both the subject and the investigator are "blind" to the treatment. Comparisons between the groups revealed significant differences between the groups. Homocysteine levels were lowered while folic acid and vitamin B_6 and B_{12} levels were higher in the group that ate the fortified cereal. Because of the rigorous design the authors could conclude that eating a fortified cereal will benefit older adults.[4] In summary, because major threats to internal and external validity were controlled, the observed differences were due to the treatment and the results may be generalized to similar groups of individuals; in other words, eating a cereal fortified with B vitamins may help older adults.

Post-Test-Only Control Group Design

The second experimental design is termed the post-test-only control group design. The subjects are randomized, given a treatment, and then the results are measured and compared:

$$R \; X_0 \; O$$

$$R \; X_1 \; O$$

Typically, this type of design is used when a pre-test is inappropriate or unavailable for other reasons. For example, an orthopedic group may be interested in the outcomes of a total hip replacement when using one particular appliance versus a second appliance. In this case, a pre-test is inappropriate because patients who acquire total hip replacements are generally lacking substantial range of motion at the hip joint, often because of pain. In this example, the outcomes such as time to ambulation, pain, and range of motion may be appropriate to measure after the surgery. Because it is impossible to know the baseline or the pre-test condition of the individuals, there might be some threats to internal validity based on preexisting conditions, but it is believed that randomization minimizes these effects.

Gallo and Staskin investigated the effect of external cues on patient compliance in performing pelvic floor exercises.[5] Because compliance is measured after a patient is educated about a treatment program, a pre-test is not appropriate. In this study 86 women with stress urinary incontinence were given a program on pelvic floor exercises and then randomly assigned to a group that received an additional audio cassette or not. They were then subsequently evaluated for compliance to the pelvic floor exercise program and compared. The women who received the audio cassette, termed an

---

[†]The astute reader will undoubtedly observe that the example used is a slight variation from the classical pre-test, post-test, control group design because the investigators used two baseline measurements and two post-test measurements, so the design was:

| R | O_1 | O_2 | $X_{not\ fortified}$ | O_3 | O_4 |
| R | O_1 | O_2 | $X_{fortified}$ | O_3 | O_4 |

Ordinarily one might also be concerned about pre-test-post-test sensitization with multiple tests but in this study the dependent variable was blood levels of homocysteine, vitamins B_6 and B_{12} and folic acid, and it should not be affected by repeated testing.

external cue by the authors, demonstrated significantly better compliance than the group who received only instruction.[5] In this case, the robust experimental design, a post-test only control group design, controlled major threats to internal and external validity allowing the authors to conclude that external cues improve compliance for women with stress urinary incontinence.

Solomon Four-Group Design

The next experimental design is the Solomon four-group design. In this design, groups with and without pre-tests are exposed to one of two treatments and subsequently tested after treatment:

$$R \; O_1 \; X_0 \; O_2$$
$$R \; O_1 \; X_1 \; O_2$$
$$R \quad\;\; X_0 \; O_2$$
$$R \quad\;\; X_1 \; O_2$$

The astute reader will note that the Solomon four-group design is actually a combination of the previous two designs: the pre-test–post-test, control group design, and the post-test-only control group design. This particular design is useful because it allows an investigator to assess whether an effect occurs because of the pre-test. On the other hand, there is a draw back to this design because it requires twice as many subjects.

Danley et al. investigated the effect of a multimedia learning experience designed to prepare dental students and dentists to recognize and respond to domestic violence.[6] The investigators were interested in assuring that observed changes in the subjects between the pre-test and the post-test were not due to the fact that the subjects completed the pre-test. When the subjects who completed the pre-test, the multimedia learning experience and the post-test were compared to subjects who completed the multimedia learning experience and the post-test, they found no significant differences between the groups. On the other hand, the two groups who completed the multimedia learning experience were more knowledgeable than the subjects who were controls.[6]

Quasi-experimental Designs

The final group of research designs is termed quasiexperimental designs. Although they are more rigorous than the pre-experimental designs, they are not as rigorous and as robust as the true experimental designs. Typically, they lack one or more of the typical character-

istics that would make them true experimental designs. Generally, randomization is lacking, or multiple measurements make testing effects a potential problem.

Nonequivalent Control Group Design

The nonequivalent control group design is similar to the pre-test–post-test, control group design, but because the groups are not randomized they must be considered nonequivalent:

$$\frac{O_1 \; X_0 \; O_2}{O_1 \; X_1 \; O_2}$$

An example of the use of this design is a hypothetical comparison of patient satisfaction with care from two clinics: one that hired a PA 6 months ago (X_1) and one with no PA (X_0). The astute reader can think of many ways in which the patients may differ and affect the outcome, such as age, years seen by the provider, and so forth. Because the groups are nonequivalent, therefore, the results obtained from studies using this particular design must be viewed with caution; preexisting conditions in the subjects may account for the changes after treatment.

Kristjansson et al. studied the effectiveness of a short duration learning experience for teenagers that focused upon preventing skin cancer.[7] Because the presentation was given in a classroom to an entire class, they compared the classes that received the presentation to classes that did not. In this example, randomly assigning students would have made the study very complex and unmanageable. Although their results suggested that the short-duration learning experience was successful, the fact that the groups were nonequivalent suggests that they should be viewed with caution. For example, it is not known if one or more classes were comprised of students who were more concerned about their health, or more motivated to accept the content presented.

Separate Sample Pre-test–Post-test Design

The separate sample pre-test–post-test design is used when the investigators suspect that the pre-test will significantly bias the post-test results:

$$\frac{O \; X}{X \; O}$$

While measuring a change from pre-test to post-test is appropriate when using a physical test such as blood level or heart rate, a pre-test of a mental, psychological, or performance variable often affects the post-test. For example, a pre-test for manual dexterity may result in some motor learning that could affect subsequent performance. If the investigator was interested in evaluating the effect of a new treatment, the observed changes could be due to motor learning from the pre-test. The separate sample pre-test–post-test design addresses concerns about the pre-test biasing the outcome.

Markert et al. used a separate pre-test–post-test design to assess the knowledge acquired by professionals who attended continuing medical education (CME) programs.[8] The investigators noted in this article that pre-testing and post-testing attendees was an inappropriate approach for assessing knowledge. They felt that a pre-test would bias performance on a post-test. Given the observation that most medical professionals are bright individuals who are committed to learning, it seems logical that they would remember items from a pre-test. Instead, Markert et al. randomly assigned attendees to either a pre-test group, which they considered a "control" group or a post-test only group, which they considered the "treatment" group. Upon comparing the groups the "treatment" group demonstrated significantly more knowledge in selected topic areas.[8]

Time Series Design

A third quasi-experimental design is the time series design. In these designs, groups are compared to each other and there are multiple tests:

$$\frac{O_1 \ X_0 \ O_2 \ O_3 \ O_4}{O_1 \ X_1 \ O_2 \ O_3 \ O_4}$$

Because there are multiple measurements, one cannot conclude that changes or differences are not a result of sensitization or learning. In other words, the threat to validity of repeated testing is of concern, as well as the threat that groups may be nonequivalent.

In a study that compared nursing and medical interventions for skin care, Pokorny et al. examined differences in patients who developed pressure sores and those who did not.[9] Data were gathered on the day of admission, the day of surgery, and the following 4 days. Because the patients were admitted for cardiac surgery, it was anticipated that a subject would average 6 days in the hospital. The investigators in this study looked for differences in the daily nursing and medical interventions between patients who developed pressure sores and those who did not. For this study, the dependent variable (what was measured) consisted of the documented interventions, and specifically differences. The authors concluded that multiple assessments of skin condition by nurses were important in preventing pressure sores.[9] Because patients were not randomly assigned to groups that received standard or optimized skin assessment, differences in patients may have affected the results.

Summary

The designs just presented are by no means exhaustive of the pre-experimental, experimental, and quasi-experimental designs found in the literature. Nonetheless, by recognizing the common designs, one can quickly focus on threats to validity. If one is constructing or designing a study, knowledge of common research designs may help avoid pitfalls. Remember, however, that although one can have a robust research design, failure to obtain reliable measurements using valid instrument may render the conclusions of the study inaccurate or erroneous. Finally, reading research critically or performing research is a learning experience that generally requires a great deal of practice.

When evaluating the Methods section of published research reports, this information should help clinicians to knowledgeably critique and evaluate the methods used in the study's results before applying them to practice. For all PAs, this information should help in interpreting new medical information presented in literature, professional conferences, and through other sources. Ultimately, designing studies is common sense—devising ways to obtain and interpret original information accurately, whether from medical journals or the bedside. Well-informed clinicians may be able to interpret and apply clinical information in new or better ways.

By definition, original research studies are unique. A few principles of research, however, apply to the breadth of studies PAs encounter throughout their professional lifetimes. Applying the principles presented in this chapter should help beginning investigators select an effective research method for a planned research study and, when necessary, communicate effectively with methodological consultants.

Acknowledgment

Dr. Bork wishes to recognize and thank the Medical College of Ohio, Physician Assistant Studies Class of 2005 for their assistance in identifying many examples of articles in the medical literature that used the designs discussed in this chapter.

References

1. Levine SM. A survey of clinical practice of lung transplantation in North America. Chest 2004;125:1–16.
2. Tourangeau AE, Lemonde M, Luba M, et al. Evaluation of a leadership development intervention. Nursing Leadership 2003;16(3):94–104.
3. Lynch DC, Pathman DE, Teplin SE, et al. Interim evaluation of the rural health scholars program. Teaching and Learning in Medicine 2001;13:36–42.

4. Tucker KL, Olson B, Bakun P, et al. Breakfast cereal fortified with folic acid, vitamin B-6 and vitamin B-12 increases vitamin concentrations and reduces homocysteine concentrations: a randomized trial. American Journal of Clinical Nutrition 2004;79:805–811.

5. Gallo ML, Staskin DR. Cues to action: pelvic floor muscle exercise compliance in women with stress urinar incontinence. Neurourology and Urodynamics 1997;16:167–177.

6. Danley D, Gansky SA, Chow D, et al. Preparing dental students to recognize and respond to domestic violence. Journal of the American Dental Association 2004;135;67–73.

7. Kristjansson K, Helgason R, Mansson-Brahme E, et al. You and your skin: a short-duration presentation of skin cancer prevention for teenagers. Health Education Research 2003;18:88–97.

8. Markert RJ, O'Neill SC, Bhatia SC. Using a quasi-experimental research design to assess knowledge in continuing medical education programs. Journal of Continuing Education in the Health Professions 2003;23:157–162.

9. Pokorney ME, Koldjeski D, Swanson M. Skin care intervention for patients having cardiac surgery. American Journal of Critical Care 2003;12:535–544.

chapter 6

Common Research Designs

Robert W. Jarski, PhD, PA-C

Chapter Overview

Chapter 5 presents the variety of designs that are typically used in quantitative studies. Add to this the qualitative methods described in Chapter 7 and the community-based participatory research in Chapter 8, and the beginning researcher will understand that there are many study designs, but the number is not unlimited. When preparing to conduct a research study, it is useful to become familiar with the range of designs that are presented in this text. This chapter will assist you, the physician assistant (PA), in getting started and selecting appropriate designs for answering research questions and testing hypotheses through data-based studies. A secondary objective is to help the researcher avoid some common pitfalls in (1) subject selection, (2) devising instrumentation, (3) developing procedures, and (4) performing the statistical analyses. The latter will address the issue of how many patients are needed for a study, a procedure commonly referred to as statistical power analysis. The sections that follow this discussion describe some designs that PAs can conduct and work with.

From Concept to Concrete

The first step in designing a study is topic selection. Topics may be identified in several ways, as described in Chapter 3, and should be in a clinical area or discipline that is of interest to you, the researcher. By properly completing a well-conducted study, the investigator becomes a relative expert on the topic. The time and dedication necessary to conduct a study should result in information that the investigator truly wishes to master.

Once the topic has been narrowed to a tentative research question or hypothesis, it is fruitful to adopt a "common sense" approach to selecting a study design. The names that are applied to the research designs are useful for the purposes of (1) classifying studies when communicating with others and (2) selecting an appropriate statistical test that matches the selected study design. A logical plan should be thought through before a design is selected. Using the schematic tools of "O, X, and R," presented in the previous chapter, is generally helpful. By comparing the conceived scheme to those listed in Chapter 5, the design can be evaluated, refined, and matched with a statistical tool. Chapter 7 outlines qualitative approaches.

This common sense approach involves thinking about the number of ways the question or hypothesis can be addressed. Should the study be prospective or retrospective? Who should the subjects be? What data are necessary? The researcher should solicit both experienced and inexperienced investigators to suggest possible ways of answering the research question or hypothesis. Although some designs may be unrealistic or impractical, ideas can usually be modified or developed to suit realities such as available resources, finances or monetary support, ethics, and the time frame allotted for completion.

Once the topic has been selected, the research question must be developed. The following six approaches have been used successfully by many beginning investigators:

1. The question may originate from an actual clinical problem observed about a patient at the bedside.

2. You may have concerns about how well a new or alternative technology compares to known techniques. For example, how well do home glucose monitoring devices compare to standardized laboratory measurement?

3. The astute clinician may observe a "gap" in clinical knowledge where a theory about patient care or evaluation is elevated from opinion to evidence supported by data.

4. A study may help resolve a controversial issue. When published studies present contradictory results, a study may be designed to help tilt the scale in one direction or the other. Most published articles include "suggestions for future investigations" in the discussion section, inviting the next step in resolving a research problem.

5. Talking with an expert in the field of interest often generates productive research ideas. He or she may describe a study that should be done although "there was never time to do it."

6. A previously published study may be duplicated. (See Chapter 3.) A creative, new approach to a previously published study may involve varying a therapeutic method or including a different demographic group of subjects.

Certain design pitfalls that could make the results inconclusive or difficult to interpret need to be avoided. Methods for identifying some of these are discussed below. The bottom line is this: the particular methods used for answering a research question or for testing a hypothesis determine the type of study design, not the other way around. As in clinical work, the presenting problem determines the approach used to help resolve it. Some investigations may involve both quantitative and qualitative approaches.

Prospective versus Retrospective Research Designs

All studies can be classified as either prospective or retrospective. As with any design, each has advantages and disadvantages. In its simplest form, a prospective study is one in which the investigator identifies subjects and plans to obtain measures following a future treatment, risk factor, or event. All true experimental designs are prospective. (See Chapter 5.) In epidemiologic studies, a prospective design is synonymous with a cohort study. It refers to investigations in which individuals who have a condition and those without the condition are identified and then later evaluated for the presence or absence of an outcome.

A retrospective study is one in which individuals both with and without a disease or condition are identified and investigated for their past exposure or nonexposure to a treatment, risk factor, or event. Chart review studies are typically retrospective. In epidemiologic studies, a retrospective study is synonymous with a case-control study.

Advantages of prospective designs include the ability to:

1. Study new or previously nonexisting phenomena, technology, or treatments.

2. Plan a design that investigates possible mechanisms as well as outcomes.

3. Decrease variability by selecting subjects on the basis of inclusion and exclusion criteria established prior to beginning the study.

4. Control treatment variables.

5. Include both individual and multiple treatments or exposures.

Disadvantages include (1) expense; (2) lack of assurance that sufficient subject numbers can be recruited and retained; and (3) problems of study duration such as attrition, change of subject's health status or comorbidities, and the investigators' time and commitment.

Advantages of retrospective designs include the facts that:

1. They are inexpensive.

2. They can be planned, and the data collected and analyzed in a short period of time.

3. Subjects or cases are often readily available and in large numbers which may help diminish the statistical effects of randomly occurring between-group differences.

4. There is no risk to patients.

5. Situations that would involve ethical concerns are minimal.

6. This design may be the only way to investigate outcomes that have been caused by dangerous or discontinued drugs and treatments.

Disadvantages include the facts that (1) data may be unstandardized or inaccurate; (2) it is often difficult or impossible to verify treatment and data collection procedures and protocols; (3) selection of control or reference groups may be difficult; and (4) extraneous variables, including the effects of unrecorded events and history, may not be known.

Although there are some obvious shortcomings, it is incorrect to automatically assume that all retrospective designs are inferior to prospective ones. The investigator must carefully weigh the various advantages and disadvantages when considering the type of design that is best suited to the research question or hypothesis. Each study's merit and the potential value of its results should be based on the logical construction of the study plan and the degree to which intervening variables and other barriers to interpretation have been controlled. Knowledge about some important topics might not occur at all without retrospective designs. Each study should (1) represent the investigator's best effort, (2) recognize the possible design limitations in the discussion section, and (3) offer suggestions for future investigations based on the experiences gained.

The adage "the perfect study has not yet been published" is a reality of biomedical research conducted in the milieu of human variables. Problems always exist when extrapolating sample data to populations, and population data to individual patients. There are also realities of time, as well as monetary and ethical constraints. Major barriers to interpreting study results should be remedied or avoided in the planning stages by conducting a pilot study. (See below.) But even studies that are less than perfect usually offer *some* contribution to knowledge in terms of feasibility and future promise, the development of methods for future studies, and pilot data. However, if the anticipated results are likely to be completely inclusive, the design should be improved or an alternative study planned.

Reference Group and Placebo-Controlled Designs

The randomized controlled trial remains the highest level of evidence for medical studies.[1] Is a placebo control always the best choice for between-group comparisons? Again, this depends on the study's research question or study hypothesis. For example, if a new cholesterol-lowering agent is being evaluated, should its efficacy be compared to that of a placebo? It would be expected that *any* comparable therapeutic would be superior to a physiologically inert substance, that is, a placebo. The more clinically relevant comparison would evaluate how well the drug compares to others among which a clinician can choose. Comparing the new agent to an alternative drug, rather than placebo, would be

preferred. The correct research question would be, "Is the new agent better than what we use now?" rather than, "Is the new agent better than an inert substance?" In addition, if the presently available therapeutic is the standard of care, it may be unethical to discontinue its use and substitute with placebo for the purpose of a clinical trial. A reference group would be required in this situation.

The Disguised Single-Case Study Design

When two or more individuals are performing data collection measurements or carrying out a clinical procedure, some degree of variability is expected among the individuals involved. To avoid this variability, some investigators have opted to use *one* person to perform measurements or procedures throughout a study. However, in effect, this would be a single-case study of the technician or operator. Although this approach may increase internal reliability, it decreases external validity. The preferred approach would be to involve several evaluators or operators whose abilities are likely to be representative. When this is done, intra- and inter-rater reliability should be calculated. A study's value includes how well the results can be generalized to other settings (external validity).

The Pre-Proposal

Written proposals are required by research advisors, sponsors, institutional review boards, and funding agencies. Specific guidelines and content may be required. In the initial stages of designing any study, it is always useful to actually *write* a brief proposal, or more accurately, a pre-proposal. By doing so, the research design can be refined and improved—rarely if ever will a researcher's first attempt be the finished product. Rather, it is a process of writing and rewriting the pre-proposal as thoughts and new ideas develop.

The process of physically writing the pre-proposal always generates a new level of clarity and reality for the researcher. Once written, it can be focused, shared with others for input, and revised. It is suggested that both inexperienced and experienced investigators participate in the development and revision. Inexperienced individuals often contribute fresh ideas and insights, and their relative unfamiliarity with research methods requires the proposal's author to present it logically and clearly. Those who are experienced in research design may detect methodologic, technical, or ethical issues that need to be addressed, and suggest ways to correct and strengthen the design.

A proposal resembles a research article abstract. Examples can be found in any medical article that reports original data. The main difference between a proposal and an abstract is that the proposal is written in the future tense and there is additional emphasis on the methods, including ethical considerations. Also, although there will be no completed results section, a proposal includes mock data or a description of the form the anticipated results will take. Research article abstracts are reports of completed studies written in the past tense.

In general, the proposal, like a completed study's abstract, begins with a brief description of the problem to be addressed or the rationale that led to the topic. The most important component appears next: the purpose of the study. It is typically one sentence that begins: "The purpose of the proposed study will be to…" The purpose statement directly addresses the study question and/or hypothesis. Some studies may have secondary purposes. These should usually be included in the proposal and, on completion of the project, also included in the abstract.

The proposal's methods section typically consists of four parts:

1. A description of the subjects that will be used,

2. The instruments (e.g., technical devices, questionnaires, an expert panel that will be used for generating data),

3. The procedures (the steps that will actually be carried out for data collection),

4. The statistical tests that will be used for data analysis. This section usually includes the power analysis which estimates the necessary number of subjects.

The Pilot Study

Most studies benefit when a pilot study is conducted. Unforeseen methodologic problems almost always appear once the physical acts of data collection and analysis begin. Many problems can be detected and remedied before actual data collection begins. The pilot run consists of carrying out all of the study's methods—from subject recruitment to statistically analyzing the pilot data. For many pilot studies, the number of patients, chart reviews, and so forth may be approximately 4 to 10, depending on the complexity of the protocol, the time allotted for completing the project, and the per-subject costs. In addition, if power analysis information is not available from a previous study, pilot data can be used for this. In some cases, the first several data sets obtained on actual subjects can be handled as part of the pilot run and retained for the final data analysis if they are free of biases and the procedures are not changed.

Statistical Analysis

This is a process that many beginning—and experienced—researchers often find intimidating. Although many small-scale research studies may contribute worthwhile information to the fund of medical knowledge, the primary benefit of conducting a study is that the PA achieves a depth of understanding of medical literature that is otherwise unattainable. Many clinicians have indicated that the "hands-on" experience of conducting their own research has increased their ability to understand, interpret, and apply medical literature to clinical practice. To remain current throughout a professional lifetime, PAs rely on new medical information generated from studies. Understanding the process of acquiring and statistically presenting new medical information is essential for keeping current. The PA and virtually all other health professions have recognized this and research knowledge is now a required component of the professional curriculum.[2]

Like the medical specialties, statistics has become a sophisticated discipline. But PAs do not need to become statisticians to conduct and interpret medical literature, nor to analyze data from their studies. However, some basic knowledge about statistics is essential for (1) communicating effectively with statistical experts, (2) conducting the data analysis, and (3) understanding medical literature in general.

Several easy-to-use statistical programs are available (e.g., Minitab, SAS, SPSS) and a number of interactive Web sites are devoted to less popular statistical tests that can be found online through the usual search engines. However, only those that are sponsored by reputable sources, usually universities, should be considered, and even these must be verified through cross-validation using trial data with known calculated values.

Because of easily accessible and user-friendly computerized statistical packages, there is a temptation to "plug in data and crunch." In some cases this has led to gross errors—when cells are filled with numbers, a result can usually be produced. However, it may not be the correct result if an inappropriate test was selected or if particular data conditions were not met. Most individuals are able to analyze their own data if they obtain statistical consultation when necessary and learn a few specific statistical principles.

Although numerous statistical tests are available for describing, comparing, and presenting study data, there are only a few prototype statistical tests. As in learning about prototype drugs in pharmacology, the PA who becomes familiar with a few prototype statistical tests will understand related ones. At a minimum, basic knowledge about the types of data that will be collected (i.e., nominal, ordinal, interval, and ratio) and four prototype statistical tests (Spearman's and Pearson's correlation, chi-square, and *t*-tests) is essential. This information may be found in a text specifically targeted toward PAs[3] and detailed information including mathematical formulas may be found in selected texts on research design and statistics.[4–6] See Chapter 9 for more direction on data analysis.

Subject Selection

When human subjects are used for research, they must be suitable for the study design and for addressing the study question in terms of their existing state of health or disease, past history, comorbidities, and demographics. For example, results from a study on evaluating the use of a new ankle splint in a sample of *healthy* subjects may not be generalized to the particular population that will be using the splint—patients with ankle injuries.

When selecting subjects for a study design, the researcher must ask: "To what degree can the results be generalized to other patients with similar conditions and in other settings?" and "What factors are likely to interfere with interpreting the results or finding a clear-cut answer to the study question?" Careful selection of the study sample will help avoid problems of generalizing to the target population. The inclusion and exclusion criteria for sample selection should be established before data are collected.

Sample Size

Once a study design has been selected, it is necessary to estimate the sample size. This is almost always required when funding is requested because cost, time, and equipment needs are related to the necessary number of patients, charts for review, specimens, and so forth. Most studies should provide some assurance that the appropriate number has been examined so the results are conclusive. The estimated sample size is derived by calculating "statistical power."

Quantitative studies are designed to test a null hypothesis, or the result of no effect. (See Chapter 3.) Ideally, the sample size would be small enough to save time and money, yet sufficiently large to test the null hypothesis using a representative sample. If a sample is fairly homogeneous for the variable being assessed, fewer subjects are needed. In fact, if the variable were perfectly homogeneous, a study could be performed on only one subject and the results generalized to the pop-

ulation! However, health sciences research is faced with human differences (heterogeneity) and we must therefore use sample sizes that are greater than one. But how large must the sample be?

Three factors are necessary for calculating sample size: (1) the effect size (which is a measure of similarity between variables in correlational studies, or the degree of difference in studies involving between-group differences); (2) level of significance (which is almost always set at 0.05 in medical studies [two-tailed]); and (3) statistical power. This refers to the probability of committing a type II or beta-error—incorrectly accepting a null hypothesis when it is actually false. The beta-error is usually set at 0.80 which means there is a 20 percent chance of committing a type II error. This is conventionally used along with a 0.05 alpha-error, which means there is a 5 percent chance of committing a type I error. In completed studies, the alpha-error corresponds to a *p*-value of 0.05.

Although the primary purpose of a power analysis is to avoid a type II error, it also provides the number of subjects that are necessary to achieve a significant *p*-value without using excessively large subject numbers that may unnecessarily increase time and expense, or artificially inflate *p*-values. The following relationship shows how the *p*-value is decreased (made to appear more significant) when large subject numbers are used:

$$p \sim \frac{\text{a measure of variability, e.g., standard deviation}}{N \text{ or the number of patients, charts, etc.}}$$

When the effect size (or means and standard deviations) are known, sample size may be calculated from the power analysis, as noted above. In most medical studies, the level of significance and desired power level are typically set at 0.05 and 0.80, respectively. Programs for calculating sample size may be found in most computerized statistical software, and formulas may be found in appropriate references.[5] Alternatively, power estimation tables may be consulted.[4,5]

When beginning a study, the effect size or the variables necessary for calculating it (i.e., means and standard deviations) may be found in similar, previously conducted studies published in medical literature. If the planned study is unlike any other or comparable studies are not available for obtaining their power analysis information, it is then necessary to conduct a pilot study for estimating subject numbers. Alternatively, the first several data sets collected may be used, assuming that the subjects who follow will be similar.

The particular objective of some studies may not require a power analysis for estimating the number of subjects needed to achieve statistical significance prior to beginning the study. This would include case series designs, methods papers (which describe a technique or method for data collection to be used in future studies), and pilot studies (whose purpose is exploratory in nature or a first attempt to determine future promise or feasibility of a new research idea). Many studies conducted by beginning investigators qualify as pilot studies. A power analysis or estimate is usually necessary for most other types of study designs.

Survey Designs

Although they are a convenient, inexpensive, and popular data collection method, survey research has all of the inherent potential problems of other forms of data collection plus some additional ones that should be considered. In addition to the advantages mentioned earlier, surveys as self-reports may be the only way to assess important albeit subjective information. For example, pain is the major presenting clinical complaint, which is subjective. But this fact alone does not diminish its importance.

Survey designs and other self-reports, like any other research method, should be used when it is the best or only way to answer a research question. If the question requires self-reports, and objective measures are unavailable (e.g., those assessing pain, mood, satisfaction), surveys are appropriate. However, if objective measures are available, they should generally be used to avoid the pitfalls and limitations of self-reported surveys. For example, if a study requires blood pressure measurements, it would be preferable to obtain objective data from measurements or medical records, rather than asking individuals for their self-report. The latter method has the obvious limitations of recall, communication, the Hawthorne effect, and other sources of error and bias.

Various methods for conducting surveys are available including mail and telephone surveys, personal interviews, Web-based surveys, and special adaptations such as focus groups and the delphi technique.[5] The quality of surveys and their results is extremely variable, ranging from well-conducted scientific surveys to ones that are fraught with flaws and unreconcilable sources of error. Poorly conducted surveys have given this potentially valuable research tool a poor reputation, and properly so. Each of the survey methodologies has well-established developmental protocols. When carefully and meticulously done, surveys may produce valuable data; when poorly done, they are useless. Attrition is a problem for any research design, but response rate is an issue for nearly all types of survey studies; there is no agreed upon number for an "acceptable" response rate less than 100 percent.[5]

When considering the use of a survey design, the investigator is advised to consult appropriate texts. In addition, well known and widely used instruments with published reliability and validity data are preferred to other instruments, especially those created exclusively for a new study. A widely used instrument allows study reports to be compared and interpreted in the context of other studies using the same instrument. A new instrument should be created only when no existing instrument satisfactorily addresses a study's purpose or hypothesis. When a new instrument is created, its accuracy is questionable until it is evaluated for validity and reliability. All instruments, new and established, should be pilot tested on a group of subjects similar to the study subjects. Specific procedures for creating and evaluating survey instruments, and for conducting survey research are available in specialized references.[5,7]

Like any research method, surveys can provide valuable information when they are properly designed and conducted. Sometimes surveys are the only way to assess certain research questions or hypotheses. To do them well involves established procedures that are as stringent as any other study design. But studies are not useful when they contain serious gaps, flaws, or other methodologic problems that make interpretation of the results impossible.

Summary

The primary guiding force behind the selection of a study design is the research question, or hypothesis. It leads to the recruitment of appropriate subjects that will allow generalization of the results outside the study setting, and the appropriate choice of instruments for collecting or generating study data. The number of subjects necessary for a study is derived from the statistical power analysis. Retrospective designs are not always inferior to prospective ones; each offers particular advantages and disadvantages. Study designs, including surveys and self-reports, have some recommended technical procedures that should be followed to help avoid errors. Although the "perfect" medical study on humans has probably not yet been completed, the best design possible based on logic and feedback elicited from others should be used to help avoid problems of internal and external validity and reliability, biases, and other factors that may make the study results difficult to apply or interpret. Most if not all studies offer some valuable contribution. It may be evidence about the promise or feasibility of an attempted idea, the improvement of methods or techniques, or suggestions for future investigators based on the experience gained.

The sections that follow outline some research designs that PAs and PA students can be involved with and conduct. We recognize that there are many many more designs and methods for conducting research. We hope that what we present helps you in getting started.

References

1. Evidence-Based Medicine Working Group. Evidence-based medicine: a new approach to teaching the practice of medicine. Journal of the American Medical Association 1992;268:2420.
2. Accreditation Review Commission of Education for the Physician Assistant Accreditation. Standards for Physician Assistant Education, 2001.
3. Jarski RW. Using the medical literature: life-long learning skills. In Ballweg R, Stolberg S, Sullivan EM (eds): Physician Assistant: A Guide to Clinical Practice. Philadelphia: WB Saunders, 2003.
4. Gall MD, Gall JP, Borg WR. Educational Research. Boston: Allyn and Bacon, 2002.
5. Neutens JJ, Rubinson L. Research Techniques for the Health Sciences. San Francisco: Benjamin Cummings, 2001.
6. Riegelman RK. Studying a Study and Testing a Test. Philadelphia: Lippincott, Williams and Wilkins, 2000.
7. Aday LA. Designing and Conducting Health Surveys: A Comprehensive Guide. San Francisco: Jossey-Bass, 1989.

Section 1
Clinical Investigations
J. Dennis Blessing, PhD, PA-C

Section Overview

This section presents a basic overview of some types of clinical investigations. Biomedical investigations of people (commonly referred to as "human subjects research") are known by many names. Regardless of the name, these investigations involve people. Those people are our patients. Clinical investigations are different from what we think of as traditional research. This section provides an overview of clinical investigations and outlines a basic approach for some types of clinical investigations. Traditional research is important to medical science and it will always be a part of medicine. However, the laboratory can be a long distance from the clinic where you have to deal with real people and situations. Adding to our problems of application is the fact that the literature contains many, many conflicting reports and results about health and illness. The development of the concept of evidence-based medicine and practice is helping to clarify many aspects of the (sometimes) confusing practice of medicine. Clinical research and investigations are one way to test interventions, applications, procedures, and so forth for outcomes and effect in people. Conducting research in humans requires the same attention to detail, planning, control, documentation, and scientific rigor in methodology and analysis as any research project. A big MUST for clinical intervention and outcome studies is the protection of human subjects and at every point attempt to maintain the principle of "Do No Harm." Clinical studies can involve drugs, devices, procedures, interventions, approaches, and almost any aspect of practice. The design of studies can take on a number of forms. Clinical studies and investigations offer PAs an opportunity to be involved in research activities that can involve their clinical practice. Almost any type of practice can identify some type of clinical investigation opportunity. Clinical research may be that perfect mix of practice and helping advance our knowledge in the better of humankind.

Introduction

The scientific process that directly involves people goes by many names. Clinical investigations, clinical outcomes, clinical trial, clinical study, and clinical applications are some of the terms used to describe this type of research project. This author prefers the term "clinical investigation" and will use that term in this section. Regardless of the nomenclature, these studies involve people. The methodology and design of clinical trials can take many forms. Clinical investigations involve people who are our patients. As such, there are added dimensions to clinical investigations that require, in some ways, more vigilance and rigor, informed consent, and subject protection. A review of the literature will give you a number of definitions for clinical investigations (or one of its synonyms). As a starting point, we will use this broad, general definition:

> **Clinical Investigation**: a research study involving patients that attempts to answer questions about new therapies,* current therapies,* or new ways of using known therapies.*

PAs, PA students, and PA faculty can be involved with and play a major role in clinical investigations. Ultimately, there is no reason why a PA cannot be the primary investigator on a clinical investigation.

First Things First

Before you undertake your clinical investigation, you must have followed the process of developing your research project as outlined elsewhere in this book. You must have defined your problems; developed your research questions, hypotheses, or null hypotheses;

---

*can be a drug, device, intervention, treatment, etc.
(Adapted from The University of Texas Health Science Center at San Antonio's Executive Research Committee at *http://www.uthscsa.edu/*)

completed your literature search and review; and made decisions about design/methodology and data analysis. There is much to do before you determine which format of clinical investigation to choose. You should always consider the Randomized Controlled Study design if possible. It is considered the "gold standard." In many instances, drug and medical device companies seek clinical practices for inclusion in clinical investigations. Above all, you must take every step possible to protect your patients and human subjects from harm. This is not completely possible, because any drug, device, or intervention involves some risk. There is no risk free clinical investigation. The other consideration is the protection of "Personal Health Information." In many institutions, there is an Institutional Review Board (IRB) or Ethics Committee that must approve all research involving human subjects and the protection of personal health information is part of their reviews and considerations. How data will be handled, used, and protected is very important to safeguarding the privacy of patients and subjects privacy. Please go to Chapter 15 for more information.

Table 6–1
Phases of Drug Trials

Phase	Description
Phase I	Initial studies to determine metabolism and pharmacokinetics of a drug in humans, including side effects associated with increasing doses and evidence of effectiveness; usually conducted in a small number of healthy people (20–100).
Phase II	Controlled clinical investigations conducted to evaluate the effectiveness and therapeutic range of a drug for a particular indication in patients with the disease or condition and to determine common side effects and risks. Usually conducted in larger group of individuals (100–300).
Phase III	Expanded controlled and uncontrolled investigations after evidence suggesting drug effectiveness has been obtained; intended to gather additional information on overall benefit–risk of drug and to provide adequate basis for labeling. May include testing against current drugs or placebo. Usually conducted in a fairly large group of people (1,000–3,000).
Phase IV	Post-release studies to delineate additional information about risks, benefits, and optimal use. Can involve very, very large numbers of people.

Adapted from The University of Texas Health Science Center at San Antonio's Executive Research Committee at *http://www.uthscsa.edu/*

Some Types of Clinical Investigations

A Brief Review of Drug and Medical Device Studies

Drug and medical device studies may be the best known type of clinical investigations or trials. They are mentioned here because they are part of the process that brings therapeutic substances and medical devices for our use. The process for drug and medical device approval in the United States is a long and rigorous one, regulated by law and under the responsibility of the Food and Drug Administration (FDA). The FDA ensures the safety and effectiveness of all drugs, biological agents, vaccines, and medical devices used in diagnosis, treatment, and prevention of illness and injury through a rigorous process of testing. Table 6–1 lists the phases of drug investigations.

PAs are most likely to be involved with Phase IV studies. Drug studies, like other clinical investigations, can follow different research designs, but fall within the phase categories. I have presented them first because the phases are similar for other clinical investigations. It is also important that as a consumer of the medical literature that you understand the phases of drug studies, particularly since you will be prescribing for your patients.

Randomized Controlled Studies

Randomized controlled studies are clinical investigations based on subject assignment to an experimental (subjects who receive the drug or device) or control group (subjects who do not receive the drug or device or who may receive placebo) based on chance (randomization). Such studies can include more than one experimental group. For example, a drug study may have one subject group assigned to a particular drug dose or schedule and another group to a different drug dose or schedule. Regardless of how many experimental groups there are, there is usually only one control group. This type of study is considered the "gold standard" for clinical investigations, particularly when the investigation is blinded or double-blinded. Many times, such investigations are "blinded" or "double-blinded" or even "triple blinded." "Blinded" means that the subjects do not know which group (experimental or control) they belong to or are assigned. "Double-blinded" means that, in addition, the investigators do not know to which group the subjects are assigned. "Triple-blinded" means that, in addition, the people doing the statistical analysis do not know the group assignments. Blinding is done to attempt to eliminate bias that may occur by the knowledge of the group assignment. In drug studies, the term "open label" is used when the drug is known to the subjects and investigators.

A number of other terms are used to describe various types of studies and their designs. These are often included in the titles of clinical investigations for descriptive purposes. In some locations, Institutional Review Boards (or similar review groups) have specific requirements for the titles of investigations.

Cohort Studies

A clinical investigation of a group of people with similar or common characteristics carried out over time. More than one cohort of subjects may be involved in the same investigation. Cohort studies involve observations across time and do not involve an intervention. Subjects do not have the condition or outcome of interest at the beginning of the study period (prospective). Cohort clinical investigation can also be retrospective and look back at risks, interventions, and behaviors in subjects who have developed the condition or disease being investigated.

Subjects are interviewed, observed, or surveyed in some fashion for the presence or absence of risks or characteristics that may be predictive of development of a condition or disease. Cohort studies are often descriptive of a disease process and its risks and conditions. Cohort investigations can be analytic, identifying risks and comparing outcomes between and within cohorts. Cohort studies involve the following steps:

1. You must identify specific problems to be studied. This is the "what" you are studying.
2. You must develop well defined research questions or hypotheses.
3. You must identify your cohort (sample or subjects) as precisely as possible. These are your inclusion criteria.

   Some possible cohort characteristics:

   a. Specific age group
   b. Gender
   c. Health (or disease) condition
   d. Particular medication need
   e. Variables

4. Define exclusion criteria. These are the things that would keep people out of your cohort.
5. Define the time interval for your investigation. Some cohort studies have been going on for years. The Framingham Heart Study began in 1948 and continues today.
6. Define your study end-points or markers.
7. Define your measurement for these end-points or study markers. You must be able to measure an ob-

servation by some means. This is usually the development of the condition you want to investigate.

A major challenge is deciding on the size of the cohort. Again, it may be useful to consult a statistician. Another thing to consider is attrition and how it will effect your investigation. It would be very rare to have a cohort that did not lose subjects for any number of reasons. Cohort studies conducted over a long period of time may not be feasible for a student, but may fit a practice very well.

Case-Controlled Studies

Case-controlled studies are a clinical investigation where subjects are selected based on whether or not they have the disease or condition you are studying. Controls for case-controlled studies are people without the disease or condition being studied. This type of clinical investigation is common in epidemiologic studies. Case-controlled studies are typically retrospective studies. The emphasis in case-controlled studies is the identification of the prevalence or exposure to known or suspected risk factors. The ultimate outcome of case-controlled studies is to define the "odds ratio" for the risk factors for development of a condition or disease. An "odds ratio" is calculated using the following formula:

$$\text{Odds ratio} = \frac{ad}{bc}$$

where:

a = subjects with the disease who have a risk factor
b = subjects with the disease who do not have the risk factor
c = subjects without the disease who have the risk factor
d = subjects without the disease who do not have the risk factor.
(risk factor can be exposure to a disease or cause of a disease)

You can calculate odds for people exposed to a disease and for those not exposed. Using the definitions from above, the odds ratio for a person exposed to a risk factor who has the disease is

$$\text{Odds ratio for exposed} = \frac{a}{b}$$

The odds ratio for a nonexposed person would be calculated as follows.

$$\text{Odds ratio for a nonexposed person} = \frac{c}{d}$$

It is these statistics, their meaning, and your interpretation that make the report.

Case Series Studies

Case series studies or a case report are certainly something that a PA or PA student can do. A case study or a case series studies involves the description of one or more patients with unusual presentations or conditions, or the outcomes from innovative interventions. These reports are usually descriptive in nature, but very detailed. If a series of cases is reported, common factors may be identified. New or unusual presentations or treatment outcomes in a case or series of cases may lead to further research and may even lead to the identification of a new disease. Many case reports or case series are interesting (unusual) presentations or clinical challenges. Case series are more than just reporting presentations, findings, and outcomes. They require a detailed investigation into risk factors, etiology, and variables of the case. Case studies require a more detailed and intensive examination than the usual medical history and physical examination. Genetic, social, and environmental factors must be considered. In a case series, common factors must be searched for that may not be readily apparent. The data collected may be subjective and objective. You must pay great attention to detail of every case in looking for common factors or variables.

Case studies can help us to understand unusual or rare conditions, presentations, or effective new treatments. Case studies may reveal unknown relationships of risk factors and disease or reveal a new condition. There is something unique in case studies that bring them to our attention. Thorough investigation leads to better understanding of our approach to a set of conditions and relationships of disease. Case studies or case series that describe new, innovative, or nontraditional treatments also help in our advancement of medical science.

Some considerations in case studies are the following:

1. What are you describing?
   a. Occurrence of a new disease
   b. Unusual presentation of a known disease
   c. Association of risk factors to a disease
   d. Outcomes of treatment
2. How unique is your case or case series?
3. What is in the literature already?
4. How will you account for the relationships of factors to disease?
5. What more is needed to establish your findings?

As stated earlier in the section, case studies or a case series studies are investigations that PAs and PA students can do. The key is to identify something out of the ordinary and investigate it.

Cross-Sectional Study

This type of retrospective study is a form of the cohort study and, perhaps, a case series. It can also be a one-time intervention. In this design, you identify a point in time to study and the variables, conditions, or characteristics that you want to study. OR you apply the intervention at one time point. The sample is usually stratified by some conditions set by the investigator. This can also be a type of population study or a study of prevalence. The problems with this type of study are that it is difficult to control confounding variables and differences in the sample may pose a threat to external validity (ages, life experiences, condition onset, etc.)

The keys are:

1. Define your population and sample.
2. Be very specific in defining what is to be studied.
3. Consider the variables and how to account for confounding variables.
4. Define the stratification of your sample.
5. Define the outcomes in which you are interested.

Your report and discussion will revolve around the points and include contrasts, support, and questions raised in other similar studies.

Section Conclusion

The study types discussed above are a sample of the many types of clinical investigations. They are presented in a simplistic manner because we believe it is important to gain and use a very basic approach as you begin your research efforts. Clinical investigations offer practicing PAs a great opportunity to include research in their clinical practices. Always remember the importance of protecting the human subject.

Section 2

Evidence-Based Medicine

Constance Goldgar, MS, PA-C

> It's not what we know that hurts us. It's what we know that ain't so.
>
> Will Rogers

> A well-used library is one of the few antidotes a general practitioner has to the premature senility that is liable to overtake him. It is astonishing with how little reading a doctor may practice medicine, but it is not astonishing, how badly he may do it.
>
> Butler, "Equanimitas," 1901

Section Overview

Research as it pertains to PAs can take many forms. This section delineates one of a few possible roads that PAs and PA students may choose as they negotiate down the research path. Although PAs certainly may choose traditional research, there are various alternatives that can enrich and encompass our clinical lives. Certainly, evidence-based medicine (EBM) is becoming the basis for medical practice in many areas. Yet, there is still so much in medicine for which we don't have good evidence. EBM offers the PA and the PA student the opportunity to contribute to the fund of knowledge in a way that has application. Table 6–2 provides a comparison of traditional research skills and EBM skills.

This list incorporates many of the skills or criteria that define graduate education in general.[1] However, the same skill set can also be interpreted in a clinically applicable manner that would allow PAs to utilize clinical practice as a means for actually honing and applying research methodology. In fact, we would hope all clinicians have the ability to use these skills on a daily basis. The clinical interpretation of these aptitudes is outlined on the right side of Table 6–2. These elements, in essence, comprise the practice of EBM.

Introduction: What Is Evidence-Based Medicine?

The best, and likely most quoted, definition of EBM is one from David Sackett: "Evidence-based medicine is the conscientious, explicit, and judicious use of current best evidence in making decisions about the care of individual patients."[2] EBM is about solving clinical problems. In 1992, EBM was described as a shift in medical paradigms. In contrast to the traditional paradigm of medical practice, EBM acknowledges that intuition, unsystematic clinical experience, and pathophysiologic rationale are insufficient grounds for clinical decision-making.[3] EBM stresses looking for evidence from clinical research and deals directly with the uncertainties of clinical medicine. The research part of EBM is really the development of a set of tools or a systematic approach to lifelong, self-directed learning so we can be the best clinicians for our patients.

How Can EBM Be Used for Research?

As presented earlier, traditional research and EBM share similar skill sets. One of the missing criteria, however, at least from the research skills, is that of writing, or providing some tangible output of the research activities. EBM is certainly practiced without the requirement of a written end product. A clinician, however, may decide to take the fruits of his or her EBM labors to the next step. The culmination of the steps of formulating a clear clinical question, locating relevant research, critically appraising the evidence against specified criteria, and synthesizing the results may be translated into something useful in the professional, academic, or personal arenas. A PA clinician may write an evidence-based review article of a common clinical problem. If taken to publication, this EBM product provides predistilled, valid information for fellow clinicians. Likewise, a student may utilize an evidence-based review paper as a capstone event, for instance, for a master's project. Or they may also have the inclination to submit it for publication. The honing of all evidence-based skills takes place in this work as well as in the critically appraised topic (CAT).[4] The POEM,[5] defined in the next section, although not explicitly requiring the searching or synthesis steps, addresses the ability to choose and appropriately critique clinically relevant research that is important to patients.

Table 6–2
Comparison of Skill Sets for Traditional Research and for Evidence-Based Medicine

Skill Set for Graduate Level Research	Skill Set for Practice of Evidence-Based Medicine
1. Be able to frame a logical, clear research question.	1. Identify an area of clinical uncertainty.
2. Access information within the discipline.	2. Formulate a relevant, focused, clinically important question.
3. Demonstrate critical thinking skills.	3. Select appropriate resource(s) and conduct a search.
4. Integrate, and synthesize knowledge from multiple sources.	4. Appraise the evidence for validity and clinical applicability.
5. Write in a clear, consistent, and logical manner.	5. Integrate evidence with clinical expertise, patient preferences and apply it to practice.
	6. Evaluate the outcomes of your actions.
	7. Write an evidence-based review article or CAT.

This section explores the three models of EBM projects mentioned earlier: (1) the evidence-based review article, (2) the CAT, and (3) the POEM (patient oriented evidence that matters). It will then take you step-by-step through the "practice" of EBM and its application to each one of these research endeavors.

How to Use EBM for Capstone Projects or Publication

In becoming proficient with the skill set of EBM, a clinician or student may decide to take the fruits of his or her labors to the next step.

There are a few formats for written evidence-based medicine endeavors: (1) an evidence-based review article, (2) the critically appraised topic (or CAT), and (3) a brief review of an article that qualifies as a POEM (patient-oriented evidence that matters).[5] Other brief written EBM formats exist, but they basically revolve around the same "ingredients." For the extremely ambitious, there is the systematic review or meta-analysis. This type of research is beyond the scope of this section, as it requires financial and time resources outside of most clinicians' or researchers' ranges, and almost

certainly those of most PA students. Therefore, we will discuss in detail how to approach the execution of these three EBM written projects.

The Evidence-Based Review Article

The evidence-based review article may take one of two forms. Although it always involves asking a focused clinical question, the question may emanate from a specific clinical scenario, or it may be a burning question the author has an interest in pursuing. The process of writing such a paper involves all of the steps in practicing EBM. It begins with the formulation of a clear, answerable clinical question. Then, it requires a thorough search of the highest quality studies as well as summarized sources of evidence-based information (at a minimum, searching PubMed, Cochrane Library, and then adding one of these: TRIP Database, InfoPOEMs, Clinical Evidence, ACP Journal Club, National Guidelines Clearinghouse). Next, the quality of each research report is critically evaluated against specified validity criteria.

Relationships between the clinical outcomes, sample characteristics, and methodological characteristics are then examined, synthesized, and discussed. Unlike a true systematic review, quantitative methods are not used to combine study results since this would require professional statistical manipulation. However, trends between the chosen studies are identified, as well as outliers, setting up the discussion of the evidence. Synthesized results can then be presented in a summary statement constructed around the questions, along with an assessment of the evidence and suitability to help answer the questions. It is not uncommon to find evidence lacking, despite a well-crafted question. Studies may be planned or are underway, with results pending. These issues enhance the discussion.

Although the ingredients of the evidence-based review paper may appear similar to a critically appraised topic (CAT, next in this section), the evidence-based review paper is a thorough treatise that demonstrates, not summarizes, mastery of EBM skills. The requirement of an exhaustive search of the literature also differentiates EBM from a CAT. The structure of this endeavor follows that of a formal scientific paper. Table 6–3 outlines the classic elements of an evidence-based review paper.

Critically Appraised Topic (CAT)

CATs were originally designed as assignments for McMaster University internal medicine fellows as a means of improving their critical appraisal and EBM skills.[4] Because they utilize all of the "tools" in the practice of EBM, they have become an important exercise for

Table 6–3
Main Elements of an Evidence-Based Review Paper

Section	Description of Contents
Introduction	• Brief presentation of the patient case that elicits the clinical question for case-based review; for review paper, introduction and background as below • Introduction that describes the impact and relevance of the clinical question and limited background information (e.g., epidemiology, pathophysiology) • Presentation of focused clinical question
Methods	• Description of the search strategy in enough detail to be duplicable • Inclusion and exclusion criteria for the final studies chosen
Results	• Brief summary of the studies (usually three to five articles with the highest level of evidence), including validity assessment of each
Discussion	• Discussion and synthesis of evidence from the studies collectively to provide an answer to the question • Includes evidence interpretation as it applies to the patient case (if case-based)

sharpening skills. A CAT contains the characteristic elements outlined in Table 6–4.[6] Box 6–1[7] provides an actual, critically appraised topic for a clinical question regarding routine screening for *Chlamydia trachomatis.*

CATs evolve from patient encounters that generate clinical questions, similar to what we have seen in the evidence-based review paper. A CAT follows the same steps as in the practice of EBM: formulating a question, efficiently and effectively searching the literature, critically appraising the literature, and applying the evidence to the patient. Unlike the previously described evidence-based review paper, a CAT is not a comprehensive review of a subject or a synthesis of all the available knowledge. It is a brief, evidence-based assessment of the one or two most relevant studies retrieved to answer a focused clinical question. It is usually written as a one-page summary. Box 6–1 provides an example of a critically appraised topic for a clinical question regarding routine screening for *Chlamydia trachomatis.*

As you can see from the CAT example, knowledge of basic statistical and epidemiologic concepts is necessary for the delivery of a clear, and useful, bottom line. This CAT appraised more than one evidence source and the author demonstrated facility with screening issues on an individual and population basis. Those working in primary care would point out quickly that testing for *Chlamydia* has changed over the past several years.

Although out of date, this is a good example of the process of using EBM tools

The limitations of CATs, however, need to be addressed. An individual CAT has limited applicability. A CAT is a single piece of evidence that is summarized and should not be considered complete or representative of the entire body of evidence on a clinical issue. Individual CATs can be wrong or contain inferior evidence or errors of fact, calculation, or interpretation. They have a short "half life" and usually become obsolete as new evidence becomes available.[8] Owing to burgeoning databases of prefiltered secondary literature (such as Cochrane, Clinical Evidence, or InfoPOEMs) that have quality standards and are continuously updated, CATs are now used primarily as an educational exercise. Many institutions have amassed various banks of CATs (Table 6–5) and databases of CATs are still available. These Web sites provide samples of well-formed clinical questions, as well as illustrate the CAT format.

POEMs

Slawson and Shaughnessy are usually credited with coining the acronym POEM, which stands for "**P**atient **O**riented **E**vidence that **M**atters." POEMs are summaries of valid research, usually focusing on primary care issues that ideally have the potential to change the

---

Table 6–4
Outline of a Critically Appraised Topic (CAT)

Element	Description
Title	Gives a declarative answer to your question.
Clinical bottom line	Describes how this evidence is used in clinical care. Will the study change or affect how you practice medicine? Why or why not? (Ask yourself if your findings are worth telling your colleagues about.)
Clinical scenario	Summary of the patient case: in one paragraph, describe the patient's age and sex, clinical and geographic setting, presenting complaint, relevant medical history, and pertinent physical and laboratory findings.
Clinical question	To achieve a focused, pertinent clinical question that leads to a well-defined literature search and pertinent results, PICO format should be used.
Search terms and strategy used	Provide the terms of your search so that others can repeat it and update it. Note how many citations were retrieved. List the one or two citations chosen and why they were chosen.
The study	Give a short summary of the study design and methods of analysis.
The evidence	In evaluating the evidence, briefly describe the paper and its major outcomes and conclusions. Note any problems with the study, assessing the validity and relevance of the study as it relates to your clinical question. Compile a table summarizing the key results. The use of evidence-based medicine concepts such as likelihood ratios, predictive values, and numbers needed to treat is encouraged here.
Comments and references	Self-explanatory
Others	Author, expiry date

Adapted from: Ball C, Phillip B. What is a CAT? Evidence Based On Call (EBOC). June, 2002. Cited date: August, 2004. Available from: *http://www.eboncall.org/* (accessed February 17, 2005).

BOX 6–1

Example of a CAT

Author: Barbara A. Porter
Date: October 31, 1997
Critically appraised topic: Chamydial screening to prevent pelvic inflammatory disease (PID)[1]

Scenario:
An asymptomatic 22-year-old female presents to clinic for a routine physical exam. She is sexually active, has had two sexual partners in the last year, and has never been treated for an STD. Will screening her for chlamydia at today's visit decrease her risk of developing PID in the future?

Clinical bottom line:
In women thought to be at increased risk for chlamydial infection, cervical screening reduced the risk of subsequent PID by 58 percent relative to women who were not screened.
Eighty-three women at increased risk for chlamydial infections need to be screened by cervical testing in order to prevent one case of PID.

The evidence:
Randomized controlled trial of 2,607 women identified as being at increased risk for chlamydial infection. Women were assigned to receive either screening for cervical chlamydial disease or usual care. The diagnosis of PID within one year of onset of study was the outcome measured, and was determined by patient report, review of inpatient and outpatient diagnostic databases, and medical record review.
    Randomization into groups occurred before inclusion/exclusion criteria sought.
    Except for marital status, the two groups were similar in baseline characteristics.

Endpoint*	Screened	Usual Care	Absolute risk reduction	Relative risk	Relative risk reduction	NNS**
PID	9/1009	33/1598	0.012	0.42	0.58	83

*Calculations based on rates expressed as cases of PID per number of women; paper's rates are per women-months.
**Number needed to screen.

Comments:

1. Results are strained by several flaws in study design:

    *Randomization style, that is, because of study design, subjects randomized to screening group were more intensely recruited, which may have introduced behavior changes in this population.
    *Thirty-six percent of women in the screening group did not receive the intervention, which seems like a large percentage; however, data was analyzed by "intention to screen."

    Subjects and health workers were not blinded.
    *Were the seven women diagnosed with chlamydia in the screened population also diagnosed with PID during the screening test, or were these subsequent diagnoses?

2. Although this study set out to evaluate the usefulness of screening for chlamydia in preventing PID, the paper did not provide a detailed evaluation of the screening tool. Is the prevalence of chlamydia known in this population? What are the sensitivity and specificity of the two screening tests? Why did they use two diagnostic tests? Is one a "gold standard"? The fact that screening required a pelvic exam makes cervical testing less attractive as a screening tool.

3. First-void urine testing with ligase chain reaction assay for chlamydia may be a more appropriate screening tool,[2] and its utility in the prevention of PID should be studied.

4. Some PID is caused by gonorrhea. Were subjects with chlamydia treated for gonorrhea as well?

5. Besides decreasing the risk of PID secondary to indolent infection, does making a diagnosis of chlamydia lead to education and behavioral changes? Is there a way to measure this?

1. Scholes D, Stergachis A, Heidrich FE, et al. Prevention of pelvic inflammatory disease by screening for cervical chlamydial infection. N Engl J Med 1996;334:1362–1366.
2. Marrazzo JM, White CL, Krekeler B, et al. Community-based urine screening for Chlamydia trachomatis with a ligase chain reaction assay. Ann Intern Med 1997;127:796–803.

Table 6–5
Current Web Sites Containing Examples/Sources of CATs

Source and Web Sites	Total no.
Centre for Evidence-Based Medicine (CATbank-Oxford, UK) *http://www.minervation.com/cebm2/cats/allcats.html*	64
Critically Appraised Topics—University of Rochester Medical Center. *http://www.med.unc.edu/medicine/edursrc/%21catlist.htm*	109
Evidence-Based Pediatrics Web Site—University of Michigan. *http://www.med.umich.edu/pediatrics/ebm/cat.htm*	141
UNC Critically Appraised Topics—University of North Carolina at Chapel Hill, School of Medicine. *http://www.med.unc.edu/medicine/edursrc/!catlist.htm*	69
BestBETs (Best Evidence Topics) in Emergency Medicine— Manchester Royal Infirmary, UK* *http://www.bestbets.org/*	487

*This database is peer reviewed, maintained regularly, with some quality control. All Web sites accessed on February 17, 2005.

way we practice.[5] Information Mastery stresses that the evidence must matter to both the clinician and the patient. There are three main questions that help determine if a study qualifies to be a POEM:

1. Did the research focus on an outcome that patients care about (e.g., morbidity, mortality, quality of life)?

2. Is the problem studied common and is the intervention feasible?

3. Does the information have the potential to change the practice of many clinicians?[9]

Currently POEMs are published as unsolicited manuscripts in the *Journal of Family Practice*. An editorial group reviews a wide range of journals in primary care, internal medicine, and in a variety of specialties and selects studies that are subsequently evaluated with international criteria for validity. POEMs are mentioned here, not as a potentially publishable entity, but rather to provide a format for enhancing EBM skills. Writing a POEM demonstrates the ability to appropriately choose an article that meets the three qualifications described in the preceding list, evaluate it with specific evidence-based criteria, and succinctly summarize its applicability to clinical practice. A POEM utilizes all of the skills of EBM, but in contrast to the evidence-based review paper or CAT, it does not require choosing and critiquing multiple articles, nor is the synthesis step required. The format, as illustrated in Table 6–6, is not dissimilar from a CAT.

Evidence-based review articles, CATs, and POEMs are tangible ways of assessing our EBM skills. They also comprise all of the steps considered to define traditional research. The remainder of this section describes the skills needed to accomplish these projects and, more importantly, those needed for making better decisions in patient care. Ultimately the practice of EBM is not just

better medicine for patients, but also better medicine for clinicians.[11] Quoting Mark Ebell: "The EBM approach to patient care is intellectually rewarding and leads you down a path of exploration and lifelong learning."[11]

Topic Selection: The Clinical Question

Step 1 in the practice of EBM is the identification of gaps in our medical knowledge base generated by specific patient cases. The skill that we need to develop in this step is the ability to formulate an answerable clinical

Table 6–6
Outline of a POEM

Element	Description
Clinical question:	One line question that captures the objective of the study
Bottom line:	One paragraph that translates results into what population results apply to, and useful statistics such as number needed to treat (NNT); includes level of evidence assignment
Study design:	For example, randomized control trial, cohort study
Setting:	Refers to the patient population studied.
Synopsis:	A few paragraphs beginning with the study objective, population, and short description of study design and conduct. Includes validity assessment and results.

Adapted from: InfoPOEM Group. Sample POEM article: Knee taping useful for osteoarthritis pain. InfoPOEMs:The Clinical Awareness System. 2004. Cited date: September, 2004. Available from: *http://www.infopoems.com/productInfo/samplePOEM.cfm* (accessed February 17, 2005).

question. It is not always as easy as it seems. Before embarking on how to select a topic and formulate an answerable clinical question for an evidence-based research endeavor, it is important to review where clinical questions come from, the types of clinical questions there are, and how to go about formulating a well-built, answerable clinical question.

Where Do Clinical Questions Come From?

The first step in the practice of EBM is asking clinical questions. Clinical questions arise in daily practice and most of them remain unsought and unanswered. But where do clinical questions come from? Every time we see a patient, we need new information or need to determine a new application of information about some element of the diagnosis, prognosis, or management. Because our time to find this information is limited, we need to develop skills for efficient searching. The first step toward achieving this efficiency is becoming skilled at asking clinical questions. Asking questions in a well-articulated way serves many purposes: it helps achieve clarity of what we are asking; it can aid in communicating to our colleagues and patients; and it also identifies areas that need revisiting in our medical knowledge base. But more importantly, a well-built question will hopefully lead directly and with more efficiency to a well-constructed search strategy, so that we may answer the question for our patient.

Background and Foreground Questions

It has been estimated that the average clinician will have about five clinical or care questions for every inpatient encounter and around two or three questions for every three outpatient encounters.[12] Certainly, as we gain clinical experience, the quality and depth and, sometimes, the number of clinical questions that occur to us changes. David Sackett et al. in their book, *Evidence-Based Medicine: How to Practice and Teach EBM*, discuss these types of questions, dividing them into two main groups: background and foreground questions.[2] Background questions typically involve general knowledge about a disorder. Background questions also have two essential components: a question root about who, what, when, how, and why with a verb, plus a disorder or an aspect of a disorder. Foreground questions, on the other hand, are questions that involve specific knowledge about how to diagnose, treat, or predict outcomes. When we begin as students to lay down our clinical and knowledge foundation, the majority of questions will be in the background category. As we gain clinical experience, there is a shift toward foreground questions. However, even seasoned clinicians, when encountering an uncommon clinical problem or presentation, or because they need to refresh information, will still raise and ask background questions.[2]

Formulating Answerable Clinical Questions

To be able to convert gaps in our knowledge into answerable questions, it is useful to have a model for constructing foreground questions. The basic elements of a foreground question are:

1. The Patient and/or Problem or Population of interest;
2. The main Intervention (defined very broadly, including an exposure, a diagnostic test, a prognostic factor, a treatment, a patient perception, and so forth);
3. Comparison intervention(s), if relevant (what are other options);
4. The clinical Outcome(s) of interest.

This structure is often referred to as PICO (*P* for patient/problem/population, *I* for intervention, *C* for comparison, *O* for outcome).[13]

For example:

P: In a patient with uncomplicated type 2 diabetes mellitus and mildly elevated blood pressure (Patient/Population)

I: how does an angiotensin-converting enzyme (ACE) inhibitor (Intervention)

C: compare to an angiotensin receptor blocker (Comparison)

O: in reducing diabetic renal disease? (Outcome)

Once you have formulated a question using the PICO approach, it is easier to sort out the type of question that you are asking. Sackett et al.[2] describe 10 areas where clinical questions arise (see Box 6–2). The categorization of type of question becomes more useful, as we will see later, when searching and critiquing the medical literature. Based on the various types of questions, there are methods of research that match specific types of questions. For example, a question about therapy is usually best answered by a randomized controlled trial (RCT). The next section, about searching the literature, will provide more detail on best levels of evidence for the various types of clinical questions.

Other Elements for Topic Selection

Almost any well-articulated clinical question can launch an evidence-based review or critically appraised topic. There are a few elements that are helpful when deciding on a topic for such efforts. Primary among these is that the topic should be one that the author is in-

Ten Common Areas for Clinical Questions

1. Clinical findings: how to properly gather and interpret findings from the history and physical examination

2. Etiology: how to identify causes for disease (including its iatrogenic forms)

3. Differential diagnosis: when considering the possible causes of our patient's clinical problem, how to select those that are likely, serious, and responsive to treatment

4. Clinical manifestations of a disease: knowing how often and when a disease causes its clinical manifestations and how to use this knowledge in classifying our patients' illnesses

5. Diagnostic tests: how to select and interpret diagnostic tests, in order to confirm or exclude a diagnosis, based on considering their precision, accuracy, acceptability, expense, safety, and so forth

6. Prognosis: how to estimate our patient's likely clinical course over time and anticipate likely complications of the disorder

7. Therapy: how to select treatments to offer our patients that do more good than harm and that are worth the efforts and costs of using them

8. Prevention: how to reduce the chance of disease by identifying and modifying risk factors and how to diagnose disease early by screening

9. Patient experience and meaning: how to empathize with our patients' situations, appreciate the meaning they find in the experience and understand how this meaning influences their healing

10. Self-improvement: how to keep up to date, improve my clinical and other skills and run a better, more efficient clinical practice

Used with permission from: Sackett D, Straus SE, Richardson WS, et al: Evidence Based Medicine: How to Practice and Teach EBM, 2nd ed. St. Louis: Churchill Livingstone, 2000. Chapter 1, p. 19.

terested in and, perhaps, passionate about. Because of the work and time involved, an area of research that sustains your interest is critical. Passion for what you are doing also infuses enthusiasm and attention in those who read your work. In addition, to generate the most interest (and passion?) the topic of the clinical question chosen should include one or more of the following aspects:

- An element of controversy, for example, if a diagnosis or therapy has multiple approaches to management that appear to be of equal value;

- When the current standard of care may be ineffective or even harmful;

- An area of care in which there is considerable variation or choice in regimens, modalities, or treatment alternatives;

- An area of care in which a new intervention is compared to existing alternatives and may change clinical practice (usually Clinical Trials);

- An area of care in which treatments have very different costs and/or outcomes.

When you finally decide on a topic, the emphasis should be to provide information that, if valid, may change clinical practice. This will take both the researcher (you) and the reader to a fruitful outcome.

Searching the Medical Literature

Need for a Systematic Approach

Reviewing and searching the medical literature was presented in Chapter 4, but the very nature of our topic makes a review and further discussion necessary in this section. Searching the medical literature can be time consuming and potentially unrewarding unless one utilizes sources of information that are efficient, targeted to the type of clinical question that is asked, and have high validity. Ideally, there will be a compendium of the most frequently asked questions in a database that can be used as we see patients. This is referred to as "information at the point of care."[14] There are currently a few quality primary care based databases that make such an attempt, for example, InfoRetriever, Up-to-Date, and Clinical Evidence. Although it is anticipated that such databases will become more and more available in the near future, what is required currently is a systematic approach to the medical literature, including familiarity with quality medical databases and facility with the use of PubMed, the mother of all medical literature (in this author's opinion).

Medical literature, as we all know, is ubiquitous and voluminous. It may be divided into two general categories: primary sources and secondary sources. Primary sources basically include all that is available through PubMed, that is, original research studies. Secondary studies include meta-analyses, systematic reviews, and other types of overviews, guidelines, and decision analyses. Secondary sources are those that, it is hoped, will save us work by having collated or reviewed the pertinent medical literature for us. Of course, that also means the secondary sources must have validity, be updated frequently, and be recognized for quality in their methodology.

Where and How to Spend Time: Information Mastery

Through "Information Mastery," Slawson and Shaughnessy help clinicians prioritize their time wading through the medical literature by identifying its clinical relevance.[15] They developed the "POEM" (patient-oriented evidence that matters) and "DOE" (disease-oriented evidence) to guide clinicians to effective and efficient ways of finding information that is relevant to clinical practice.[5] For example, although it may

be interesting to read an article about how statins reduce atherosclerotic plaques and improve blood flow on angiography, the POEM that looked at patient outcomes such as reduced frequency of anginal episodes and mortality as a result of taking statins would be more relevant and more applicable to patients—and, perhaps, have more worth for the time it takes to read and critique the POEM. There are still many areas in the medical literature in which DOE exists, but the important POEM has not yet been studied for the area. An example of this would be understanding that prostate-specific antigen (PSA) screening detects prostate cancer at an earlier stage, but what hasn't been studied yet is if PSA screening, because of the nature of prostate cancer, reduces mortality or improves quality of life (at the time of this writing).

When searching the medical literature, in either primary or secondary sources, it is useful to know what types of original research or what secondary literature sources have the most validity. Figures 6–1 and 6–2 depict the hierarchy of levels of evidence with regard to primary and secondary literature.[16] The "levels of evidence" concept is discussed further in the "Critical

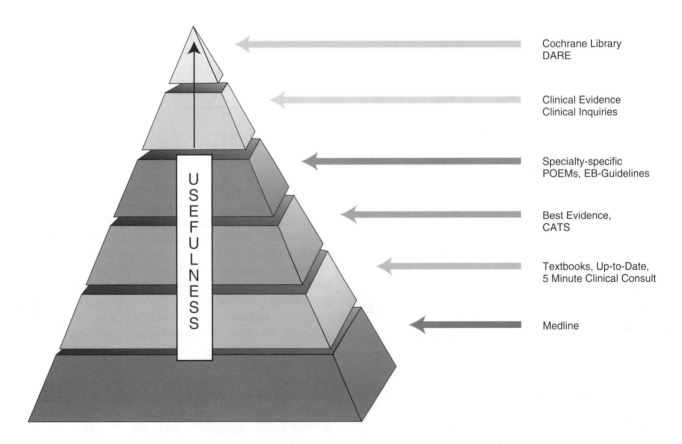

Cochrane Library
DARE

Clinical Evidence
Clinical Inquiries

Specialty-specific
POEMs, EB-Guidelines

Best Evidence,
CATS

Textbooks, Up-to-Date,
5 Minute Clinical Consult

Medline

FIG. 6–1. Pyramid of levels of evidence in the secondary literature. Adapted with permission from: Wagoner B, Mellish M, Hyman C, Doherty M, Markinson A. SUNY Downstate Medical Center Evidence Based Course. Guide to Research Methods: the Evidence Pyramid. 2002. Cited date: July, 2004. Available from: *http://servers.medlib.hscbklyn.edu/ebm/2100.htm*

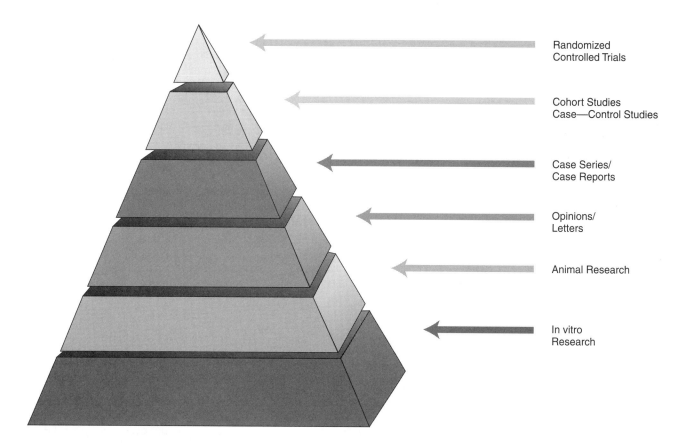

Randomized
Controlled Trials

Cohort Studies
Case—Control Studies

Case Series/
Case Reports

Opinions/
Letters

Animal Research

In vitro
Research

FIG. 6–2. Pyramid of levels of evidence in the primary literature. Adapted with permission from: Wagoner B, Mellish M, Hyman C, Doherty M, Markinson A. SUNY Downstate Medical Center Evidence Based Course. Guide to Research Methods: the Evidence Pyramid. 2002. Cited date: July, 2004. Available from: *http://servers.medlib.hscbklyn.edu/ebm/2100.htm*

Appraisal" step. The emphasis again is to spend your time most efficiently searching in areas where the highest levels of evidence are likely to be found.

Secondary Literature Databases

Unfortunately, all that is published is not necessarily up-to-date, valid, or properly done. Also, not all databases and resources are free. Currently, however, there are several databases that are accepted as having high validity and relevance. Many of these, as you might expect, require subscriptions for access. Some databases that require subscriptions also allow you a free trial of their databases. Table 6–7 summarizes several current valid sources of secondary medical literature.

Types of Clinical Questions and Searching the Medical Literature

As mentioned in the previous section, knowing the type of clinical question asked will help identify the best study methodology and enable an efficient approach to searching the literature. Table 6–8 illustrates matching

of question type in primary studies and Table 6–9 depicts questions type matched with quality secondary literature sources or Medline filters.[17]

Developing a Search Strategy

There are a myriad of approaches to finding articles in the medical literature. If one "Googled" this query alone, he or she would find a plethora of tutorials to help in this endeavor. Librarians can be very helpful in offering advice and direction. It is imperative, however, to develop some expertise in developing search strategies and to create a systematic method of approach. This will decrease your frustration and increase the yield in quality evidence.

If we go back to the section about clinical question formulation and combine the PICO approach with what we have learned about question type and best matching study design, the following elements will likely be used in most search strategies:

- Question Type
- Patient/Population

Table 6-7
EBM Literature Resources

Category Name	Description	Subscription
Journal		
ACP Journal Club *http://www.acpjc.org* 800-523-1546, ext. 2600	Bimonthly journal that analyzes the content of more than 100 clinical journals and summarizes those articles found to have scientific merit and relevance to medical practice	$78/year includes print version and on-line access. Publisher/Sponsor: American College of Physicians
American Family Physician *http://www.aafp.org/afp* 800-274-2237 ext. 5168	Twice-monthly clinical review journal that contains evidence-based components, such as POEMs (patient-oriented evidence that matters), Cochrane for Clinicians, and Point-of-Care Guides	Free online access; free print subscriptions are available to family physicians. Publisher/Sponsor: American Academy of Family Physicians
Bandolier *http://www.jr2.ox.ac.uk/ bandolier*	Monthly journal that searches PubMed and the Cochrane Library for systematic reviews and meta-analyses published in the recent past and summarizes those that "are both interesting and make sense." Often offers "tutorials" on EBM topics.	Free online; £72/year for print version. Publisher/Sponsor: Pain Research at Oxford University with multiple sponsors
The Journal of Family Practice *http://www.jfponline.org* 1-800-707-7040	Monthly clinical review journal that contains evidence-based components, such as its online archives of POEMs.	Free subscriptions are available to family physicians. Publisher/Sponsor: Dowden Health Media
Secondary Literature Sources		
Clinical Evidence *http://www.clinicalevidence. com*	A compendium of systematic reviews, gathered from Cochrane, MEDLINE, and other sources, updated and expanded every six months	Primary care clinicians can receive free copies of Clinical Evidence Concise with access to the full text online and on: *http://www.unitedhealthfoundation.org/registration.cfm* Publisher/Sponsor: BMJ Publishing Group
The Cochrane Database of Systematic Reviews *http://www.cochrane.org/*	Arguably the most extensive collection of systematic reviews. Reviewers discuss whether adequate data are available for the development of EBM guidelines for diagnosis and management.	Free online access to abstracts; £140 for full-text online access. +44 (0)1243 779777
DARE abstracts The York Database of Abstracts of Reviews of Effectiveness (DARE) *http://www.york.ac.uk/inst/crd/ darehp.htm*	A collection of abstracts of systematic reviews. Abstract summaries review articles on diagnostic or treatment interventions and discuss clinical implications.	Free online. Centre for Reviews and Dissemination, Also part of the Cochrane Library.
Effective Health Care* *http://www.york.ac.uk/inst/crd/ ehcb.htm*	Bimonthly, peer-reviewed bulletin for medical decision-makers. Based on systematic reviews and synthesis of research on clinical effectiveness, cost effectiveness, and acceptability of health service interventions.	Free online CRD receives core funding from the Department of Health's NHS Research and Development Programme.
Evidence-Based Medicine* *http://www.evidence-basedmedicine.com*	Bimonthly publication with article summaries include commentaries by clinical experts. This JFP newsletter features up-to-date POEMs and tests approved for Category 1 CME credit.	Subscription is required.
Evidence-Based Practice Newsletter (including JFP POEMs*) *http://www.ebponline.net*	This JFP newsletter features up-to-date POEMs and tests approved for Category 1 CME credit.	Subscription is required.

(continued)

Category Name	Description	Subscription
Search Engines/Databases		
INFORetriever *http://www.infopoems.com*	A search engine with access to evidence-based sources such as POEMs, Cochrane, clinical rules, a diagnostic test database, practice guideline summaries and Griffith's Five-Minute Clinical Consult; subscribers also receive Daily POEMs via e-mail.	$249/year for online, CD or hand-held computer versions. *orders@infopoems.com* Free trial
SUMSearch *http://sumsearch.uthscsa.edu/*	A search engine that gathers evidence-based clinical information from MEDLINE, DARE, and the National Guideline Clearinghouse.	Free online
TRIP Database (Turning Research Into Practice) *http://www.tripdatabase.com*	A search engine that gathers evidence-based clinical information from MEDLINE, DARE, the National Guideline Clearinghouse, BestBets, and many other evidence-based Web sites.	Five free visits per week online; Deluxe unlimited version requires subscription *subs@tripdatabase.com*
First Consult (formerly PDxMD) *http://www.firstconsult.com*	A database of evidence summaries drawn from Cochrane, Clinical Evidence, the National Guideline Clearinghouse, and others.	$149/year for online, CD or hand-held computer versions. Free trial
DynaMed *http://www.dynamicmedical.com*	A database of summaries of the evidence drawn from sources such as Clinical Evidence and the Cochrane Library.	$200/year for online access; a CD version is also available. Free trial
National Health Service (NHS) Centre for Reviews and Dissemination (CRD) *http://www.york.ac.uk/inst/crd/*	Searches CRD Databases (includes DARE, NHS Economic Evaluation Database, Health Technology Assessment Database) for EBM reviews. More limited than TRIP Database.	Free online CRD receives core funding from the Department of Health's NHS Research and Development Programme.
UpToDate *http://www.uptodate.com*	A database of topic reviews by content experts. New topic reviews undergo a rigorous editorial process, which involves a review of the available evidence including consensus statements, synthesis with existing material in UpToDate, and assessment of completeness and clinical relevance.	Individual rate: $495 (renewal rate $395); Trainee rate: $195 (proof of status required; renewal rate $195) No commercial support UpToDate is an official educational program of, or produced in cooperation with major medical societies in the United States. Free trial
BestBets (Best evidence topics) *http://www.bestbets.org/*	BETs initially had an emergency medicine focus, but there are a significant number of BETs covering cardiothoracics, nursing, primary care and pediatrics issues. BestBETs represents a modified version of critically appraised topics (CATs). Provide rapid evidence-based answers to real-life clinical questions, using a systematic approach to reviewing the literature.	Free online. Sponsor: Accident and Emergency Department, Manchester Royal Infirmary
Clinical Guidelines		
National Guideline Clearinghouse *http://www.guidelines.gov*	Comprehensive database of evidence-based clinical practice guidelines from government agencies and health-care organizations. Describes and compares guideline statements with respect to objectives, methods, outcomes, evidence.	Free online Publisher/Sponsor: The Agency for Healthcare Research and Quality
US Preventive Services Taskforce (USPSTF) *http://www.ahrq.gov/clinic/uspstfix.htm*	Recommendations for clinical preventive services based on systematic reviews by the U.S. Preventive Services Task Force	Free online

(continued)

Table 6-7
EBM Literature Resources *(Continued)*

Category Name	Description	Subscription
Clinical Guidelines		
Primary Care Clinical Practice Guidelines *http://medicine.ucsf.edu/resources/guidelines*	Web site that includes links to NGC, CEBM, AHRQ, individual articles, and organizations	Free online University of California, San Francisco
Institute for Clinical Systems Improvement (ICSI) *http://www.ICSI.org*	Guidelines for preventive services and disease management developed by ICSI, an independent, nonprofit collaboration of health care organizations.	Free online Publisher/Sponsor: Institute for Clinical Systems Improvement
EBM Guidelines *http://www.ebmguidelines.com*	Main sources of evidence are Cochrane reviews and Database of Reviews of Effectiveness (DARE) abstracts, which are evaluated as they are published. If they bear relevance to topics in EBM guidelines, they are abstracted as evidence summaries.	£99 for Internet, CD-ROM, or mobile handheld, £130 for Internet and CD-ROM, or £150 for Internet, CD-ROM, and handheld. Institutional pricing is available. A free 14-day trial

All Web sites in this table accessed on February 17, 2005.

- Intervention/Exposure
- Outcome(s)
- Best Feasible Study
- Suitable Database(s)
- Best Single Search Term for Study Type

In the PICO example given earlier, the question, "In a patient with uncomplicated type 2 diabetes mellitus and mildly elevated blood pressure, how does an ACE-inhibitor compare to an angiotensin receptor blocker in reducing diabetic renal disease?" could translate into the following approach:

- Element   Response
- Question Type   Therapy

Table 6–8
Clinical Question Type Matched with Best Study Design for Primary Literature

Type of Question	Type of Study/Methodology
Therapy	Double-blind randomized controlled trial
Diagnosis	Controlled trial
Prognosis	Cohort studies, Case control, Case series
Etiology/HARM	Cohort studies
Prevention	Randomized controlled trial, cohort studies

Adapted from Dorsch J. Evidence Based Medicine—Finding the Best Clinical Literature. Applying Clinical Search Filters. December, 2003. Cited: September, 2004. Available at: *http://www.uic.edu/depts/lib/lhsp/resources/levels.shtml*

- Patient/Population   Middle-aged type 2 diabetic patients
- Intervention/Exposure Antihypertensive ACEI versus ARB
- Outcome   Renal disease
- Best Feasible Study Design   Meta-analysis RCT
- Suitable Databases   Cochrane, PubMed
- Best Single Search Term   Meta-analysis RCT

A Step-by-Step Approach to Searching the Literature

It is not within the scope of this section to go into detail regarding Medline search strategies. However, the steps below are some suggestions for effective searches in Medline/PubMed, as well as for the use of other valid databases.

1. Begin with a precisely structured question (see earlier examples). With a good, clear question, there is a better chance of finding a matching result.
2. Break the question down into its various concepts. A question that uses the PICO structure already includes these elements. Once the question is broken down to components or concepts, some additional steps may be necessary.
   a. Identify synonyms. For example:
      -Generic and trade names for drugs
      -Variant spellings (i.e., estrogen OR oestrogen)

Table 6–9
Evidence-Based Secondary/Filtered/Synthesized Literature

Filtered/Synthesized Information	Description/Definition	How to Find
Systematic reviews	• Differ from traditional review articles in that conclusions are evidence-based rather than commentary. • Start with a clearly articulated question. • Use explicit, rigorous methods to identify, critically appraise, and synthesize relevant studies. • Appraise relevant published and unpublished evidence before combining and analyzing data. • Include description of how primary data sources are identified. • Individual studies are assessed for validity.	Cochrane Collaboration -Cochrane Database of Systematic Reviews -York Database of Abstracts of Reviews of Effectiveness -Cochrane Controlled Trials Register -Cochrane Review Methodology Database In MEDLINE: -Review (pt) AND medline (tw) -(Quantitative OR Systematic OR Methodologic) AND (Review OR Overview)
Meta-analyses	• A specific methodologic and statistical technique for combining quantitative data • A type of systematic overview	Cochrane Databases -In MEDLINE: -Meta-analysis (pt) -meta-anal* (tw) OR metaanal* (tw)
Evidence-based practice guidelines	• Gather, appraise, and combine evidence systematically. • Statements designed to assist practitioner and patient decisions. • Developed by professional groups, government agencies, and local practices. • Structured abstract: objective, option, outcomes, evidence, values, benefits/harms/costs, recommendation, validation, sponsors	National Guidelines Clearinghouse *http://www.ngc.gov* Agency for Health Care Policy Research US Preventive Services Task Force MD Consult *http://www.uic.edu/depts/lib/restricted/md-consult.html*

Adapted from Dorsch J. Evidence Based Medicine—Finding the Best Clinical Literature. Applying Clinical Search Filters. December, 2003. Cited: September, 2004. Available at: *http://www.uic.edu/depts/lib/lhsp/resources/levels.shtml*

-Abbreviations (SLE OR systemic lupus erythematosus)
b. Use special database features. For example:
-Check to see if any of the concepts to be searched can be translated to MeSH subheadings (PubMed).
-Use a thesaurus or vocabularies to translate individual concepts into valid subject headings.
-PubMed provides animated tutorials to help use these features.
c. Use truncation (allows you to search for the root word and its variant endings). An asterisk (*) is the most common truncation symbol. For example:
-"diabet*" retrieves "diabetes, diabetic, diabetics, etc." (truncating too soon will give you inaccurate results (e.g., "diab*" can retrieve words such as "diabolical").
d. If no appropriate subject headings are found, consider conducting a keyword search using truncation.

3. Construct a clear search strategy with the concepts you have identified.

You can search for one concept at a time. Or, combine the concepts using "AND" or "OR" appropriately.
a. Using "AND"
-Requires that ALL terms are present in the article.
-Narrows your search (you get fewer articles than are in each set).
-Example: a search for "diabetes AND hypertension" will retrieve articles containing both terms.
b. Using "OR"
-Allows EITHER term to be present in each article.
-Broadens your search.
-Example: a search for "inflammatory bowel disease OR Crohn disease" retrieves articles that mention either condition.

4. Identify the most appropriate or relevant database(s) to begin the search.
This step involves being able to match the type of question being asked with the best type of study that would answer the question. Databases such as

PubMed allow for limits by study type (e.g., meta-analysis, randomized controlled trial, or clinical trial).

PubMed has another searching mode called "Clinical Queries" that automatically uses filters for question types—for example, for a therapy question Clinical Queries will ask for a sensitive (broad) search or a specific (narrow) search. A sensitive search will filter with "trial" OR "clinical trial" OR therapeutic use. A specific search filters with "randomized controlled trial" OR "randomized" AND "controlled" AND "trial." Clinical Queries creates filters for therapy, diagnosis, etiology, and prognosis type questions.

The Cochrane Library is often utilized primarily for the systematic reviews it contains. However, this database also includes searches for randomized controlled trials in its Controlled Trials Register.

TRIP database and SUMSearch (see Tables 6–2 through 6–6, Box 6–2) have search engines that link to evidence-based resources as well as PubMed and list results in descending order of quality of evidence. Their search engines are not as complicated or robust as PubMed, but certainly worth becoming acquainted with.

5. Refining/revising the search strategy
   a. Use special database features.
      -If focusing on a particular population (e.g., gender, age group), these can be applied in limits in PubMed.
      -It is nearly always helpful to check the "abstract" box in PubMed or you won't know what the article is about.
      -Many databases allow searching for articles over specific time periods, for example, last 5 years.
      -It is always helpful to limit to "human" as we are thinking POEM.
      -Articles may be specified in particular languages, for example, English.
      -If searching for a particular type of publication (e.g., review articles, meta-analyses, clinical trials), this can be specified in PubMed.
   b. Narrow your search if you retrieve too many citations.
      -Add additional concepts to your search by adding search terms using "AND."
      -Limit your search (e.g., by publication date, publication type, language, etc.).
      -In MEDLINE and CINAHL: In the MeSH browser, add subheadings to subject heading, for example, instead of searching for all articles on calcium channel blockers, add the subheadings "adverse effects," & "contraindications," & "poisoning," & "toxicity."
   c. Broaden your search if you retrieve too few citations.

-Eliminate peripheral concepts.
-Identify additional search terms.
-If you can identify one good article on your topic, examine the subject headings assigned and revise your search using those subject headings to find additional relevant articles.
-Use "related articles" in PubMed, although often this may over broaden the search (caveat: limits will not apply when using this feature).
-Add synonyms or related terms to your search using "OR."
-Apply fewer limits or no limits to your search.
-In MEDLINE and CINAHL: Use the "EXPLODE" command to retrieve general as well as specific subject headings. Choose "all subheadings."

How to Save and Describe a Search Strategy

For any publishable evidence-based review paper or CAT, it is critical to keep track of your search strategy. This includes terms used in the search, limits, and all of the databases in which these were employed. Ideally, the description of the search strategy should be duplicable in the sense that someone else could get to the same evidence that you did. PubMed, luckily, also has a feature that will automatically track where and how the search, up to that point, has been conducted. The feature "History" does this for the continuous time period you use PubMed. Other databases do not provide this feature and you need to track this by hand.

Narrowing the Evidence

Once sufficient evidence is located (and "sufficient" will certainly vary depending on the nature of the question), the collection of studies will need to be winnowed to the best ones to answer the question. This can be accomplished in a number of ways, but usually includes devising targeted inclusion and exclusion criteria for the clinical question. When there is a large amount of evidence, more criteria will be applied. On average, a relatively common clinical question with a reasonable search strategy may elicit somewhere between 50 and 100 studies. How do you separate the wheat from the chaff? Table 6–10 depicts the steps involved in a review and in narrowing the evidence.

Developing Inclusion and Exclusion Criteria

Once a body of literature has been gathered, the next step is to devise appropriate inclusion and exclusion cri-

Table 6–10
An Approach to Sorting Through the Evidence

Accept	Reject
Abstracts found matching search terms	Abstracts rejected at title stage
Articles identified through alternative means (i.e., hand searching references)	Articles rejected at abstract stage
Articles accepted at abstract stage	Articles rejected at first reading
Articles accepted at first reading	Articles not meeting inclusion/exclusion criteria
Articles meeting inclusion/exclusion criteria	Articles rejected at critical appraisal stage
Articles with highest level of evidence	

teria so that the studies can be narrowed more specifically to the elements of the PICO question, especially pertaining to the patient. Inclusion criteria may relate to specific level of evidence required to answer the clinical question. For example, for a therapy question, the choice may be to restrict evidence to only randomized controlled trials or meta-analyses of randomized controlled trials. For a prognosis question, included studies would need to have a large prospective cohort. Further inclusion criteria would hopefully reflect the characteristics of the patient or population specified in the clinical question. For instance, a question regarding the use of statins in treating a middle-aged female with hypercholesterolemia would not be answered adequately if the population studied were male elderly VA patients. Table 6–11 provides additional examples of possible inclusion criteria.

Once inclusion and exclusion criteria have been developed and applied uniformly, the articles can then be critically appraised, which is the final step in accepting or rejecting the chosen study.

All of the work regarding the search strategy and creating inclusion and exclusion criteria constitute the "Methods" section of an evidence-based review paper. Box 6–3 gives two examples of well-written search strategies. It cannot be emphasized enough that being able to provide a clear and duplicable description of this process makes your review a valid and reliable effort.

Critical Appraisal (or Now that I Have the Evidence, What Do I Do with It?)

What do you do with the final studies you have found? Chapter 2 of this book discusses in detail interpretation of the medical literature. This section discusses how to winnow the found evidence to the "best" evidence and then critically appraise the selected studies. The "science of trashing papers"[18] will be approached from two perspectives: (1) utilization of specific worksheets or checklists, and (2) the assignment of levels of evidence.

Ideally, a comprehensive search is narrowed to the three to six studies that best answer the question. Once you have completed a thorough search and sorted the studies to the most valid and relevant ones, what happens next? Before spending the time and effort critiquing each study it is critical to be certain that:

- The studies chosen are indeed POEMs (deal with patient-oriented outcomes);
- The study populations applies to the patient in your clinical question as much as possible;
- The studies may change your practice.[9]

If at all possible, you would like your search for information to have led to secondary, pre-filtered literature sources that help answer your question. Familiarity

Table 6–11
Examples of Inclusion Criteria

1. Whether the study includes enough information for analysis (i.e., standard deviation or standard error in addition to point estimate)
2. The year of study, for example, if technology or dosing changes have occurred recently (for example, include studies since 1984 on dyspepsia only if you're interested in *Helicobacter pylori*).
3. The dosage used in the study (to ensure that an effective dose was used)
4. An adequate time period to conduct the study and follow the subjects, for example, for SSRI treatment, would like >16 weeks of continuous medication.
5. The language of the article—you or a colleague should to be able to read it!
6. The minimum sample size—very small studies may be unrepresentative and/or not worth the effort
7. The patient age (adults only, >60 only, children, etc.)
8. The study setting (emergency department, outpatient, inpatient)

BOX 6–3

Sample Descriptions of Search Strategies

Sample 1.
Search strategies:
Inclusion and exclusion criteria:
Studies were included if they were systematic reviews, meta-analysis or randomized controlled trials comparing International Classification of Diseases (ICDs) with conventional therapy in people at high risk of sudden cardiac death. This produced 133 "hits" and these abstracts were inspected for relevance. Smaller controlled trials were hand searched specifically looking at ICD versus antiarrhythmic therapy for treatment of ventricular tachyarrhythmias. Trials with over 100 patients were chosen to give adequate power.

Inclusion criteria:
Included were all RCTs involving patients "at risk" for sudden cardiac death or ventricular arrhythmia that had evidence of heart failure and CAD. Outcomes had to include sudden cardiac death or all-cause mortality. Only studies regarding ICD use in primary prevention were included.

Exclusion criteria:
Excluded were any studies evaluating ICDs for secondary prevention and trials for patients with inherited arrhythmic disorders such as long QT syndrome and Brugada syndrome or nonischemic cardiomyopathies. Two primary prevention trials were excluded: the CABG Patch and CAT trials. Participants in the CAT trial had severe heart failure but did not have coronary artery disease, thus was not representative of my patient. The CABG Patch trial was also excluded because it studied a population that had just undergone revascularization, giving them a potential advantage over the participants in the other three studies.

Methods
A PubMed search was completed in May 2002 using the search terms "posttraumatic stress disorder AND drug therapy," yielding 377 articles. The following search limits were then applied and constitute the inclusion criteria: Clinical trials, adults, 19+ years old, and publication dates from 1997 to 2002. These limits narrowed the yield to 50 articles.

Articles were then excluded based on the following criteria: (1) open label studies, (2) non-SSRI class medications, (3) studies that did not use the CAPS-2 and CGI-I assessment tools as primary or secondary outcome measures, (4) studies that were less than 12 weeks in duration, and (5) studies that treated only combat veterans or refugees. Five published studies were identified using the above criteria. These studies were then individually evaluated for relevance and validity using standardized criteria and each study was assigned a level of evidence rating (Oxford Centre for Evidence-based Medicine). The primary outcome measurements for the purposes of this review is response to treatment as measured by the Clinician Administered PTSD Scale, Part 2 (CAPS2 total and cluster ratings) and the Clinical Global Impressions-Improvement (CGI-I) scale.

Similar searches were also performed on the following databases: Cochrane Library, InfoPoems, and TRIP database. No additional clinical trials meeting the aforementioned criteria were found.

---

with quality databases, such as the Cochrane Library, or finding systematic reviews or meta-analyses, can help decrease your work. Unfortunately, however, these resources will not answer the majority of clinical questions.

Using Checklists to Help Critique

Critiquing original research articles may seem daunting at first. For those who would like a firmer grip on this art, a variety of user-friendly resources exist. Primary among these is the JAMA Users' Guides to the Medical Literature.[18] This series began in 1992, with the first article in the series helping clinicians make sense of articles on treatment. Since 1992, more than 25 articles in the series have been published dealing with a multitude of types of medical articles. The British Medical Journal,

likewise, began the "How to Read a Paper" series in 1997 by Trish Greenhalgh.[19] Although not as specific as the JAMA Users' Guides,[18] this series helps readers sort through basic statistics and study design issues that are needed for critiquing a paper. Many evidence-based resources, based on the JAMA Users' Guides, have developed structured checklists to walk us through the validity assessment of different types of articles. As a shortcut to a full epidemiology or research design course, we can learn the terminology and concepts that are crucial in judging validity. Although not a substitute for more in-depth knowledge of statistics or study design concepts, checklists help to organize an approach to critiques and help avoid leaping from one part of the study to another. Checklists are also handy until you become familiar with the main criteria for each type of

BOX 6–4

Example of Validity Assessment Questions for Therapy

Study design

1. Was it a controlled trial?

2. Were the subjects randomly assigned?

3. Are the patients in the study similar to typical primary care patients so that the results will apply?

4. Were steps taken to conceal the treatment assignment from study personnel entering patients into the study?

5. Were patients and study personnel "blind" to treatment?

Study conduct

1. Were all patients who entered the trial properly accounted for at its conclusion?

2. Was follow-up complete? How long and how thorough was the process?

3. Were patients analyzed in the groups to which they were randomized, that is, "intention-to-treat" analysis?

4. Were the intervention and control groups similar?

Study results

1. What were the results?

2. Are the results clinically as well as statistically significant?

3. Was the power of the study adequate?

4. Were there other factors that might have affected the outcome?

5. How will the results change your practice?

study. An example of validity questions from a checklist for a study about therapy, for example, can be found in Box 6–4.

The checklists are quite practical; however, two issues arise that present a challenge. One challenge is deciding which checklist is most appropriate. Although the JAMA Users' Guides have specific questions for a myriad of article types, there are a few checklists that should be considered a priority because they cover the most common types of clinical questions. These would include the following areas: etiology/harm, diagnosis, therapy, and prognosis checklists for original research

studies, and systematic review/meta-analysis and guideline checklists for secondary studies.[20–28] From the BestBets Web site, you can download checklists that specifically match the study design type, for example, cohort, randomized controlled trial, as opposed to the type of clinical question.[29] Table 6–12 illustrates three potential sources of critiquing checklists and their accompanying Web sites.

When using the study design checklists it is important to keep in mind which study design affords the best evidence for that particular type of question. For example, a therapy question is best matched with either a meta-

Table 6–12
Web Sites and Sources of Critiquing Checklists

Source and Web Site	Comments
JAMA User's Guide to the Medical Literature *http://www.usersguides.org/textbooks.asp*	The guides are available either as individual articles in JAMA or can be found collated into this textbook: Users' guides to the medical literature: essentials of evidence-based clinical practice. Gordon Guyatt and Drummond Rennie (editors).
BestBets *http://www.bestbets.org/cgi-bin/public_pdf.pl*	Downloadable worksheets in pdf format are provided based on study designs or question type: Case-control, Cohort, Decision rule, Diagnosis, Economic, Educational intervention, Guideline, Prognosis, Qualitative, Randomized control trial, Review or meta-analysis, Screening, Survey
InfoPoems *http://www.infopoems.com/productInfo/ methodsValidity.html*	Provide validity criteria used for evaluating POEMs: structure similar to JAMA Users' Guide.

Table 6-13
Rudimentary Statistics Providing Foundation for EBM Application

Treatment Related	Diagnosis Related	Other
Relative risk (RR)	Sensitivity	p value
Absolute risk reduction (ARR)	Specificity	Confidence intervals
Relative risk reduction (RRR)	Positive predictive value	Power/sample size
Number needed to treat (NNT)	Negative predictive value	Intention to treat principle (ITT)
Number needed to harm (NNH)	Likelihood ratios	Test for heterogeneity
Odds ratio (OR)	Number needed to diagnose/screen (NND/NNS)	Fixed effects model and Random effects model

analysis of randomized control trials or a high-quality randomized control trial. It may help to refer again to Tables 6–8 and 6–9, where highest levels of evidence are matched with their study question counterpart in both primary and secondary sources of evidence.

If you have had the chance to peruse a sample of the checklists mentioned in the preceding, you will note that they require understanding of some basic statistical and epidemiologic concepts. The ability to define these concepts is certainly useful, but ultimately it will behoove a critical reader to have a firmer foundation in these areas.

It is not necessary to be a statistician to practice EBM; clinicians should, however, be users of statistics. It is worth the time to master a few statistical terms and applications to become a discerning reader, capable of deciding which articles are worthy affecting clinical practice and which ones might be misusing statistics. Table 6–13 outlines the bare minimum of statistical terms and analyses that enable appropriate use of the checklists. Chapter 9 provides a base for data analysis and the flow diagrams provide basic statistical decisions.

Likewise, epidemiology is considered to be another scary facet of EBM. Knowledge of study designs, types

of bias, sample selection methods, and allocation is useful to separate the wheat from the chaff in clinical studies. Table 6–14 offers some basic terminology necessary for critiquing the literature.

Many useful tutorials on EBM can be found on the Internet to supplement and increase your knowledge base in this area. At the end of this section you will find a summary of EBM resources including Web urls for EBM tutorials, reading materials (even books!), and other useful materials. A glossary of the terms is presented in Table 6–15.

Levels of Evidence

About 20 years ago, David Sackett and Suzanne Fletcher created "levels of evidence" for ranking the validity of evidence regarding the value of preventive strategies for the Canadian Task Force on the Periodic Health Examination.[30] "Grades of recommendation" were assigned to aspects of the health exam as a way of summarizing the strength of evidence for performing these. Today there are various descriptions of rankings of evidence. The gold standard for evidence ranking is the Oxford Centre for Evidence-Based Practice Levels of Evidence Table (Table 6–15).[30] This table can be downloaded as a rich text format document at the following Web site: *http://www.cebm.net/levels_of_evidence.asp*

Other grades of recommendations exist in the literature, especially as reported in evidence-based guidelines. These may also be used as models for providing a hierarchy of evidence (Table 6–16).

Recognizing that quality sources of secondary literature report various levels of evidence will help the searcher retrieve the highest levels of evidence. The searcher, however, will also need to designate levels of evidence for the original research that is located and critiqued. The ability to attribute a level of evidence for a particular clinical question accomplishes a number of goals. It helps the reader understand whether a change in clinical practice is advisable given the levels of

Table 6-14
Basic Epidemiological Concepts Providing Foundation for EBM Application

Types of Studies	Types of Bias	Other
Randomized control trial	Selection	Incidence
Cohort study	Self-selection	Prevalence
Case-control study	Recall	Blinding
Systematic review/ meta-analysis	Information	Concealment of allocation
Case series	Lead time	Randomization
Case report (N of 1)	Interviewer	Confounding
	Publication	

Table 6-15
Oxford Table of Levels of Evidence and Grades of Recommendation

Level	Therapy/Prevention, Etiology/Harm	Prognosis	Diagnosis	Differential Diagnosis/ Symptom Prevalence Study	Economic and Decision Analyses
1a	SR (with homogeneity*) of RCTs	SR (with homogeneity*) of inception cohort studies; CDR† validated in different populations	SR (with homogeneity*) of Level 1 diagnostic studies; CDR† with 1b studies from different clinical centers.	SR (with homogeneity*) of prospective cohort studies	SR (with homogeneity*) of level 1 economic studies
1b	Individual RCT (with narrow confidence interval)	Individual inception cohort study with >80% follow-up; CDR† validated in a single population	Validating** cohort study with good††† reference standards; or CDR† tested in one clinical center	Prospective cohort study with good follow-up****	Analysis based on clinically sensible costs or alternatives; systematic review of the evidence; and including multiway sensitivity analyses
1c	All or none§	All or none case-series	Absolute SpPins and SnNouts††	All or none case-series	Absolute better-value or worse-value analyses††††
2a	SR (with homogeneity*) of cohort studies	SR (with homogeneity*) of either retrospective cohort studies or untreated control groups in RCTs	SR (with homogeneity*) of level >2 diagnostic studies	SR (with homogeneity*) of 2b and better studies	SR (with homogeneity*) of level > 2 economic studies
2b	Individual cohort study (including low quality RCT; e.g., <80% follow-up)	Retrospective cohort study or follow-up of untreated control patients in an RCT; Derivation of CDR† or validated on split-sample§§§ only	Exploratory** cohort study with good††† reference standards; CDR† after derivation, or validated only on split-sample§§§ or databases	Retrospective cohort study, or poor follow-up	Analysis based on clinically sensible costs or alternatives; limited review(s) of the evidence, or single studies; and including multiway sensitivity analyses
2c	"Outcomes" research; ecological studies	"Outcomes" research		Ecological studies	Audit or outcomes research
3a	SR (with homogeneity*) of case-control studies		SR (with homogeneity*) of 3b and better studies	SR (with homogeneity*) of 3b and better studies	SR (with homogeneity*) of 3b and better studies
3b	Individual case-control study		Nonconsecutive study; or without consistently applied reference standards	Nonconsecutive cohort study, or very limited population	Analysis based on limited alternatives or costs, poor quality estimates of data, but including sensitivity analyses incorporating clinically sensible variations.
4	Case-series (and poor quality cohort and case-control studies§§)	Case-series (and poor quality prognostic cohort studies***)	Case-control study, poor or non-independent reference standard	Case-series or superseded reference standards	Analysis with no sensitivity analysis

(continued)

Table 6-15
Oxford Table of Levels of Evidence and Grades of Recommendation *(Continued)*

Level	Therapy/Prevention, Etiology/Harm	Prognosis	Diagnosis	Differential Diagnosis/Symptom Prevalence Study	Economic and Decision Analyses
5	Expert opinion without explicit critical appraisal, or based on physiology, bench research or "first principles"	Expert opinion without explicit critical appraisal, or based on physiology, bench research or "first principles"	Expert opinion without explicit critical appraisal, or based on physiology, bench research or "first principles"	Expert opinion without explicit critical appraisal, or based on physiology, bench research or "first principles"	Expert opinion without explicit critical appraisal, or based on economic theory or "first principles"

Notes

1. Users can add a minus-sign "−" to denote the level of that fails to provide a conclusive answer because of:

2. EITHER a single result with a wide Confidence Interval (such that, for example, an ARR in an RCT is not statistically significant but whose confidence intervals fail to exclude clinically important benefit or harm)

3. OR a Systematic Review with troublesome (and statistically significant) heterogeneity.

4. Such evidence is inconclusive, and therefore can only generate Grade D recommendations.

*By homogeneity we mean a systematic review that is free of worrisome variations (heterogeneity) in the directions and degrees of results between individual studies. Not all systematic reviews with statistically significant heterogeneity need be worrisome, and not all worrisome heterogeneity need be statistically significant. As noted earlier, studies displaying worrisome heterogeneity should be tagged with a "−" at the end of their designated level.

†Clinical Decision Rule. (These are algorithms or scoring systems that lead to a prognostic estimation or a diagnostic category.)

‡See note 2 for advice on how to understand, rate and use trials or other studies with wide confidence intervals.

§Met when all patients died before the Rx became available, but some now survive on it; or when some patients died before the Rx became available, but none now die on it.

§§By poor quality cohort study we mean one that failed to clearly define comparison groups and/or failed to measure exposures and outcomes in the same (preferably blinded), objective way in both exposed and nonexposed individuals and/or failed to identify or appropriately control known confounders and/or failed to carry out a sufficiently long and complete follow-up of patients. By poor quality case-control study we mean one that failed to clearly define comparison groups and/or failed to measure exposures and outcomes in the same (preferably blinded), objective way in both cases and controls and/or failed to identify or appropriately control known confounders.

§§§Split-sample validation is achieved by collecting all the information in a single tranche, then artificially dividing this into "derivation" and "validation" samples.

††An "Absolute SpPin" is a diagnostic finding whose Specificity is so high that a Positive result rules-in the diagnosis. An "Absolute SnNout" is a diagnostic finding whose Sensitivity is so high that a Negative result rules-out the diagnosis.

‡‡Good, better, bad, and worse refer to the comparisons between treatments in terms of their clinical risks and benefits.

†††Good reference standards are independent of the test, and applied blindly or objectively applied to all patients. Poor reference standards are haphazardly applied, but still independent of the test. Use of a nonindependent reference standard (where the "test" is included in the "reference", or where the "testing" affects the "reference") implies a level 4 study.

††††Better-value treatments are clearly as good but cheaper, or better at the same or reduced cost. Worse-value treatments are as good and more expensive, or worse and the equally or more expensive.

**Validating studies test the quality of a specific diagnostic test, based on prior evidence. An exploratory study collects information and trawls the data (e.g., using a regression analysis) to find which factors are "significant."

***By poor quality prognostic cohort study we mean one in which sampling was biased in favor of patients who already had the target outcome, or the measurement of outcomes was accomplished in <80% of study patients, or outcomes were determined in an unblinded, nonobjective way, or there was no correction for confounding factors

****Good follow-up in a differential diagnosis study is >80%, with adequate time for alternative diagnoses to emerge (e.g., 1–6 months acute, 1–5 years chronic)

Grades of Recommendation

A   consistent level 1 studies

B   consistent level 2 or 3 studies or extrapolations from level 1 studies

C   level 4 studies or extrapolations from level 2 or 3 studies

D   level 5 evidence or troublingly inconsistent or inconclusive studies of any level

References

1. Canadian Task Force of the Periodic Health Examination. The periodic health examination. CMAJ 1979;121:1193–1254.

2. Sackett DL. Rules of evidence and clinical recommendations on use of antithrombotic agents. Chest 1986;89 (2 Suppl.): 2S–3S.

3. Cook DJ, Guyatt GH, Laupacis A, et al. Clinical recommendations using levels of evidence for antithrombotic agents. Chest 1995;108(4 Suppl):227S–230S

4. Yusuf S, Cairns JA, Camm AJ, et al. Evidence-Based Cardiology. London: BMJ Publishing Group, 1998.

Used with permission from: Ball C, Sackett D, Phillips R, et al. Levels of Evidence and Grades of Recommendations. Centre for Evidence Based Medicine (Oxford). 2001. Cited: September, 2004. Available at: *http://www.cebm.net*

Table 6–16
Two Examples of Grades of Recommendation

Grade		Description
A	Good evidence to support	Consistent level 1 studies
B	Fair evidence to support	Consistent level 2 or 3 studies or extrapolations from level 1 studies
C	Insufficient evidence to recommend for or against.	Level 4 studies or extrapolations from level 2 or 3 studies
D	Fair evidence to exclude	Level 5 evidence or troublingly inconsistent or inconclusive studies of any level
E	Good evidence to exclude	NA

evidence. It will also identify gaps in the literature with regard to the clinical question at hand, especially if the level of evidence is consistently poor. High levels of evidence, unfortunately, do not exist for all clinical questions. This is likely to continue for the foreseeable future owing to the nature of medical problems, the nature (and cost) of clinical research, as well as study design ethical limitations.

Often, when we begin to develop critical appraisal skills, there is an early period of "article nihilism." We now have the dissecting knife for articles and we mean to use it! Although this sharpness of critique is common early on, we must remember the goal of critiquing the literature—that is, to examine the study for its strengths and weaknesses as well as its clinical applicability. Nearly every study will be flawed in some manner, but the best question to ask yourself is—"Is it fatally flawed?"[31]

Abstracting and Synthesizing the Evidence

The studies have all been thoroughly read with a checklist critique for each one. How do you go about putting all of the validity assessments and results together in a way that makes sense? Various strategies can be used to collate and synthesize materials from the chosen evidence. The main objective is to devise a way to present it in a clear and organized fashion that is either easy to read, or easy to explain, or preferably both. The inclusion and exclusion criteria that were employed in selecting studies for your clinical question will hopefully have garnered you the ability to combine and compare "apples and apples" with regard to the data gathered in the studies.

Although the data used to compare studies certainly depend on the type of clinical question, there are usually three main areas in which data can be effectively pooled and sorted. The first area is the description of characteristics, and sometimes the conduct, of each study. We will use an example of a therapy question to

illustrate this assessment: In a 24-year-old woman (non-combat veteran, non-refugee) are SSRIs effective in reducing the frequency and severity of post-traumatic stress disorder symptoms? One might construct a table cross-referencing the studies for the following: (1) similarity to primary care population, (2) total number of subjects, (3) type of SSRI used, and (4) adequate SSRI dosing. The reader would immediately have an idea of whether the information might apply to his or her patient case and if the studies were reasonably conducted.

A second compilation that is integral to an evidence-based review article is the synthesis of validity assessment information used for the evidence. Using the same clinical question on therapy above, assuming all studies that were chosen were randomized controlled trials, one might formulate the following validity categories: (1) blinding, (2) adequate timeline, (3) patient accounting, (4) data analyzed by intention-to-treat, and (5) power. At this point in the data gathering, the author assigns a level of evidence for each study. The reader can then decide that the combined strength of the evidence is sufficient for considering change. Figure 6–3 demonstrates how these can be combined in a clear and logical fashion.

Lastly, the results of the various studies must be illustrated and discussed in a way that allows the reader to observe the trends, or lack thereof, of the chosen studies. With the same clinical question, the outcomes of interest should be accounted for. In this case, a gold standard tool for PTSD, the Clinician Administered PTSD Scale (CAPS) and subscales were reported for the studies. Figure 6–4 depicts a table of results for this outcome measurement tool.

The author of this table chose to simply denote whether statistically significant decreases in these particular symptoms were demonstrated in each of the studies. If studies use the same statistical measures, for example, p values or relative risks, the actual values for the statistics may be put in the table instead. In fact, this would provide a more accurate way to allow the reader

Study (SSRI)	Blinding	Adequate Timeline (>12wks)	Patient Accounting	Intention to Treat Analysis	Power Adequate
Marshall et al (Paroxetine)	A	A	A	A	A
Tucker et al (Paroxetine)	A	A	M	A	A
Davidson et al (Sertraline)	A	I	A	A	M
Brandy et al (Sertraline)	A	I	A	A	M
Martenyi et al (Fluoxctine)	A	S	I	A	I

A=Adequate M=Marginal I=Inadequate

FIG. 6–3. Example of summary table of a validity assessment. A = Adequate; M = Marginal; I = Inadequate.

Study	CAPS2-Total	CAPS2-Reexperiencing	CAPS2-Avoidance/Numbing	CAPS2-Hyperarousal
Marshall et al (Paroxetine)	S	S	S	S
Tucker et al (Paroxetine)	S	S	S	S
Davidson et al (Sertraline)	S	NS	S	NS
Brandy et al (Sertraline)	S	NS	S	S
Martenyi et al (Fluoxetine)	S	S	NS	S

S=Significant difference between treatment group versus placebo
NS=No significant difference between treatment group versus placebo

FIG. 6–4. Example of a table of compiled study results. S = Significant difference between treatment group versus placebo; NS = no significant difference between treatment group versus placebo.

to analyze trends. All studies that you find on a clinical question, however, may not use the same statistical methods, and you may need to be creative (and correct) in portraying the results.

The use of statistical terms previously discussed, for example, likelihood ratios and predictive values for diagnostic issues, and numbers needed to treat (NNT) for treatment articles, is encouraged. The concepts of numbers needed to treat, numbers needed to screen (NNS), and even numbers needed to diagnose (NND) are readily calculable from relative risk data. This terminology allows one to communicate benefit or risk more easily to both patients and colleagues.

The advantage of providing this type of information in table form cannot be overemphasized. All of the important elements of the studies are immediately sorted in one place when providing tables in an evidence-based review paper. The tables, and the trends within them, can then be discussed in detail. This visual aid improves comprehension of what will be the bottom line answer to the clinical question. In a presentation, the tables serve as the main discussion areas of the studies' designs, validity assessments, and results as well. The same exercise in compiling data needs to be done if the author is constructing a CAT, although this work is not included in the final written endeavor; however, the clinical bottom line is derived from it.

The Clinical Bottom Line

All three of the evidence-based medicine processes discussed return to the clinical question, as well as the patient, and pronounce "the clinical bottom line." In both the CAT and POEM formats, the answer immediately follows the question; the author proceeds then to summarize in outline form how they got there. As seen in both the CAT and POEM formats previously outlined, the bottom line is a succinct statement that sums up the work in total, including strengths and weaknesses, and answers the clinical question. The evidence-based review article, likewise, returns to the clinical question, and if the question is case based, specifically applies the evidence to that patient. This provides a full circle of reasoning to the evidence-based medicine and clinical decision-making processes that should be practiced in evidence-based medicine.

The penultimate step in the practice of evidence-based medicine is applying the evidence to the patient case. The decision whether to implement evidence depends on a number of factors that have already been reviewed in terms of relevance and validity. Application must also incorporate consideration of how the benefits outweigh the risks or adverse effects of an intervention. Application may include whether the benefits justify

the costs with regard to population-based issues such as screening or setting priorities with regard to resources.

It is often a challenge to apply evidence from a study or compilation of studies to an individual patient. Study results are typically reported as "average" effects of that study population, and even with confidence intervals that illustrate a reasonable range of application or effect. Individual patients are bound to differ from the subjects studied in some way. The concept of numbers needed to treat (or numbers needed to harm, diagnosis, or screen) is more readily applicable in many situations. This concept, although more user-friendly to clinicians, will still require some tailoring such as stratification of risk to the individual patient. Individual risk stratification can be estimated, for example, from a patient's comorbidities, known physiological characteristics, or cointerventions (e.g., other medications the patient is taking).

Other important and very individualized factors regarding the patient also need to be addressed. These factors include socioeconomic, ethnic, cultural, compliance, and value-laden aspects of the patient and his or her "environment." For example, when considering an antihypertensive agent for some patients, a beta-blocker would not be the first-line choice for that population compared to a diuretic. One must consider not only integrating evidence with one's clinical experience, but also the rights and expectations of the patient involved. As we form alliances with our patients for their care, so are we responsible for providing information regarding risks and benefits and how a particular intervention may affect them.

In an evidence-based review paper that revolves around a particuar case, it is important to incorporate in the discussion the various factors in the decision-making process that make the evidence applicable, or not. Likewise, the strength of the evidence, in terms of validity, is integrated into the decision. The clinical bottom line should be answered with these aspects in the discussion.

The CAT may or may not include all of the patient data, but definitely should include all of the important aspects of the validity assessment in providing a more succinct bottom line. The POEM is not case based and will provide a validity assessment of strictly one study after clearly establishing the clinical question.

The final step in the practice of evidence-based medicine is to evaluate the outcomes of your actions: that is, what is it that has been learned from the experience? The CAT, because of its abbreviated format, does not usually return to the application of the evidence. The POEM, since it is not case based, will also not demonstrate this step. A case-oriented evidence-based review paper should involve this step. Either in presentation or written form, the circle of clinical reasoning is complete when one can evaluate the results of the action they decide to take or not take with the patient that elicited the question. This gives the entire endeavor context and makes it a true learning experience for both the reader and the author.

Section Summary

Mastering the skills of evidence-based medicine offers the PA and the PA student a multitude of benefits. It provides skills that promote lifelong, self-directed learning that ultimately makes clinical practice more fulfilling. EBM helps us to become aware of the gaps in our medical knowledge and to approach the medical literature without fear. But most of all, it makes us feel more confident in utilizing information to provide the best care for patients.

EBM also provides a research methodology that tracks closely with traditional research objectives, yet it is clinically relevant and practical without the "ivory tower" aspects. As medical literature increases exponentially, as modern medicine becomes more complex, and as our time becomes more limited, EBM provides a framework to:

- Help stay up to date with the current literature (and remove the "stale" information).
- Communicate effectively with colleagues and patients.
- Make better use of resources, including time.
- Avoid common pitfalls of clinical decision-making.

But beyond achieving facility with all of the "steps" of EBM practice, it fosters an attitudinal shift toward reflection, observation, and evaluation of the daily practice of medicine.

Section References

1. Council of Graduate Schools. CGS policy statement on master's education: a guide for faculty and administrators. Washington, DC: CGS Publications, 1996. p. 4.
2. Sackett DL, Straus SE, Richardson WS, Rosenberg W, Haynes RB. Evidence-Based Medicine: How to Practice and Teach EBM, 2nd ed. St. Louis: Churchill Livingstone, 2000, Chapter 1.
3. Guyatt G, Haynes RB, Jaeschke R, et al. 1A. Introduction: the philosophy of evidence based medicine. In Guyatt G, Rennie D (eds): Users' Guides to the Medical Literature: Essentials of Evidence-Based Clinical Practice. Chicago: AMA Press, 2001, p. 6.
4. Sauve S, Lee HN, Meade MO, Lang JD, Farkouh M, Cook DJ, Sackett DL. The critically appraised topic: a practical approach to learning critical appraisal. Ann R Soc Phys Surg Canada 1995;28:396–398.
5. Slawson DC, Shaughnessy AF. Becoming an information master: using POEMs to change practice with confidence. Patient-Oriented Evidence that Matters. Journal of Family Practice 2000;49(1):63–67.
6. Ball C, Phillip B. What is a CAT? Evidence Based On Call (EBOC). June, 2002. Cited date: August, 2004. Available from: *http://www.eboncall.org/*
7. Porter BA. Critically-appraised topic: Chamydial screening to prevent pelvic inflammatory disease. UNC Critically Appraised Topics. Online CAT Bank. October 31, 1997. Cited date: August, 2004. Available from: *http://www.med.unc.edu/medicine/edursrc/welcome*
8. Badenoch D. What is a CAT? NHS Research & Development—Centre for Evidence Based Medicine. 2002. Cited date: August, 2004. Available from: *http://www.minervation.com/cebm2/docs/cats/catabout.html#limitations*
9. InfoPOEM Group. What is a POEM. Patient-Oriented Evidence that Matters.™ InfoPOEMs:The Clinical Awareness System. 2004. Cited date: September, 2004. Available from: *http://www.infopoems.com/resources.html*
10. InfoPOEM Group. Sample POEM article: Knee taping useful for osteoarthritis pain. InfoPOEMs:The Clinical Awareness System. 2004. Cited date: September, 2004. Available from: *http://www.infopoems.com/productInfo/samplePOEM.cfm*
11. White B. Making Evidence-based Medicine Doable in Everyday Practice. Family Practice Management, February, 2004. Cited date: July, 2004. Available from: *http://www.aafp.org/fpm*
12. Covell DG, Uman GC, Manning PR. Information needs in office practice: are they being met? Annals of Internal Medicine 1985;103:596–599.
13. Centre for Evidence Based Medicine (Oxford). Focusing Clinical Questions. Centre for Evidence Based Medicine. 2004. Cited date: August, 2004. Available from: *http://www.cebm.net/focus_quest.asp*
14. Ebell M. Information at the Point of Care: Answering Clinical Questions Journal of the American Board of Family Practice 1999;12(3):225–235.
15. Slawson DO, Shaugnessy AF. Information mastery: feeling good about not knowing everything. Journal of Family Practice 1994;39:489–499.
16. Wagoner B, Mellish M, Hyman C, Doherty M, Markinson A. SUNY Downstate Medical Center Evidence Based Medicine Course. Guide to Research Methods: The Evidence Pyramid. 2002. Cited date: July, 2004. Available from: *http://servers.medlib.hscbklyn.edu/ebm/2100.htm*
17. Dorsch J. Evidence Based Medicine—Finding the Best Clinical Literature. Applying Clinical Search Filters. December, 2003. Cited: September, 2004. Available at: *http://www.uic.edu/depts/lib/lhsp/resources/levels.shtml*
18. Guyatt G, Rennie D (eds). Users' Guides to the Medical Literature: Essentials of Evidence-Based Clinical Practice. Chicago: AMA Press, 2001.
19. Greenhalgh T. How to Read a Paper. London: BMJ Publishing Group, 1997, Chapter 1, Section 1.3.
20. Guyatt GH, Sackett DL, Cook DJ. Users' guides to the medical literature. II. How to use an article about therapy or prevention. A. Are the results of the study valid? JAMA 1993;270:2598–2601.
21. Guyatt GH, Sackett DL, Cook DJ. Users' guides to the medical literature. II. How to use an article about therapy or prevention. B. Are the results of the study valid? Evidence-Based Medicine Working Group. JAMA 1993;59–63.
22. Guyatt GH, Sackett DL, Cook DJ. Users' guides to the medical literature. II. How to use an article about therapy or prevention. B. What were the results and will they help me in caring for my patients? Evidence-Based Medicine Working Group. JAMA 1994;271:59–63.
23. Jaeschke R, Guyatt G, Sackett DL. Users' guides to the medical literature. III. How to use an article about a diagnostic test. A. Are the results of the study valid? Evidence-Based Medicine Working Group. JAMA 1994;271:389–391.
24. Jaeschke R, Guyatt GH, Sackett DL. Users' guides to the medical literature. III. How to use an article about a diagnostic test. B.

What are the results and will they help me in caring for my patients? The Evidence-Based Medicine Working Group. JAMA 1994;271:703–707.

25. Levine M, Walter S, Lee H, Haines T, Holbrook A, Moyer V. Users' guides to the medical literature. IV. How to use an article about harm. Evidence-Based Medicine Working Group. JAMA 1994;271:1615–1619.

26. Laupacis A, Wells G, Richardson WS, Tugwell P. Users' guides to the medical literature. V. How to use an article about prognosis. Evidence-Based Medicine Working Group. JAMA 1994;272: 234–237.

27. Oxman AD, Cook DJ, Guyatt GH. Users' guides to the medical literature. VI. How to use an overview. Evidence-Based Medicine Working Group [see comments]. JAMA 1994;272:1367–1371.

28. Hayward RS, Wilson MC, Tunis SR, Bass EB, Guyatt G. Users' guides to the medical literature. VIII. How to use clinical practice guidelines. A. Are the recommendations valid? The Evidence-Based Medicine Working Group. JAMA 1995;274:570–574.

29. Mackway-Jones K, Morton R, Carley S. BETS Critical Appraisal Worksheets. BestBETS. Best Evidence Topics. 2004. Cited: August, 2004. Available at: *http://www.bestbets.org/cgi-bin/public_pdf.pl*

30. Ball C, Sackett D, Phillips R, et al. Levels of Evidence and Grades of Recommendations. Centre for Evidence Based Medicine (Oxford). 2001. Cited: September, 2004. Available at: *http://www.cebm.net*

31. Mackway-Jognes K, Carley SD, Morton RJ, Donnan S. The Best Evidence Topic (BET) Report: A modified CAT for summarising the available evidence in emergency medicine. Best Evidence Topics. Cited: August, 2004. Available at: *http://www.bestbets.org/background/betscats.html*

Section 3
The Clinical Review
Richard W. Dehn, MPA, PA-C

Section Overview

This section covers the clinical review. Clinical reviews are one of the most common types of articles found in medical journals and, probably, the most common article type found in the journals that specifically target PAs. Clinical reviews are also a common form of scholarship done by PA students and, for some programs, the educational capstone. Clinical reviews can summarize what is known, present new data or information or theory and serve PAs and all health-care professionals in a number of ways. Clinical reviews are a form of scholarship that all PAs can do.

Introduction

Clinical reviews are a common form of scholarship in the medical professions. The purpose of a clinical review is to improve the knowledge and understanding of practicing clinicians, and ultimately to improve the overall quality of how medical care is delivered by summarizing what is known about a disease entity. Successful clinical reviews address clinical conditions that are encountered frequently or of interest to medical providers. Often clinical reviews emphasize diagnosis and treatment of commonly seen, or important diseases, or of particularly challenging clinical dilemmas. Typically a clinical review takes the form of a written manuscript that is intended for publication in a professional journal or supplemental issue targeting practicing clinicians. However, a clinical review can also be delivered as a formal presentation or multimedia production.

Clinical reviews are not experimental or investigative research, but instead are a discrete process directed toward educating clinicians. Unlike research processes, clinical reviews do not seek to answer a specific research question, but instead intend to educate the clinician concerning a specific aspect of medical practice. Clinical reviews are sometimes based on a specific clinical question; however, in the clinical review process; this question does not, in itself, lead to an experimental or observational process, but instead a review of the existing literature on the topic.

Clinical reviews can be divided into four subcategories:

1. A general review of a clinical topic;
2. A summative review of a clinical topic;
3. A systematic review of the literature on a specific topic;
4. The case or case series report.

These types of clinical reviews differ primarily in the degree to which the source information is grounded in the literature.

The General Clinical Review Article

The successful general clinical review article addresses a common or particularly vexing problem that would be of interest to a sizable number of practitioners.[1] Thus, narrow topics or those of only curious value are best avoided. Since many clinicians utilize the contents of clinical review articles as practice recommendations, authors should pay careful attention to factual accuracy and make efforts to avoid personal bias. A clinical review that is well referenced with the most recent data is the key to accuracy and quality. Often the clinical review article is structured similarly to the way a topic would be presented in a medical textbook with defined sections that review basic facts and concepts relating to the topic or disease entity. Clinical review articles often are called update articles because their purpose is to bring the reader's practice knowledge and skills up to date in the topic area. Often general clinical review articles are structured to contain the following sections[2]:

Introduction and Background: This section typically includes a definition of the disease, a historical background of the disease, and the prevalence of the disease. Here, early in the manuscript, the author tries to justify the importance of the topic to the practicing clinician as well as pique interest. Thus, the introduction should be written in a way that will convince the reader to invest the time and effort to read the rest of the article.

Review of Anatomy, Physiology, and Pathophysiology: This section should review the basic anatomy, physiology, and pathophysiology as it applies to understanding the disease being discussed. In addition, this review can provide information that encourages the reader to understand how clinical and physical findings and other aspects of the topic interrelate and are the result of changes in human functioning.

History and Physical Exam Findings: In this section the signs and symptoms associated with the topic are reviewed. Risk factors and historical data commonly associated with the disease should also be included in this section, as well as information that may facilitate the recognition and interpretation of pertinent history and physical findings. In this section any directed physical examination necessary and any specific techniques required should be carefully described and explained. Unique physical findings that allow differentiation of this disease and the ruling-out of competing diagnoses should also be discussed.

Laboratory and Diagnostic Testing: This section should include the selection and interpretation of the most appropriate studies that help in the recognition and management of the disease or problem. Explanations of when studies are indicated or not indicated, cost effectiveness, relative value of the test for a specific condition, and the studies or procedures most likely to establish the diagnosis or rule it out are often helpful and should also be included in this section.

Assessment and Differential Diagnosis: This section should cover the reasoning processes that lead to the correct diagnoses of the disease or condition. It is helpful to provide a broad differential diagnosis and highlight the history, physical findings, and laboratory or diagnostic testing results that point to the correct diagnoses. Your reasons or reasoning for selecting the correct diagnoses over other possible diagnoses should be provided and explained in this section. You want the reader to understand how to move to this important point from all that has gone before.

Treatment and Follow-up: This section should include the prioritization of the management and medical interventions necessary for treatment. It is important to include the need for referral, consultation, hospital admission, or necessary emergent or acute care, and the reasoning used to come to these decisions, and include detailed descriptions of these actions, if appropriate. Emphasize well-accepted treatments, including potential complications, appropriate aftercare guidelines, pharmacotherapy, and drug interactions. Provide a follow-up plan and monitoring regimen, including signs of relapse and treatment failure.

Prevention and Patient Education: In this section, emphasize an approach to the patient most likely to elicit information to allow early identification of those at risk. Be sure to provide patient education guidelines and handout materials where appropriate. Identify patient groups at greatest risk and be sure to include preventive agents or techniques. Include and explain common screening tests for this condition including the relative value of each test. In today's litigious society, patient education is a must. Patient education must become part of the treatment of every disease condition.

The Summative Review of a Clinical Topic

The summative review of a clinical topic is much like a general review article. However the topic area is typically narrower and an effort is made to review the existing literature more thoroughly than with the general clinical review. Summative reviews are characterized as qualitative, where the inclusion criterion is determined by the author based on a subjective determination of the quality of the reviewed data and publications. Thus the overall quality of a summative review is subject to the author's biases and choice of sources.[3] Summative reviews are also known as summative review articles or summative reviews of the literature.

The Systematic Review of the Literature on a Specific Topic

Systematic reviews can be defined as concise summaries of the best available evidence designed to address carefully defined clinical questions. This type of review is a type of evidence-based medicine (EBM) review (see other sections of this chapter). The substantial increase in the quantity, quality, and complexity of clinically oriented experimental and observational data in recent years has led to a growing need for articles that review as much information as possible about a topic and distill it into a conclusion understandable by clinicians.[4,5]

The systematic review is a contribution of EBM philosophy, and many journals and Internet sites, dedicated to EBM, offer systematic reviews. Systematic reviews are generally quantitative, meaning that a system is devised that is then used to determine which data and publications are included in the review. Authors should specify inclusion criteria, outcomes of interest, and criteria used for determining the quality and validity of individual articles chosen for review. In addition, authors should also indicate how the search for research articles was conducted, including what databases were used, and whether unpublished articles or those written in foreign languages were actively sought out and included. The overall quality of a systematic review is dependent on the effectiveness of the systematic search approach utilized to find the best data available. Biases found in systematic reviews are often inherent in the selection system. One example is publication bias, in which only data showing significance are published and data demonstrating other conclusions are not, resulting in the exclusion of nonsignificant data from the analysis. Another potential bias in systematic reviews is selection bias, in which the selection criteria produced the skewing of data selected. Also complicating systematic reviews is the effect of the existence of duplicate publications that magnify the impact of a single data set that is reported in multiple publications. The most difficult part of systematic reviews is finding data from different studies that are similar enough to be combined and analyzed without a "comparing apples and oranges" effect.

Both the summative and systematic review processes require that the author possess several unique skills. Included in this skills set are:

- The ability to search the medical literature. Since summative or systematic reviews of good quality require that, ideally, all data and information that exist on a specific clinical question be located and reviewed, the author will need to have good information searching skills. With the digitalization of scientific libraries, the organization of scientific research databases, the increasing power of search engines, and the growing availability of information via the Internet, good searching skills include a combination of general library science knowledge, competence in medical informatics, and practical skills in operating various search engines within various information databases. The best quality selection processes include unpublished data, however such data may be difficult to obtain, or the fact that unpublished data exists may not even be known to the author.

- Critical skills to accurately deconstruct and critique a research article. This process requires a good understanding of the research process, such as the principles of scientific and medical study design, an understanding of basic statistics commonly used in research studies, an appreciation of the problems commonly associated with clinical research, as well as the limits of what conclusions can be derived from studies.

- Statistical and data manipulation skills. If the review is systematic and quantitative in nature, the author will need sophisticated data skills to determine the quality of available data and to determine how best to combine it. In addition, substantial statistical analysis skills will be required to determine the best methods to analyze the combined data sets.

The Case or Case Series Report

As the quantity and quality of experimental data have increased over time, the popularity and perceived usefulness of the case or case series report have declined as clinicians become more aware of the potential bias produced by the small sample sizes inherent in case series reports. However, the case or case series report will always have an important role in alerting the medical community of new diseases, or in describing diseases so rare that traditional study designs cannot, for all practical purposes, be used to investigate them.[6] Case study and case series reports are presented elsewhere in this text.

Section References

1. American Family Physician, Authors Guide, available at *http://www.aafp.org/x13554.xml*, accessed 9/27, 2004.
2. The Journal of the American Academy of Physician Assistants, JAAPA Submission Guidelines, available at *http://www.jaapa.com/be_core/MVC?action=free_pages&mag=j&name=submission_guidelines.xml*, accessed 9/27/2004.
3. Cook DJ, Mulrow CD, Haynes RB. Systematic Reviews: Synthesis of Best Evidence for Clinical Decisions. Annals of Internal Medicine 1997;376–380.
4. Mulrow CD, Cook DJ, Davidoff F. Systematic Reviews: Critical Links in the Great Chain of Evidence. Annals of Internal Medicine 1997;126:389–391.
5. Siwek J, Gourlay ML, Slawson DC, Shaughnessy AF. How to write an evidence-based clinical review article. American Family Physician 2002;65:251–258.
6. Henley CE. Writing for Publication, available at *http://www.healthsciences.okstate.edu/college/fammed/workshops/Writing%20for%20publication.pdf*, accessed 9/27/2004.

Section 4

Survey Research

J. Dennis Blessing, PhD, PA-C

Section Overview

Surveys are one of the most commonly used methods to gather information and data in the world. Surveys are used to gather data on topics ranging in importance from the U.S. Census and practice characteristics of PAs to the kind of dishwashing soap we use, our favorite movie, and who we plan to vote for in the next election. Surveys can reveal trends, attitudes, opinions, lifestyles, needs, expectations, knowledge/information, behaviors, demographics; the list could on go almost to infinity. Surveys can be used in almost every aspect of our lives and health care is no different. They can gather a large amount of data from any number of people on a wide variety of subjects and issues. Surveys can be delivered and conducted in several formats. They can be long or short, simple or complex, can use words or symbols, require written responses or simple choices, and can collect quantitative or qualitative data. Despite their almost eclectic nature, survey research must still conform to the exacting requirements of research design and methodology to have true value, meaning, and impact. This section presents the basic concepts of survey research including design, item construction, data analysis, and conducting the research. Emphasis is placed on designing items and developing concepts that are valid to survey research in health care and the PA profession. A short discussion of sample size is presented.

Introduction: What Surveys Can and Cannot Do

Surveys can be used to gather almost any type of information and data. Demographics, opinions, preferences, expectations, descriptive data, knowledge, and some forms of outcomes can be measured or obtained by surveys. Surveys can be conducted by mail (including e-mail), in person, via telephone, and through the Internet. Surveys can collect quantitative data or qualitative information. Survey samples can consist of very specific selected individuals, groups of individuals, or people who are part of the general population. Sample subjects can be defined by almost any characteristic. Samples can be randomized or assigned, stratified or open, well defined or ill defined, or a sample of convenience. Surveys can be relatively easy, inexpensive, fast,

and a consistent research tool (Table 6-17). Despite these advantages, disadvantages do exist. One major disadvantage is difficulty in establishing causality.[1] Causation involves manipulating a variable and looking for the effect on another variable. This is very difficult to do with a one time survey. However, well designed surveys can be used as the pre-intervention and post-intervention assessment tools in experimental and quasi-experimental designs. You must ensure that your survey measures the variables and outcomes being studied.

Other challenges to surveys revolve around reliability on respondent self report and response, respondent interpretation of survey items, extrapolation to a population, nonrespondent influence, and respondent bias (Table 6-18). Although there is no way to completely avoid these challenges to survey research, good design and item construction should help to limit the impact and influence on outcomes.

Types of Surveys

Surveys can be delivered in different manners. The choice of delivery format (distribution) is considered in the research design stage of planning and preparation for the investigation. Surveys can be conducted by mail, telephone, Internet, and interview. Each format has its advantages and disadvantages, and these are presented later in the chapter (Table 6–19). The research purpose(s), population to be studied, and sample size are factors that must be considered in the decision on the survey delivery form. We concentrate on mail surveys because they are the most common form of survey research that PAs and PA students have done. We also touch on Internet surveys because of their gaining popularity. Telephone and interview surveys are briefly discussed.

Table 6–17
Some General Advantages of Surveys

Advantage	Reasoning
Costs	Relatively low cost, but depends on survey and methodology.
Sample size	Can vary from small to extremely large, can be targeted.
Issues	Can gather information on single or multiple issues or topics.
Format	Can vary; mail, internet, interview, telephone.
Impact	Results can be very influential.

Table 6–18
Some General Disadvantages of Surveys

Disadvantage	Reason
Respondent self report	There is no way to ensure individuals will respond to surveys or choose to participate.
Respondent interpretation	There is a risk that respondents will interpret survey items in a manner different from investigator intent.
Respondent bias	There is a risk that people who choose to respond may be different from the population being studied.
Extrapolation to non-responders	Can the response of a few be extrapolated to the population?
Item bias	Can the data be generalized?
	Is there bias in the way an item is worded?

Table 6–19
Comparison of Survey Methods

Characteristic	Mail	Telephone	Interview	Internet
Cost	Relatively low	Low to moderate, depends on local versus long distance	Relatively high	Variable
Cost examples	Printing, postage	Telephone costs, personnel training and expense to conduct interview	Personnel training and expense to conduct interview	Professional help with Web design
Response rate	Potential to be low	Dependent on willingness of subject to participate	Relatively high; only willing subjects are interviewed	Variable, but instant; respondents must have computer
Investigator time	Relatively limited	Requires training of interviewers and/or conduct of interviews	Requires training of interviewers and/or conduct of interviews	Relatively limited
Respondent time	Completed as convenient	Telephone time	Interview time	Completed as convenient
Study time	Relatively long; must allow for mail and response times	Relatively short, but subject contact time may be long	Relatively short, but subject contact time may be long	Relatively short, dependent on subject time to respond
Anonymity	Survey form can be completely anonymous.	Phone number is known	Person to person interaction	Web address can be identified
Sample size	Can be very large.	Usually small to medium	Limited, usually small	Can be very large
Respondent bias	Respondent item interpretation	Interviewer influence by voice	Interviewer influence—high	Must be computer literate
Investigator bias	Generally very limited except for item construction	Voice influence; interpretation of survey items	Influence by voice, facial expression, body movement; interpretation of survey items	Generally very limited except for item construction
Other	Requires mailing lists	Multiple interviewers conducting survey	Multiple interviewers conducting survey	Computer access

Planning Is Key

Doing a survey investigation or study is not a matter of thinking up some questions, putting them on paper, and sending them out. You must be meticulous with your planning, just as for any other type of research effort. One of the first things you need to do is to define what you want to achieve in your study. You really cannot do much beyond your literature review until you have conceptualized what you want to achieve and learn. Once you have the goals of your project defined, everything else that follows will reflect your effort to meet your goals and answer the research questions, hypotheses, or null hypotheses that you will test.

Mail Surveys

Mail surveys are likely the most common method used to gather data on PAs, PA students, and PA education

(author observation). The use of mail surveys offers a number of advantages and disadvantages. Two key advantages to mail surveys are that the sample size can be large and dispersed and a large amount of data can be collected. Major limitations to mail surveys are potential for low response rate, respondent misinterpretation of items, and time of return to investigator. Table 6–20 lists some of the positives and negatives of mail surveys.

Response rates are a threat to mail surveys and, generally, response rates tend to be low, particularly when used without a well-defined target population or sample. Here are some points the author has found helpful in surveys of PAs, students, and educators.

1. A cover letter should accompany the survey. Use a personal salutation if you know the subject; otherwise use Mr., Ms., Mrs., or professional title such as Dr.

2. The survey instrument must be well designed in its content (items) and visually appealing.

Table 6–20
Aspects of Mail Surveys

Aspect	Comment
Cost	Low; primarily printing and postage costs, data entry may be costly.
Personnel	Investigators only; requires no training of interviewers or field workers.
Sample size	Can be very large; can be general or to a specific population set; can be geographically wide or distant from investigator; requires a name and address.
Response rates	Potential to be low and/or slow return to investigator; a response rate greater than 30% is rare.[1]
Data	Potential for quantity, but quality is limited by respondent interpretation of survey items; only survey item data can be collected.
Bias	Relies on respondent interpretation of survey items; nonrespondent bias is high.
Subjects	Not under pressure to respond; less intrusive than person to person contact.

3. A respondent should be able to complete the survey in a short period of time. The longer it takes to complete the survey, the less likely it will be completed.

4. A return, addressed, postage paid/stamped envelope should be enclosed with the survey. The respondent should not incur any cost in completing and returning your survey.

5. Some sort of inducement or gift can be included. This adds to the study expense, however, and there is no guarantee that the response rate will be increased.

6. A follow-up request may spur some respondents. A postcard reminder may suffice and is less expensive than a letter. You may want to send another survey to nonrespondents.

An excellent reference published in 2003 by Cui, goes further in its recommendations based on classical survey research methods.[2]

1. Let the interesting questions come first.

2. Use graphics and various question-writing techniques to ease the task of reading and answering the questions.

3. Print the questionnaire in a booklet format with an interesting cover.

4. Use capital or dark letters.

5. Reduce the size of the booklet or use photos to make the survey seem smaller and easier to complete.

6. Conduct four carefully spaced mailings: the questionnaire and a cover letter for the original mailing; a postcard follow-up one week after the original mailing; a replacement questionnaire and cover letter indicating that the questionnaire has not yet been received four weeks after the original mailing; and a second replacement questionnaire and cover letter to nonrespondents by certified mail seven weeks after the original mailing.

7. Include an individually printed, addressed, and signed letter.

8. Print the address on the envelopes rather than use address labels.

9. Use smaller stationery.

10. Let the cover letter focus on the importance of the study and the respondent's reply.

11. Explain that an ID number is used and the respondent's confidentiality is protected.

12. Fold the materials in a way that differs from an advertisement.

One other item to consider is the sending of an advanced notice. This could be a postcard that informs your subjects that a survey is coming. Whether or not you can use every point for increasing response rates depends on your timeline, fiscal resources, and your sample. There is a lot of literature on survey research. You may want to do a literature or web search or purchase a text on survey research to help further develop your skills.

THE COVER LETTER

Introduction to a mail survey can be accomplished in two ways. One is to include the introductory information as part of the survey on page 1 at the beginning of the survey. It is the author's opinion that a separate one-page letter of introduction is better. Regardless of the manner of the introduction, there are certain basic points that must be included. A well-worded, informative introduction (or cover letter) should help increase response rate. If subjects understand the purpose and

Table 6–21
Key Points for the Cover Letter

Key Point	Example
1. Who you are	a. Use letter head or
	b. Describe yourself/organization/business in the opening paragraph.
2. Background for study	In our practice, we have been using an appointment system...
3. Purpose of the study	We want to learn...
4. What will be done with the data	The information you provide will help us to...
5. Why they were chosen	We are asking you to take part because...
6. Assurance of confidentiality	a. You do not have to identify yourself in any way...
	b. All information will be reported in aggregate.
	c. All responses will be coded for study purposes.
7. What respondents need to do	Please take a few minutes to complete the survey. Please follow the instructions for each question.
8. Who respondents can contact is they have questions	If you have any questions or concerns, please contact...
9. Approvals for the survey, if applicable	This study has been approved by the Institutional Review Board of ...
10. Return deadlines	If possible, please return the survey in the enclosed stamped, addressed envelope by ...
11. Statement of importance	The information you provide will be helpful in determining...
12. Acknowledge support	a. This study is supported by a grant from ...
	b. This study is being conducted for ABC, Inc.
13. Statement of appreciation	We greatly appreciate your help in this matter and for taking the time to ...
14. Closing	Sincerely,
	Your name, degree, titles
	Co-investigators, degree, title
15. Signature	Your signature

need for their input or information, they will be more likely to respond. An example of a cover letter used by the author and coauthors is presented in the chapter appendix. If an introductory statement rather than a cover letter is used, the same information that would appear in a cover letter needs to be included in that statement.

The key points for an effective cover letter are summarized in Table 6–21. A well written and informative cover letter may induce subjects to participate by appealing to their sense of responsibility and the importance of their information or input. The cover letter is an information tool. The cover letter should be concise, well-written, informative, and easy to understand. The level of wording, grammar, and writing style should fit the sample to be surveyed. Unless you are dealing with highly educated professional people, your cover letter should target an audience with middle school reading ability.

Proofreading and editing are essential to ensure the letter serves the function that the investigator(s) desire. It is a good idea to have individuals read and interpret the letter who are not part of the investigation or in any way representative of the subject sample. One way to achieve this is to include the cover letter in any prestudy evaluations or pre-tests of the survey instrument and pilot studies (Table 6–22).

FOLLOW-UP

Follow-up notices or reminders to complete and return surveys may help increase responses. A follow-up letter can be used, but a post card reminder is probably just as good and less expensive. A letter is a much better reminder if the survey dealt with very personal or sensitive information, which would be reflected by the title of the investigation. For example: You are studying the rate of sexually transmitted diseases (STDs) in corporate executives who travel frequently. It will not help you to send a postcard stating, "This is to remind you to take a few minutes to complete and return our study of the risks of STDs." Such a reminder would raise questions of ethical conduct and risks to confidentiality. Better wording for a postcard reminder would be, "This is to remind you to take a few minutes to complete and return the survey we recently sent you." In the follow-up you can add or use language that will encourage a response such as, "Your opinion is very valuable to us and we want to include your input in our study." The wording of reminders should be general and neutral or encouraging survey return or completion. Do not threaten or even appear to be threatening. For example, do not write: "If you do not complete and return the survey, no one will care what you think or know about STDs."

Table 6–22
Construct of the Cover Letter

Construction Point	Explanation
1. Limit to one page.	The longer the letter is, the less likely it is to be read.
2. Use common block format.	Script, certain serif fonts, calligraphy, etc. are hard to read.
3. White or beige or light gray paper, black print	Reading ease; visually pleasing
4. Common language	Readability and ease of understanding are key

---

A follow-up or reminder should have enough information for the recipient to identify the survey. OR, you may want to resend your survey with a reminder letter. If you use the postcard as a reminder, contact information should be included in the event that the survey has been lost and another form is needed or there are inquiries. When to send and how many reminders should be sent are part of the decision making that is done in the methodology planning for the research project. Although there are no hard and fast rules for follow-ups, 10 to 14 days seems reasonable. Subsequent reminders can be sent at 4 weeks. Sending more than two reminders is probably a waste of time.

You can use follow-up reminders in a couple of ways. One way is to send a reminder to everyone who was mailed a survey. The other way is more economical if surveys have identification codes. If the survey is coded, the investigator can identify who has returned a survey and send follow-up reminders only to those subjects who have not responded. You must explain any codes that appear on a survey or a reminder. Tell your subjects what the number is and how it will be used. Remember, if you use some type of code, the respondents are not anonymous, but confidential. An example of a postcard reminder used by the author can be found in the chapter appendix.

Internet Surveys

An Internet (or electronic) survey can look just like a mail survey, except that it is completed on the Internet. An obvious advantage is that an Internet survey can have many "bells and whistles" that are difficult to reproduce in print, such as photographs, illustrations, and so forth. The survey can be longer without increasing the costs of delivery. In fact, the cost of delivering an Internet survey is your access fee and not dependent on the amount of activity. A number of commercial Internet companies will design surveys and help with data collection. Typically, these are user friendly and economical if the investigator does not have the skill or tools to develop his or her Internet surveys. Intuitively, it would seem that Internet surveys are more cost efficient, but some analyses bring this into question.[3] Some certain advantages for Internet surveys are the following:

1. Data are immediately available when the respondent submits the survey.
2. Results can be loaded directly loaded into a data base for analysis.
3. High-quality graphics and detail can be used.
4. Respondents can be "skipped to" appropriate items based on responses.

Of course, the big disadvantage to Internet surveys is that respondents must have a computer. One report in 2002 stated that 70 percent of adults have access to a computer.[4] One limiting factor is that these tend to be younger adults (under age 54). So, a consideration in using the Internet in survey research is the demographics of the study population. Sampling may also be a problem because you will need access to Internet addresses or some way to notify subjects to "log-on" to an internet survey. E-mail may be one way to contact subjects and provide a URL or you may have to contact subjects by direct mail. Whether or not response rates are higher with Internet surveys is open to question and studies of Internet survey responses are mixed.[3] The Internet and computer skills of the investigator may have a large effect on costs.

Telephone Surveys

Political parties and polsters seem to love telephone surveys, particularly near election time. Interviewing by telephone can provide very timely information. Table 6–23 presents some key aspects of telephone interviewing as a survey format. One obvious limitation is that subjects must have a telephone. Telephone interviews allow for some personal contact between the respondent and the interviewer while maintaining a moderate amount of anonymity. This may be very valuable when dealing with sensitive or personal information. Speaking directly with a subject allows the

Table 6–23
Aspects of Telephone Surveys

Aspect	Comment
Cost	a. Actual telephone costs, such as long distance b. Training costs of interviewers c. Interviewer time costs
Personnel	a. May require multiple interviewers b. Interviewers can telephone from one location c. Skilled interviewers get better and more complete responses
Sample size	a. Subjects must have a telephone b. Size determined by investigator and funding c. Can be large d. Can be geographically dispersed
Response rates	a. Vary, due to willingness of subjects b. Timing of call may influence willingness of respondent to participate
Data	a. Potential for moderate amount and quality of data based on number of subjects willing to participate
Bias	a. Interviewer's manner, voice inflections, interpretation of survey items may influence subject responses
Time	a. Study can be conducted over a short period of time b. Responses immediately available

interviewer (or investigator) to interpret survey items, to move through a survey easily based on responses, and to clarify responses. Cost may be a major factor in telephone surveys because interviewers have to be trained and paid. Telephone costs increase if long distance is needed or a large number of subjects must be contacted. The "annoyance factor" must also be considered. Individuals may not want to be called or to have their routines interrupted by the phone ringing. The length of time a respondent will be on the phone will influence his or her response. The longer the subject is on the phone, the more likely he or she is to hang up.[1]

You must also consider what type of responses you will allow in a telephone interview. Are subjects asked to respond to specific choices or allowed to respond in an unrestricted manner? You must also consider how you will record and handle these open-ended responses. Quantifying open-ended responses may present some difficulty; such responses can be categorized for quantification. You must be careful to ensure you are using the right methods.

Personal Interview Surveys

Person-to-person, face-to-face interviewing has a number of advantages and disadvantages. Interviews must occur where people are (in the PA's office, at the mall, hospital room, patient's home, etc.) or where they go. Special sites can be utilized, but something must bring the subject/respondent there, such as a scheduled appointment to come to the interview site. What all this means is that contact must occur between the subject and the investigator or interviewer (Table 6–24). Unlike a telephone respondent, who can be influenced by the interviewer's voice, a personal interview respondent can be influenced by the physical being and bearing of the interviewer and the site of the interview. In addition to voice inflections, facial and body movements may influence responses. Interviewer personality and animation will also influence responses. For these reasons,

Table 6–24
Aspects of Personal Interviewer Surveys

Aspect	Comment
Cost	High; takes time and people.
Personnel	Requires training.
Sample size	Tend to be relatively small because of time needed to conduct interviews.
Response rates	Can be high once respondents agree to be interviewed; face-to-face encounter may improve or facilitate response and allow for clarification of responses.
Data	Varied, time may limit amount.
Bias	Interviewer bias
Time	Training and interviews take time.

interviewer training may need to be more exact and extensive. Supervision of interviewers may be required. Interviewer bias may be high. The time to train interviewers and the required time for interviews are always factors to consider in both telephone and personal interviewer study methodology and costs.

Interviews can be used to collect qualitative and quantitative data. Interviews can allow for greater exploration of subject responses and can add detail that may help interpret or understand responses. Certainly, if a product is being investigated, subjects can handle it or see it. You must consider what types of responses you will allow in a personal interview. Are subjects asked to respond to specific choices or allowed to respond in an unrestricted manner? You must also consider how you will record and handle open-ended responses. How you handle responses is something that should be planned for as part of your methodology. You cannot decide after you have collected the data.

Survey Item Construction

Survey items must provide data that will answer the research questions, hypotheses, or null hypotheses. Before any survey can be constructed, much less delivered, the purposes of the study must be defined by the research questions, hypotheses, or null hypotheses. Generally, this author has found the best format for survey research is to use the research question(s) or hypotheses format. This does not mean that null hypotheses cannot be used (Table 6–25). Without a well developed and defined research question, hypothesis, or null hypothesis, a well designed survey that can provide accurate and reliable data cannot be developed. As you construct a survey item, ask yourself, "How does the information or data gathered by this item help me answer my research question or hypothesis, or null hypothesis?"

Remember that most survey research is driven by a research question or hypothesis.

Demographic Data

It is a rare survey that does not collect some type of demographic data. In many instances, it is the demographic data that provide the basis for comparison groups. Some common types of demographic data are age, gender, occupation, education, and so forth. For PAs, some types of demographic data are practice location, practice specialty, length of time in practice, number of patients seen, procedures performed, and so forth. Demographic data is the information that describes or characterizes the subject or sample or population in some way. Most demographic data are nominal data. In the past, demographic information was usually collected at the beginning of the survey, but there is no reason that it cannot be collected at the end. It may be best to get to the heart of your survey at first and save the routine material (demographics) for the end.

Demographic survey items should be straightforward questions about the information sought. Examples include the following:

1. What is your gender?
2. What is your age?
3. What degree did you receive from your PA program?
4. What is your practice specialty?
5. How long have you been in practice?

When constructing these survey items, a direct response is probably better than using a range as a choice. An example is age. You may want to group respondents by age, but it is better to have each respondent give his or her exact age and then group the responses if that fits your needs. For example:

Table 6–25
Definitions

Type	Definition	Example
Null hypothesis[5]	A negatively worded statement about the relationship among or between variables. It does not necessarily mean or refer to zero or no difference, but provides a hypothesis that is to be "rejected" or "accepted."	There is no difference in 5-year myocardial infarct rates between angina patients treated with a calcium channel blocker and those treated with a beta-blocker.
Hypothesis[5]	A statement about the relationship among or between variables. This statement may be a conjecture or prediction of a relationship or outcome.	Patients with angina who are treated with a CCB will have a lower number of myocardial infarctions after 5 years than patients treated with beta-blockers.
Research question	Similar to a hypothesis, but is constructed as a question.	Will angina patients treated with a CCB have less myocardial infarctions in 5 years than patients treated with a beta-blocker?

- What is your age in years? _____

  versus

- What is your age group in years?

  a. 21–25   b. 26–30   c. 31–35   d. 36–40   e. >40

There are instances when grouping of response values may be a better format, such as for sensitive or private information. One example is salary. Respondents may be more willing to provide salary data in a range rather than their exact salary. This provides some degree of privacy. It may also be useful when respondents cannot recall information precisely. For example:

- What is your annual salary? _____

  versus

- What is your annual salary?

  a. <$50,000   b. $50,000–59,999
  c. $60,000–69,999   d. $70,000–79,999
  e. >$80,000

Some points to remember when gathering demographic data are

1. Be specific with your statements or questions. Specify your unit of use. Do you want time related information in weeks, days, months, years?

2. When using ranges, make sure they do not overlap. This could lead to respondent confusion. Using salary ranges again as an example, the following options could be confusing because of the overlap of choices:

   - What is your annual salary?
     a. $50,000 or less
     b. $50,000–60,000
     c. $60,000–70,000
     d. $70,000–80,000
     e. $80,000 or more

3. Avoid asking for the same data in more than one statement or question.

4. Use short to-the-point, but understandable statements or questions.

5. Ask only for the information you need that is relevant to your study. It should be clear to you and the respondent why a piece of data is needed for the investigation. You do not want to be overly invasive.

The Survey Instrument

The heart of your survey is the survey items that provide the data for your investigation. The construct of these items will influence respondent rates, willingness to answer, and quality of the data for analysis. Survey items that provide unequivocal data help ensure reliability and validity. *Survey items must be short, clear,*

exacting, understandable, and answerable. They must be designed to provide the data needed to answer the research questions, hypotheses, or null hypotheses. You must also decide on a format for your questions. However, it is not unusual for surveys to have a variety of item formats.

FIRST THINGS FIRST

Developing survey items is a process that goes from very general to very specific. One approach is to sit down and write down every question you can think of that is even remotely related to your investigation. You are developing a list of considerations for your survey. It does not have to be neat, orderly, grammatically correct, or even very specific. It is the beginning of the critical thinking for the development and building of your survey. This list should be very expansive, far longer and greater than what will be your final result. Seek consultation on ideas and points, if needed. It is the author's opinion that very little successful research is the result of one person's efforts. Once you have gotten your general thoughts down, you can begin to edit, define, delete, combine, categorize, and develop your specific survey items. The process of refining your survey and its items is continuous and always aimed toward improving your survey. While there is always room for improvement, at some point you have to stop and be happy with what you have. One question that may help you decide you are ready to go forward is to ask yourself, "Does each survey item reflect some aspect of the answer to my research question?"

ITEM FORMAT

Survey item format is dependent on the information you seek. There are two basic forms of survey items: structured and unstructured (or open-ended).[1] Some examples of "open-ended" questions are given below.

- What do you think are the benchmarks for a quality medical practice?

- What do you do to stay up-to-date on medical practice?

- What is the best way to deal with noncompliant patients?

These types of questions may remind you of the essay questions you disliked in school. Open-ended questions certainly have their value, but may be difficult to quantify or interpret. Structured survey items allow the investigation to control responses to a large degree as well as define the responses in values useful to the study. The formats of structured survey items are varied and examples are presented in Table 6–26. The choice of format depends on the data sought. An important point to

Table 6–26
Examples of Other Survey Item Formats[1,2,7]

Item Format	Example
List Responses	A checklist of responses, multiple choices
Semantic Differential Scale	A scale defined by its extremes with a range between the extremes
Comparison Scale	Choice between two or more items
Visual Analogue Scale	Used to indicate the intensity of a subjective experience along a continuum
Picture Scale	Use of series of pictures/drawings to indicate a response. May be useful for children or people who cannot read.
Forced Ranking	Respondent must rank items.
Ranking versus	Usually ranks items with the ranking value only used once.
Rating	Rating values may be repeated for different items.

remember when constructing your survey items and the possible responses to them is to state whether or not more than one option can be selected. This will help prevent misunderstanding on the part of the respondents. The following is an example.

- What activity do you prefer for earning CME?

(*check all the apply*)

    a. _____ Formal lectures.
    b. _____ Hands on exercises.
    c. _____ On the job experiences or consultations.
    d. _____ Patient/case studies.
    e. _____ Seminars/expert panels.

    versus

- What activity do you prefer for earning CME?

(*check only one*)

    a. _____ Formal lectures.
    b. _____ Hands-on exercises.
    c. _____ On-the-job experiences or consultations.
    d. _____ Patient/case studies.
    e. _____ Seminars/expert panels

You can also include specific wording in the item stem. The wording below could be used in the example given above.

- Check all the activities you prefer for earning CME.

    versus

- Check your one preferred activity for earning CME.
You want to eliminate errors in interpretation of the item stem as much as possible. You cannot guess how people will interpret what you have written or asked. It may be clear to you, but not to them. A pilot test will help reduce interpretation errors.

Rankings

The ranking of responses is valuable in many cases. An example using the question from above may look like this:

- Rank each activity in the order of your preference for earning CME?

(1 = Most preferred, 2 = next most preferred to 5 = least preferred) Rank all items.

    a. _____ Formal lectures.
    b. _____ Hands-on exercises.
    c. _____ On the job experiences or consultations.
    d. _____ Patient/case studies.
    e. _____ Seminars/expert panels.

In this case, you want to be sure that you define the ranking numbers (1–5) and whether or not all items should be ranked. This example could state, "Rank in order of preference those items you use for CME. 1 = most preferred, 5 = least preferred. Do not rank items you do not use." This may be a long statement, but it clarifies what you want the respondents to do. In some instances, it may be desirable to rate some items with the same value. The following is an example of a rating approach:

- Rate the value to you of each of the following CME delivery formats.

1 = Preferred, 2 = Acceptable, 3 = Not preferred
    _____ a. Lecture
    _____ b. Workshop
    _____ c. Video
    _____ d. Computer program
    _____ e. Monographs

OR

- Rate the value of each of the following CME delivery formats.

(Rank all items 1–5 with 1 being the most valuable to 5, least.)
    _____ a. Lecture
    _____ b. Workshop
    _____ c. Video
    _____ d. Computer program
    _____ e. Monographs

Be sure to define your ranking or rating system clearly. Using the number "1" is common as a format for the most preferred or highest value, but sometimes a reverse rating (for example, 10 as the most preferred to 1 as the least preferred) may be useful or desired. Be very clear in your instructions to the respondents. Be very consistent with your item format. If you use more than one item format, group similar format items together. This will be efficient for space and survey presentation. It will also be less likely to confuse respondents.

The Likert and Verbal Frequency Scales

Verbal Frequency Scales are very common tools in survey research. One of the most common types of verbal frequency scales is the Likert Scale. This is an "ordinal" scale used to gather information about respondent's opinions or positions on the subject under investigation. The true Likert Scale uses the following values:

- Strongly Agree, Agree, Neutral, Disagree, Strongly Disagree

The descriptor order can be reversed with "Strongly Disagree" first. The descriptors can also be numbered. For example:

- 1. Strongly Agree   2. Agree   3. Neutral
  4. Disagree   5. Strongly Disagree

OR

- 1. Strongly Disagree   2. Disagree   3. Neutral
  4. Agree   5. Strongly Agree

Remember the number does not matter because these are "Ordinal" data, not continuous data. However, you will see these types of scales treated as interval data in large samples with normal distribution. You need to consult a statistician on handling ordinal data as continuous. Investigators will sometimes use a scale similar to this, but with different descriptors or an increase in the number of descriptors. In these cases, the scale should be termed a "Likert-like Scale" or, more accurately, a "Verbal Frequency Scale"[1] rather than a "Likert Scale." An example of a "Verbal Frequency Scale" is below.

- How often do you prescribe an angiotensin-converting enzyme (ACE) inhibitor as first drug hypertension therapy?
  a. Always   b. Often   c. Occasionally
  d. Infrequently e. Never

Regardless of the descriptors used, Likert Scales or Verbal Frequency Scales are very powerful and popular research tools.[1] Table 6–27 provides keys to using a Likert or Verbal Frequency Scales. In constructing your items for a Likert Scale you are asking respondents to state their level of agreement to that item. A Verbal

---

Table 6–27
The Likert and Verbal Frequency Scales Keys

Key

1. Be clear in your instructions.
2. Use direct statements.
3. Avoid redundancy.
4. Each item should only address one element.
5. Grouping of survey items in groups of 5–10.
6. Scale responses should be logical. Make sure the word responses are appropriate for the item statement or question.
7. Allow for neutral responses if possible.
8. Use easily understood terms.
9. Be consistent in format as much as possible.
10. Responses should be logical responses for question asked. Avoid overlap of grouped responses.
11. Have survey pilot tested or reviewed by expert.
12. Always proofread everything you distribute to subjects.
13. The shorter the survey, the more likely it will be completed. Make it short and simple.
14. Number the pages; 1 of 4, 2 of 4, etc.
15. Allow respondents to comment at the end of the survey.

Frequency Scale may indicate some responses other than agreement. Likert and other scales are generally used with a series of related survey items. Instructions for respondents should lead with a direction statement along the lines of "Indicate your level of agreement or disagreement to the following statements." Figure 6–5 is an example from the author's research.[6]

Another point to remember in your instructions is to ask respondents to respond to all the survey items. Unanswered items lead to questions of validity, extrapolation, and analysis. You should plan on how to handle nonresponses in your analysis.

When constructing your items, be sure that the statement can be answered by using the scale. Avoid redundancy. Also, each item should address only one idea or concept. An example of a conflicting statement from Figure 6-5 could be as follows.

- Ranking programs will benefit society and should be part of accreditation.

This statement contains two components. A respondent may agree that ranking benefits society, but disagree that ranking should be part of accreditation. Item clarity is a key to accurate responses and sound interpretation of results. When using Verbal Frequency Scales be sure that your choices reflect the relationships that you want your subjects to respond to.

Some examples of descriptors used in Verbal Frequency Scales follow.

- Very Satisfied   Satisfied   Neutral   Dissatisfied
  Very Dissatisfied

For each of the following items, indicate your degree of agreement or disagreement using the following Likert Scale:

	Strongly Agree 5	Agree 4	Neutral 3	Disagree 2	Strongly Disagree 1
Concerning the Ranking of Programs.					
1. Physician Assistant Programs should be ranked.	5	4	3	2	1
2. Ranking programs will benefit society.	5	4	3	2	1
3. Ranking programs will help ensure the quality of PA education.	5	4	3	2	1
4. Only the top 25 ranked programs should be published.	5	4	3	2	1
5. All programs' ranking should be published.	5	4	3	2	1
6. Program rank should be a component for accreditation.	5	4	3	2	1
7. Ranking will create ill-will or loss of collegiality among programs.	5	4	3	2	1
8. Ranking will create unnecessary competition among programs.	5	4	3	2	1

FIG. 6–5. An Example of a Likert Scale from the author's research.

- Very Good   Good   Neutral   Poor   Very Poor
- Highly Positive   Positive   Neutral   Negative   Highly Negative
- Excellent   Good   Fair   Poor   Very Poor
- Very Important   Important   Somewhat Important   Not Important

For some surveys, choices of "Not Applicable" "Unsure" "No Answer" "Unknown" etc. may be needed. Also, in some instances more than five responses may be needed and in still others fewer than five. Regardless, it is necessary to be certain that there is a consistency in your options that provides adequate choices along a continuum for your subjects and will allow you to perform appropriate analysis and draw accurate conclusions. Another key is that you should have an equal number of positive and negative responses with a neutral response if possible, although this is not always necessary. An example of when you would not use a "neutral" response is when you want to force the respondent to make a choice in the Verbal Frequency Scale. One risk of this approach is that respondents who are neutral may not answer. You have to decide if the risk is worth it or if a "neutral" or noncommittal response is acceptable. Another option is to have a choice that is "not applicable" or "no experience" or "no knowledge," and so forth.

Putting the Survey Together

Once you have asked or developed your research question, done the appropriate literature search, developed your methodology, and constructed your survey items, you are ready to put it all together. Your letter of introduction or survey introduction paragraph should be first, followed by the survey. (Remember, telephone and personal surveys will have these elements, but they will be presented verbally.) Plain, block, easily read, black print on white paper is probably best. If you want to use colored paper, light beige or gray may be acceptable. Organize your survey so that like items are grouped, particularly if you are using some type of scale. In the past, demographic questions were usually presented first, but recent trends have been to place them at the end of the survey.

Assess the visual quality of your survey. Does it appear organized with well defined borders, sections, and so forth? You want your survey to look neat. Proofread your letter and survey and then have someone else proofread them. It is often difficult to proof our own work, particularly if we have been going over it time and again. Pilot test your survey. You do not need a large group of subjects, but a pilot test is an excellent way to ensure that your survey is understandable and your survey items get the information you want. Ask pilot test subjects to evaluate your survey, that is, give you feedback on their feelings, interpretations, and suggestions for improvement. You may want to have a focus group review the survey and provide feedback and critical comment. Do not take critical review personally. It is a step to make your survey as perfect as possible. Make sure you obtain institutional approval, if needed. You should have that approval in writing in your study files. If Institutional Review Board, Ethics Committee, and so forth are required, do not conduct your survey until you have approval in hand. To do so, even if approval is forthcoming, would be an ethical violation. Once all these small but important steps are taken care of, you can start.

When results begin to return, work on your investigation and study regularly. I suggest setting aside a specific period of time each day or each week for working on your study. Keep good records, protect confidentiality, do your follow-ups, and set a deadline when no further data will be accepted. At some point you must start your data analyses and you cannot continually be adding data. Once analyses are completed, your conclusion can be developed. REMEMBER: If your methodology is sound, you chose the correct analyses, and you have controlled the confounding variables and study biases; the results are the results. As a researcher you search for that truth in the universe, not for what you hoped would be the outcomes. Ultimately, the most that the majority of us can hope to contribute is just one very small piece to the universe of our knowledge.

How Many Subjects?

How many people should I survey? This is a simple question, but a difficult one to answer. If the population of interest is small, you may want to survey the entire population. One good example of a fairly easy population to sample is PA programs. At this writing there are 134 programs, so it is feasible to survey all programs. Another example is all the PAs working in Dermatology, a relatively small number. In these cases, your sample and population are the same. In some instances, a convenience sample may be desired or used. The name implies the sample; the subjects are convenient to survey for the investigator. Some examples are surveys of students conducted by faculty members or surveys of PAs who practice in the investigator's county. The key thing to remember is that the convenience sample may *not* be representative of the population (in our examples, all PA students and all PAs). This presents problems with extrapolation to the larger population. Convenience samples are of very limited benefit. Beyond the convenience sample, you have to make decisions about how many people to sample.

You want your sample to represent the population you want to study. However, you must consider costs and logistics in setting your sample size. In other words, you have to be able to afford the costs of the study and handle the survey distribution and analysis. Remember, having a larger number of respondents does not necessarily increase the accuracy of the results. A good response rate from a smaller sample may be better. Your survey instrument must be valid and reliable. Your sample must represent your population. Smaller samples are more likely to be different from the population than larger samples.[1]

You have to accept the fact that there is always a chance of error. There are some ways to try to control these inherent errors. First set a confidence level and a confidence interval.

- Confidence Level: A desired percentage of scores that would fall within a certain range of confidence limits. It is calculated by subtracting the alpha level from 1 and multiplying the result by 100.[6]
- Confidence Interval: A range of values of a sample statistic that is likely to contain a population parameter. The wider the interval, the higher the confidence level.[6]

The Confidence Level is usually set at 95 percent or 99 percent. This means that you can state with 95 percent or 99 percent confidence that your results are within the margin of error. The Confidence Interval is the margin of error, usually expressed as a range (for example, 3–4). You also need to know the size of the population you want to survey. With these pieces of information, you can calculate your sample size. Many statistical texts will have tables for determining sample size. Some statistical computer programs will do the job. This author's experience is that most samples should be in the range of 100 to 1,000 subjects. If you have difficulty in determining your sample size, consult a statistician.

What Statistics to Use?

Chapter 9 presents data analysis. Again, it may be wise to consult a statistician for the best statistical tests to use for analysis of your results. Statistical tests can be bewildering and most of us need help from an expert. However, make your test decisions as part of your planning and methodology, not after you get your data. Consult a statistician early in your planning. Demographic data can be presented as percentage and, if needed, compared to known population data. This is a good way to demonstrate that your sample is similar to the population of interest.

Another key is to understand what your statistical tests mean and demonstrate. Use statistical tests that fit your data and meet your study needs. The question about evaluating ordinal data with interval or continuous data analysis is one that you need to discuss with a statistician. Chapter 9 has flow charts that can help.

Section Summary

Surveys can provide a wealth of powerful information. Survey research requires the same attention to detail as any research project. You go through the same process in survey research as you would for any type of research project or study. Survey construction is the key to success.

Section References

1. Alreck PL, Settle RB. The Survey Research Handbook, 2nd ed. Boston: Irwin McGraw-Hill, 1995.

2. Cui WW. Reducing error in mail surveys. Practical Assessment, Research & Evaluation, 8(18). Also at *http:// PAREonline.net/ getvn.asp?v=8&n=18* (2003).

3. Sharp K. White papers: Public Sector use of internet surveys and panels. *http://www.decisionanalyst.com/publ_art/PublicSector.asp.* (2002).

4. Rea LM, Parker RA. Designing and Conduction Survey Research: A Comprehensive Guide, 2nd ed. San Francisco: Jossey-Bass, 1997.

5. Fricker RD Jr, Schonlau M. Advantages and disadvantages of internet research surveys: Evidence from the literature. Field Methods 2002;14(4):347–367. *http://www.schonlau.net/publication/ 02fieldmethods.pdf*

6. Vogt WP. Dictionary of Statistics & Methodology, 2nd ed. Thousand Oaks, CA: Sage, 1999.

7. Blessing JD, Hooker RS, Jones PE, Rahr RR. An investigation of potential criteria for ranking physician assistant programs. Perspective on Physician Assistant Education 2001;12(3):160–166.

Appendix: Example of a Cover Letter from the Author's Research

(On author's letterhead)

Dear Program Director,

The ranking of various educational programs has been done for years. However, this is a new phenomenon for physician assistant education. For the past three years *U.S. News and World Report* has ranked master's level PA programs. The basis for these rankings is opinion based and subjective, although done by well-intentioned people who may or may not be knowledgeable about all PA programs. In addition, this activity ignores the majority of PA programs, which are not graduate level programs. Many PA faculty have expressed the opinion that ranking should be based on measurable, comprehensive, objective criteria developed by PA educators. Ranking is a reality that will occur. Those who are most knowledgeable of what PA education entails should be at the forefront of deciding what criteria are used. This study's investigators strongly believe that if PA education does not take a major role in identifying the factors used to rank programs, then rankings will be done based on criteria and data that may not reflect a program's contributions and true position.

Enclosed you will find a survey of characteristics that could be used to develop a ranking system and provide an objective base for program ranking. Please take a few minutes to complete this survey and return it to us. A stamped, addressed return envelope is enclosed for your convenience. If possible, we would like to have the survey returned to us within 2 weeks. We will send a reminder postcard in about 10 days. PLEASE complete the survey whether or not you agree with the concept of program rating. One of the first questions deals with your agreement on ranking, so your opinion is not lost. Your completion of the survey will provide us the opportunity to do comparisons and other analyses based on the demographic information you provide. There is a section on the survey for your comments. The development of a fair and accurate ranking system depends on these comments.

The Research and Review Committee of the Association of Physician Assistant Programs and the Institutional Review Board of The University of Texas Health Science Center at San Antonio have approved this investigation. If there are any questions, please feel free to contact me at any time by phone, fax, e-mail, or letter. All information will be kept anonymous. You do not have to identify yourself or your program. Results and data will be reported in aggregate only.

It is our intention to present the study data at a meeting of the Association of Physician Assistant Programs. We hope to submit a final manuscript for publication. Your help in completing this survey will contribute valuable information for PA education, the profession, and the public. This study is supported, in part, by a grant from the President's Council of The University of Texas Health Science Center at San Antonio to the School of Allied Health Sciences.

Thank you for your time and best wishes for your endeavors.

Sincerely,
J. Dennis Blessing, PhD, PA-C
Professor & Chair

For: Co-author A
Co-author B
Co-author C

Example of a Postcard Reminder

Reminder

A few weeks ago you received a "Learning Assessment Survey" from me. It was distributed through your program. If you have not completed the survey, please take a few minutes to do so and return them to me. If you need another form, please contact me at the address or phone number below. The information you provide through this survey will be helpful to me in my study of how students learn and, hopefully, to the education of PAs in the future.

Thank you for your time.
Dennis Blessing, PA-C
State University
(123) 555–9876

chapter 7

Qualitative Research

Anita Duhl Glicken, MSW

Chapter Overview

This chapter provides an overview of qualitative research. All of us recognize that there is information that we need to discover that does not lend itself to hard numbers or manipulation of variables. Qualitative research has been described as interpretive, constructive, and naturalistic or "real world." From its beginnings in the social sciences, qualitative research has evolved into a methodology used across many disciplines, including medicine. In this chapter we examine the philosophy of qualitative research and describe its techniques and applications. Included is a discussion on research that combines qualitative and quantitative methods. Data, analysis, and management issues are also discussed. Qualitative research techniques have a place in physician assistant (PA) and medical research, but have not reached their true potential as tools for better understanding medicine and the work of PAs. This chapter will help readers identify indications for using a qualitative study design; identify the methods, data, and goals of qualitative analysis; describe the process of qualitative data analysis; and describe the use of an integrated approach to research methods, designs, and purposes in health-care research.

Introduction

Rapid advances in medical technology and practice, an increase in patient information and expectations, as well as the size and diversity of the health-care system all contribute to a new level of complexity in health-care services. There are no easy solutions to improving the quality of patient care. The concept of quality in health care is multidimensional, and traditionally most of the questions we wanted to answer were best explored through quantitative research. Quantitative research (reviewed in other chapters of this book) assists us in identifying new approaches to care based on randomized controlled trials, case–controlled and cohort studies, and a number of experimental and quasi-experimental designs. Research has also shown us, however, how difficult it can sometimes be to implement these findings in effective and reliable ways. In part this is because views of quality often depend on the perspectives of the patients who use the treatments and the attitudes and behaviors of the professionals who function as part of the health-care system. Qualitative research provides a variety of methods that help us identify patient and provider preferences as well as obstacles to changing practice. There is growing recognition of the unique contributions qualitative methods make to the development of contextually grounded, culturally sensitive research projects that form and inform clinical practice. Qualitative methods have traditionally been seen as a means to enhance the quality of a quantitative project. Now these methods are seen as ends in themselves, providing valuable information to inform the treatment process. This chapter discusses the role and functions of qualitative research methods in medicine. On completion of this chapter the reader will be able to:

1. Identify indications for using a qualitative study design.
2. Identify the methods, data, and goals of qualitative analysis.
3. Describe the process of qualitative data analysis.
4. Describe the use of an integrated approach to research methods, designs, and purposes in health-care research.

Philosophy of the Method

As described in previous chapters, traditional, quantitative research is based on the belief that a single, objective reality exists. This reality is governed by a set of laws and can be examined in terms of fragmented parts (facts) that can be understood with the accumulation of high-quality research. Quantitative research begins with an idea (usually stated as a hypothesis) that is then measured, generating data that by deduction allow a conclusion to be drawn.

Qualitative research is based on a different philosophy. It operates on the premise that although there may be an objective reality, individuals assign complex meanings to their perceived reality, and it is on the basis of these subjective meanings and interpretations that decisions are made. Qualitative methods, therefore, attempt to make sense and understanding of phenomena in terms of the meanings people bring to those phenomena. Qualitative research is generative in that it is designed to offer description and explanation to the topic at hand. Qualitative research begins with this intent to explore a particular area, data are collected (often through interviews and observations), and ideas and hypotheses are generated from these data largely through inductive reasoning. Because of this shift in philosophical perspective, qualitative research can be seen to differ from quantitative endeavors in three ways.

1. The purpose of the research
2. The use of the literature review and relationship between theory and data
3. The level of investigator involvement in the imposition of specific procedures and steps throughout the research process.

Indications for Using Qualitative Research

Once a research topic is identified, it is often the literature that provides the assistance needed to refine and formulate specific research questions. As indicated in Chapter 4, there are many reasons to conduct a literature search; the most obvious one is to explore what previous research, if any, has been conducted on the topic. Another reason is to clarify the level of theory and knowledge development with respect to the topic. For example, is the current body of information descriptive, explanatory, or predictive? As an illustration, if you are considering an experimental study design, you should find research that identifies a theoretical framework and assists in the development of a hypothesis and variables that might predict the outcome of your intervention using that design. Thus, the level of knowledge uncovered during the literature search establishes a rationale for your study design. What if this is not the case, however? What if you find little or no research that is directly related to your study? This lack of literature for the background and base of your study helps establish a rationale for your selected research strategy and is a strong indication that qualitative methods may be appropriate.

Qualitative methods are often used as the first step in a new area of inquiry. Using techniques such as semi-structured interviews, focus groups, and participant observations, researchers can develop a perspective that allows them to identify previously unrecognized variables, clarify the role of the variables in a particular relationship, and form the construction of the experimental study designs. For example, in an attempt to improve the quality of health care provided to gay and lesbian adolescents, focus groups were formed to uncover variables perceived by the recipients (subjects) as affecting the quality of their health care. The effects of these variables were explored and an experimental study design ensued based on variables provided by the initial participants.

Qualitative methods can also be used to augment and enhance a study when used in conjunction with other methods. This mixed methods strategy, which is addressed in greater detail later in this chapter, is increasingly visible in health-care research, particularly in studies that emphasize new treatment protocols. For example, in evaluating the impact of preventive interventions, we gain a great deal from asking participants to tell us what they did and did not find useful. Similarly, we can explore why they chose not to participate or what obstacles led them to drop out of the intervention prior to completion. In summary, indications for using qualitative approaches might include:

- No previous existing literature; either the question has not been asked, or the problem is still poorly understood or very complex.
- Studying "real" phenomena outside the formal laboratory, for example, any field research or that conducted in a naturally occurring setting
- Program evaluation; accountability to the population you service or to funding resources.
- Conduct a needs assessment.
- Strengthen quantitative research designs.

Research Techniques

There are essentially three basic data collection techniques in qualitative research: observation, interviews, and document review. All of these techniques have several variations, suggesting the potential complexity of relatively simple strategies.

OBSERVATION

Since behavior of people is a central aspect of all inquiries, a natural technique is to observe what they do and then describe, analyze, and interpret what has been observed. You do not ask people about their feelings and attitudes and how these might affect their behavior; you actually record what they do in response to a situation. This direct method is often a useful complement to other methods. For example, questionnaire or interview responses are often discrepant between what people say that they have done or will do and what they actually did or will do.

Observational methods can be seen to vary in four distinct ways. First, in "classic" fieldwork, an individual who actually participates in the situation under study collects data. For example, an investigator interested in the barriers to health-care delivery for a rural population might live in the rural community for an extended period of time. The investigator lives the life of the subject, enabling him or her to simulate the subjective experience of the participants and develop relationships with the informants.

Second, observation also varies based on the length of time the researcher is involved. Observations have been conducted for months, even years, while many recent qualitative studies rely on much briefer exposures to the research context. Depending on the research questions to be answered, more limited observations and involvement can provide sufficient data. A researcher conducting an observational study of patient utilization of health education reading materials in a clinic waiting room may collect sufficient data from a limited exposure across several days.

Third, observations may be conducted with or without the subject's awareness or permission. Although covert observation is politically and ethically controversial, the nature of the data collected by observation is often greatly influenced by the degree to which the researcher informs participants on the nature of the project. The Hawthorne effect is an example of subjects being influenced by being observed.

Fourth, observation may be limited to a specific area of inquiry as in the example cited earlier, or may be extended to include a more comprehensive view of the area under study.

INTERVIEW

The second data collection method is the interview. A number of different interview strategies may be used, varying in approach from casual to formal. Individual interviews can also range from highly structured and directed to unstructured and nondirected. Similarly, the investigator can utilize a number of strategies in conducting the interview that will affect the quantity and quality of the information obtained—for example, the number and nature of the questions asked or the use of recall strategies, active listening, and probes for content. There is also variability across a given set of interviews in the degree to which the investigator attempts to standardize the information obtained from all respondents. Most often, qualitative interviews are typically unstructured during exploratory phases of the project, with more standardized and formal interviews during later stages of investigation.

The focus group interview is becoming an increasingly popular research technique. A focus group session is a discussion in which a small number of people (usually 6 to 10) discuss a topic introduced by a moderator or facilitator. In this case, the researcher sets the agenda for the meeting and attempts to keep the group focused on the topic, often using a series of probes to be sure the key questions are covered. The session is typically very open; group members may express their own views and ask questions meaningful to them as well as comment on what someone else has said. There are some clear advantages to this method, including the generation of a much broader and richer exploration of the topic under study. As mentioned previously, focus groups are a good way to identify variables that may be used to study a specific topic, particularly if little or no information about that topic is available.

DOCUMENT REVIEW

The third data collection technique is document review. Generally, document review involves organizing and evaluating a body of existing information for combination with other data or as a stand-alone data source.

Documents can range from formal to informal. For example, objective reports, patient records, and so forth represent formal documentation. Informal documentation may be gleaned from sources such as personal notes or calendars. Clearly, documents also vary with respect to their relationship to the research question. A patient record may have direct statements related to a research question, leaving little need or room for interpretation. Other comments expressed in less formal documents or not directly related to the research question may require conceptual translation and mandate a more critical attitude on the part of the investigator.

DATA MANAGEMENT

Qualitative methods are iterative and inductive; therefore, qualitative research requires continuous recording of data for constant review. Typically, when one utilizes an interview or observational strategy, "field notes" provide a vehicle for constant recording of data. "Trigger notes" are often recorded during interview observations that later are expanded into a more comprehensive record of the interaction, including quotes.

The researcher should also record his or her subjective experiences during data collection. These "field notes" might refer to the researcher's specific thoughts or ideas about how the data might later be interpreted or form future data collection strategies. These notes are often as critical to the data analysis as the content of the interview itself, and demand organized strategies for management and control.

Some researchers choose to use electronic means to capture an observation or interview. Although this method has obvious benefit in terms of reliability and completeness, it does have limitations as well. For example, a camera may capture only one angle or perspective and the recording setting may "influence" the experience as well. An audio transcript cannot capture the rich detail that occurs in the nonverbal interactions of participants. Both audio and video recordings also generate volumes of raw data, which may be difficult for the researcher to manage. Transcribing audio recordings can be extremely expensive in terms of time and money and often requires the researcher to be selective about the data chosen for analysis. The criteria used for this selection must represent a well thought out and explicit approach to data management.

Data Analysis

Unlike quantitative studies, which often rely on total data collection to be completed before the analysis process begins, data analysis of qualitative studies can begin quite early. Data analysis requires an approach much different from that of quantitative research and is

an interative process of constantly cycling and reviewing the data. Preliminary data analysis consists of the dual process of segmenting the data and developing early concepts or categories that will later evolve into theoretical models.

Assuming the data have been recorded in an accessible way, the first step of analysis consists of segmenting the data. The researcher might first read the transcripts and memos of the observations or interviews and begin a process of coding whereby initial categories and themes are identified. The researcher often identifies parts or pieces of information indicated by words or phrases that are seen to represent something that appears to be significant. The researcher's personal experience and background often heavily influence these categories. For example, categories may come from clinical practice, existing theory, or may be generated from a high level of abstraction such as concepts of time or space. In reporting their experiences, the participants might also suggest categories. In any case, these categories evolve and subsequently relate in ways that might suggest the germination of potential interpretative theories.

The next step in the analysis process consists of reorganizing and resorting the bits of information contained in the transcripts and notes into the categories or themes that have been generated. Data are often literally cut and pasted into different "theme bins" or computer programs are used to facilitate this process. The researcher utilizes a process of "constant comparison" in sorting and recategorizing the data in various ways. Once data have been categorized, the researcher begins to explore how the categories may link to each other. In this "contextualizing process" you are essentially building theory. One explores not only sets of concepts, but also the relationships between them and the process that takes one from point A to point B. Discrepant cases and alternative explanations are also considered. Occasionally, a researcher will begin with a contextualizing approach. Rather than seeing categories and contexts only, one looks for the connections between the events, as is the case in some types of linguistic analysis.

As various theories emerge, the literature is consulted as new information is identified and related to the data. As stated earlier, this inductive method places a major emphasis on theory that is developed progressively as the data analysis is completed. The generation of new theory or understanding is the goal of qualitative inquiry and, as such, use of the literature may become much heavier at the end of the project as the researcher seeks a broader understanding and application of the data.

In the cyclical process of working with raw data and abstracting new theory, the analysis proceeds until the researcher feels that a "goodness of fit" has been established. Data analysis continues until such a time that the researcher feels the theory that has been developed adequately fits the data and conceptual framework.

Validity

The validity of qualitative analysis has been the subject of debate in the medical literature. It is important to recognize that our definitions of validity and reliability have evolved in the context of a quantitative research paradigm grounded in a different philosophical perspective. At the same time, qualitative methodologies do offer some safeguards to researchers.

Triangulation, as it has been used in naturalistic inquiry, refers to a multistrategy approach. The purpose of this approach is to combine different methods to reveal an additional piece of the puzzle or to uncover varied dimensions of the same phenomena. This is referred to as the "completeness function" in which different methods are purposely chosen because each assesses a different aspect of the dimension of the problem under study. For example, a researcher might combine open-ended interviewing with direct observation or chart extraction to achieve a complete understanding of recovery issues associated with a cerebrovascular accident. Each data collection strategy provides an understanding of the total experience of recovery. Possibilities for triangulation are often limited by logistics and the range of options available for sources of data and the methods available to research a particular question.

An additional strategy or "validity check" has been referred to as "informant review." In this case, participants are asked to review and comment on various categories, themes, and conclusions drawn by the researchers. They provide feedback on whether or not the inferences the researcher has drawn matches their experience or understanding of the situation. This process may be initiated either early in the data analysis process or later, when some theories or conclusions have been generated in a more global way. Interpreting this feedback is often problematic. Participants might offer valid criticisms of the interpretive theories or might provide new data with respect to the issue at hand. In addition, informants may be resistant to theories that are unsympathetic or critical of their experience. This type of feedback, however, is still recognized as an important component in checking the authenticity of the researcher's conclusions.

A third strategy is based on the researchers' use of their own critical appraisal skills throughout the process. Researchers should be constantly looking for alternative explanations in the data as well as systematically testing their theories for where they might be wrong in their interpretations. This involves monitoring their data for discrepant information or negative cases that don't fit their theory.

Similarly, colleagues may be called on to review the data and analysis on many levels. In a general way, colleagues may offer their own speculations about the experiences or may consult on the generation of categories and contexts for data analysis based on their own limited experience with the project. More specifically, they might be asked to independently review the data and generate themes and contexts from their own perspective. Colleagues might also be provided with the categories generated by the researcher and portions of raw data and asked to do a separate analysis based on these categories. This attempt to demonstrate some degree of "inter-rater reliability" also may serve to inform the analysis process through clarification of existing categories and the generation of new ones.

Finally, qualitative investigators are also obligated to describe, often in rich detail, the process they used to collect, analyze, and interpret their data. In quantitative research, such descriptions are often truncated by the use of commonly understood terms referring to things like randomized controlled trials or simple linear regression. In qualitative analyses it is often necessary to describe the process in greater detail, including information about attempts to ensure validity of the procedure through the use of triangulation or informant or colleague review.

A Mixed Methodology—Combining Qualitative and Quantitative Methods

There is great debate in the medical literature as to whether qualitative and quantitative methods should be combined in an overall research strategy. In part, this is the result of the discordant philosophical approaches and assumptions inherent to both. Proponents of using a mix of methodologies argue, however, that both approaches offer different tools designed to address different tasks and that both are potentially necessary in order to do a complete job of exploring the issue at hand.

This perspective has become more common in the field of needs assessment and program evaluation, in which this form of "triangulation" has become very popular. Qualitative methods often are used extensively in the hypothesis-generating phase of the research. A mix of qualitative and quantitative methods often is used simultaneously to test the hypothesis and refine the methodology as the study progresses. Finally, a qualitative investigation is often used to help the investigator explain the findings of the quantitative research. In this way, qualitative methods can be used in a study to extend and complement quantitative findings.

Quantitative studies that answer questions of "how many" or "how much" can be complemented by qualitative explorations of "how" related to the process under research. For example, quantitative studies might tell us how many children are given prescriptions for oral antibiotics and in what quantity, but qualitative studies might tell us how these antibiotics are actually administered by parents and the reasons they comply or do not comply with their health-care provider's recommendations.

To use such a combination of methods requires a wide range of expertise and skills and often a team approach to research design, data management, and analysis. Despite the potential problems of attempting to merge two disparate paradigms, there are many benefits to utilizing this type of synergistic approach.

Summary

Mastering the art of qualitative research offers the practicing PA, student, or educator the additional benefit of improving clinical skills. The approach reinforces good clinical interviewing and problem solving through the use of strong listening, open-ended questions, and an objective attitude. Qualitative interviewing utilizes these skills and forces the investigator to revisit interview content and understanding from several perspectives. Interviewers become adept at uncovering themes and categories of information which are then related to a broader context. This ability to "contextualize" data trains the student to see not only isolated facts and events, but also the process and relationship of these facts or events to each other. In fact, it is this process of "theory building" that is continuously utilized by skilled clinicians in complex diagnostic problem solving and decision making.

In medical research, the debate about the scientific legitimacy of the qualitative research paradigm will continue. Much of this debate will center on the strengths and weaknesses of alternative research models. Researchers should continue to focus their attention on the issue of strengthening project design by selecting methodologies that most accurately reflect the philosophy and scope of their inquiry. Qualitative methods can be an important approach to understanding that can greatly enhance medical practice. Qualitative research requires new skills and perspectives beyond those of quantitative efforts. In some ways, qualitative research demands a rigor that surpasses that of quantitative research, as the methods are less defined and more open to interpretation. Although data collection strategies and subsequent analysis appear straightforward, the three major strategies presented in this chapter illustrate the degree of complexity that this process often entails.

chapter 8

Community-Based Participatory Research: An Introduction for the Clinician Researcher

Scott D. Rhodes, PhD, MPH, CHES and Debra L. Benfield, MEd, RD, LDN

Chapter Overview

Despite the strides that have been made in overall health status in the United States, not all communities are benefiting equally from current medical and health advances. In fact, many of the complex health problems that persist in the United States have proven to be ill suited for traditional "outside expert" approaches to health research, health improvement, and intervention development and implementation.[1–6] To decrease the growing gaps in health status among vulnerable communities such as minority (e.g., racial/ethnic, sexual orientation) and economically disadvantaged communities, alternative approaches to health research, health promotion, and disease prevention are being explored and promoted. Community-based participatory research (CBPR) is an approach to research designed to promote community health through the establishment and maintenance of community partnerships.[7] Rather than a clinician researcher coming into a community "knowing" what is best for a community, a partnership approach to research benefits community partners, community-based organizations (CBOs), and researchers alike.

A partnership approach promotes health and aids in disease prevention because, among its strengths, it creates bridges between communities and researchers; incorporates local knowledge and local theory based on the lived experience of members of the communities involved; ensures the development of appropriate research design and methods; and lends itself to the development of culturally relevant measurement design and instrumentation. Partnerships enhance both the quality of data collected and the validity of findings and their interpretation.[3–9]

In this chapter we define and describe the advantages and processes of CBPR. We also describe why CBPR is an appropriate approach to research within the historical context of the physician assistant (PA) profession. We then introduce four research methods and describe how a CBPR approach may be applied and incorporated. Finally, we offer a case example of the application of CBPR in an ongoing research study.

Introduction: Community-Based Participatory Research Defined

Emerging evidence suggests that through a process of partnership that includes lay community members, community representatives, and clinician researchers, advances in health and reductions in health disparities can occur as health promotion and disease prevention approaches, strategies, and efforts increase in authenticity.[7,10,11] To truly understand community health, community members participate in the research process to guide the study and intervention design, ensure the accuracy of measurement, and support the interpretation of results. However, partnership is not easy; clinician researchers must establish and maintain trusting, authentic co-learning partnerships with community members if partnerships are to function well and improvements in health are to occur within communities, especially the most vulnerable among them.

CBPR is an approach to health and research intended to increase the value of studies for both community members and researchers. CBPR is a collaborative research approach that is designed to ensure and structure participation by communities affected by the issue being studied, by representatives of organizations, and by researchers in all aspects of the research process (Box 8–1).

CBPR emphasizes co-learning and the reciprocal transfer of expertise, decision-making power, and the ownership of the processes and products of research. This approach involves a strong partnership in which all parties (e.g., lay community members, CBO representatives, health department representatives, and researchers) participate and share control over *all* phases of the research process. These research phases typically include:

- Identifying research questions;
- Assessing community strengths, assets, and challenges;
- Defining priorities;
- Developing research and data collection methodologies;
- Collecting and analyzing data;
- Interpreting findings;
- Disseminating of findings; and
- Applying the results to address community concerns through action or intervention.

BOX 8–1

CBPR

CBPR is a collaborative research approach that is designed to ensure and structure participation by communities affected by the issue being studied, by representatives of organizations, and by researchers in all aspects of the research process.

While participation of the affected community in all research steps is critical to CBPR, another hallmark of CBPR is the transformation of findings into action. The accumulation of knowledge is important for the progression of science and understanding; however, the priority for most community members and CBO and health department representatives is the application of findings to improve the health status of community members, including friends, neighbors, families, consumers, patients, and clients. Furthermore, growing concern exists that the pendulum has swung too far toward "research for research sake" without the application of new knowledge to effect change to improve the health outcomes of populations and community members.[4,5,10] Actions may include individual-level change interventions, community-level interventions, and policy advocacy and change interventions.

CBPR relies on community participation to ensure that the research questions asked are important not only to the clinician researcher for accumulation of knowledge, but also to the community members themselves. CBPR helps to ensure that the methods used are reasonable and authentic to existing community structures and experiences, and as noninvasive as possible. Finally, the increased validity of findings from CBPR yields more effective actions or interventions in health care because of its base in community participation. Table 8–1 illustrates the advantages of using a CBPR approach, as summarized from the literature.

Research Paradigms

All research approaches, including the design of a study and the methods selected, reflect a specific research *paradigm.* Research paradigms are defined as a set of basic beliefs about the nature of reality that can be studied and understood.[12] These basic beliefs are accepted simply on faith, and, however well argued, no way exists to establish their ultimate truth. The *positivist* and *post-positivist* research paradigms, for example, hold that a single reality on how things really are and really work exists to be studied and understood. The *positivist* research paradigm posits that this single reality can be fully captured; this paradigm is reflected in *experimental* research designs and methods, which are used most often in the basic sciences. The *post-positivist* research paradigm, in contrast, holds that this single reality can only be *approximated* and is reflected in *quasi-experimental* research designs and methods, used most often in the social and behavioral health sciences. Both experimental and quasi-experimental methods require objective detachment between researchers and participants so that any influence in either direction (i.e., threats to validity) on what is being studied can be eliminated or reduced.

Table 8–1
Advantages of Community-Based Participatory Research

- Enhances data relevance, usefulness, and use
- Improves the quality and validity of the research by engaging local knowledge and local theory based on the lived experiences of the people involved
- Recognizes the limitations of the concept of value-free science and encourages a self-reflexive, engaged, and self-critical role of researchers
- Recognizes that knowledge is power, and thus knowledge gained can be used by all partners involved to direct resources and influence policies that will benefit the community
- Overcomes the fragmentation and separation of the individual from his culture and context
- Aims to increase health and well-being of communities involved, both directly through examining and addressing identified needs and indirectly through increasing power, control and skills

- Joins partners with diverse skills, knowledge, expertise, and sensitivities to address complex issues
- Strengthens the research, program, and problem-solving capacity of partners
- Creates theory grounded in social experience, and creates better informed and more effective practice guided by such theories
- Increases the possibility of overcoming the understandable distrust of research on the part of communities that historically have been the subjects of such research.
- Has the potential to bridge "cultural gaps"
- Involves communities that have been marginalized on the basis of, for example, race, ethnicity, class, gender, and sexual orientation in examining the impact of marginalization and attempting to reduce or eliminate it

CBPR is often aligned with a *constructivist* research paradigm, which holds that multiple realities exist to be studied and understood.[12] Each reality is an intangible construction; rooted in people's experiences with everyday life, with how they remember and make sense of them. Individual constructions of reality are assumed to be more or less "informed," rather than more or less "true," because they are always alterable. This means that as researchers and participants encounter and consider different perspectives, they will alter their own views. The result is a *consensus construction of reality*[12] that is mutually formed by variations in preceding constructions (including those of the researchers), and that can move both participants and researchers toward communicating about action, intervention, and change.[13] The methods of constructivist research require researchers and participants to be interactively linked so that the consensus construction of reality is literally created as the study proceeds. Researchers using a CBPR approach, therefore, are cast in the dual roles of participant and facilitator.

Physician Assistants and CBPR

Initially developed for the deployment of well-trained ex-military corpsmen into rural primary care practices to utilize their unique training and experiences from their service, the PA profession was designed to improve the health and well-being of vulnerable communities that faced the interrelated challenges of a dramatic undersupply of physicians and an increase in health-care costs. This commitment to community health and the provision of services to those communities that often fall through health-care cracks aligns it-

self well with CBPR. Creatively working to improve the health and well-being of vulnerable communities that initially were rural, PA clinician researchers are well positioned to take on increasingly more community-based and participatory approaches to scientific inquiry and discovery to positively affect the health and well-being of minority (e.g., racial/ethnic, sexual orientation) and economically disadvantaged communities to reduce health disparities.

Common Research Methods

Successful use of CBPR relies on various partnership principles and values that include:

- Building and maintaining trust between community members and researchers;
- Establishing formal and informal partnership networks and structures;
- Committing to transparent processes and clear and open communication;
- Agreeing on the values, goals, and objectives of the research;
- Building research upon each partner's strengths and assets;
- Balancing power and sharing resources;
- Sharing credit for the accomplishments of the research; and
- Disseminating findings to research audiences, community members, and policy makers.

Often, the clinician researcher feels that she or he must make decisions on behalf of the community. This is a natural inclination given the years spent in school, in training programs, or in the field. The clinician researcher may be motivated to apply and use her or his resources for the benefit of the community. After all, the clinician researcher is armed with intellectual resources, training and experience in the reduction of bias and the traditional approaches to increase validity with the hope of increasing generalizability, and perhaps financial resources or, at the minimum, increased access to financial resources, among other tools. Thus, the clinician researcher may forget that community members and representatives from CBOs have perspectives that will be useful for inclusion during the research process.

It has been said that for community members "the textbook of life is living." With this axiom in mind, clinician researchers must recognize that community members have a perspective that can greatly enhance all phases of the research process. Community members have firsthand knowledge of the health issue of concern. They contribute to identifying and understanding the most salient health needs of their community, giving context to epidemiological data and building theory about needs, challenges, and potential solutions that may have not occurred to or be easily understood by outsiders. Each of these points can strengthen research and intervention design through the interpretation of data and the evaluation and revision of intervention strategies.

Although their training and experiences may or may have not been learned in formal educational or training programs, representatives from CBOs and local agencies who are on the frontlines also may have an understanding of the community that is also not readily available or apparent to the clinician researcher. These individuals may include service providers, educators, providers of medical and mental health services, and counselors. They know systems and may have a wealth of experiences providing services to community members on the frontlines or at the grassroots level. However, their perspectives may lack detail and they may miss insights that have not been well discovered or explored.

Many clinician researchers might conclude that they themselves are on the frontlines in their capacity as clinicians; yet they may truly know very little about the lived experiences of their patients or clients, especially once patients or clients leave the clinician's office. To illustrate; having access to care and medications does not ensure that a patient will adhere to prescribed medication regimens for diabetes management. Patients and clients (and providers themselves) live in complex social contexts that cannot be easily understood or teased apart by outsiders. Thus, although representatives from CBOs or community agencies such as the health department have useful knowledge, experiences, and theories, alone their insight is insufficient.

CBPR can be infused into any research methodology; however, the following section highlights four research methods and briefly describes how CBPR can be applied. These methods include *action-oriented community diagnosis* (AOCD), *focus groups*, *photovoice*, and *in-depth interviews*. Although this discussion is not meant to be exhaustive, it is intended to serve as an initial "starting point" for clinician researchers who want to understand and explore the use of CBPR.

Action-Oriented Community Diagnosis

The purpose of AOCD is to understand the health status, the collective dynamics and functions of relationships within a community, and the interactions between community members and broader structures that can impede or promote the conditions and skills required to assist community members in making decisions and taking action for social change and health status improvement.[10] AOCD can be a critical first step in program planning, intervention, and evaluation because it provides the foundation for:

- The establishment of baseline data from which objectives, intended outcomes, and measures of change can be derived;

- The selection of intervention methods and delivery that are most appropriate based on the community's structure, including formal and informal power dynamics and community assets and strengths; and

- A collaborative relationship between professionals and communities, who can begin "closing the gap between what we do not know and what we ought to know."[14]

AOCD may serve as a process for *needs assessment* but actually goes beyond traditional interpretations of needs assessment. While needs assessment is defined as a systematic examination and appraisal of the type, depth, and scope of needs for the purpose of setting priorities, AOCD also identifies and explores community assets on which intervention can be based. CBPR utilizes a *strengths-based approach* to research to identify both the needs and challenges faced by communities, and just as importantly, the assets and strengths within the community. To forego the identification of community assets and strengths is to use a *deficits-based approach* that may miss key information vital to understanding the community's reality and lived experience and the strengths and resources on which intervention strategies can be based (Box 8–2).

Like all research methods that adhere to a CBPR approach, AOCD begins with the establishment of a working collaborative relationship with community members. Representatives from the community, CBOs,

BOX 8–2

Needs Assessment

Needs assessment is the systematic examination and appraisal of the type, depth, and scope of needs for the purpose of setting priorities. It is the process of identifying and measuring gaps between what is and what ought to be.

and clinician researchers come together to determine a research plan. Usually existing community-specific data are reviewed. These may include epidemiological data usually available from public health departments at the local or state levels as well as other reports and resources available from local CBOs such as faith-based service providers and other agencies.

A *windshield tour* of the community is an important initial step in the AOCD process. If the community consists of a geographical location, a clinician researcher will explore the community guided by community members to gain an appreciation of the community's geography, size, physical characteristics, and important community venues (e.g., a corner store where people gather or a house of worship). This windshield tour is meant to be an introduction to the community and its context through simple observation and community member guidance and commentary. If the community is less geographically defined such as a community of elderly shut-ins, for example, a windshield tour may include the agencies and organizations that visit and offer support to these community members. A windshield tour for a virtual community might include exploring the chat rooms, list serves, bulletin boards, and newsgroups visited and used by the community and visiting sites that are advertised on popup and pop-under screens.

After the windshield tour and throughout AOCD, clinician researchers document their experiences using *field notes*. Frequently kept in various study methodologies and often informal, field notes are documentation of details about the community that are interesting or noteworthy and when combined with other data might well prove to be important. Field notes may serve several purposes including

1. Providing the clinician researcher the opportunity to document first impressions about a community;

2. Assisting the clinician researcher to remember experiences encountered in the field;

3. Recording names of individuals and places that may prove key in the execution of the AOCD process; and

4. Documenting unusual characteristics within a community.

Field notes also allow the clinician researcher to track her or his own perspectives, impressions, feelings, and frustrations during the AOCD research process. Field notes can be simply reflective writings while the research "event," such as a windshield tour, is still fresh in the mind of the clinician researcher. It is wise to keep field notes of all research efforts because field notes serve as a documentation source for decisions made that affect the research process and subsequent data interpretation.

Because clinician researchers tend to be very different from the communities they study, clinician researchers need to gain an *emic* or insider's perspective on how people live and the issues facing the community.[15–17] An insider's perspective is privileged knowledge that only members of a particular community have. Outsiders can guess and hypothesize, but those assumptions are not value free and may not be accurate or complete. Because no researcher can completely remove her- or himself from the research, an emic perspective provides the clinician researcher insight into the perspectives of community members. For example, a homeless individual understands aspects of the lived experience of homelessness better than any outsider. Members from a disabled community can provide insights that may not be understood or correctly interpreted by an outsider.

Furthermore, one's social position in a community affects the "truth" of the experience of community life. For example, all African-American gay men do not share a truth; in fact, among other influences, perception of truth is affected by the position within the community. Thus, AOCD allows for distinctions and differences to emerge that may be lost through other approaches. This is a challenge for clinician researchers who must work with community members to merge varying—perhaps contradictory—data and perspectives and make useful sense of findings.

Of course, although the emic perspective is important, a hallmark of AOCD (and in fact CBPR) is to move toward change through some type of action or intervention. Action may include a behavioral intervention to promote medication adherence, or policy change to increase access to care, as examples. Such movement requires an understanding of *etic* or outsider perspectives. Outsiders, who usually comprise representatives from CBOs and other service providers such as the local public health department, and clinician researchers, provide perspectives on the health and well-being of communities, their access to resources, and community strengths, as well as support for subsequent action or intervention. Like community members themselves, outsiders have a story to tell based on their experiences.

After reviewing and incorporating secondary or extant data and collecting, analyzing, and interpreting emic and etic data, the clinician researcher helps the community disseminate the findings. AOCD relies on a *community forum* to present to *influential advocates* the findings of a research process. This forum highlights issues, may propose solutions, and allows the community to dialogue with influential advocates who are supporters, but who may also benefit from increased awareness and greater understanding of the situation. The forum is an opportunity to initiate dialogue and for participants to come together during a facilitated discussion to explore potential action or intervention. Without the forum, AOCD merely explores root causes, but does not move to improving health status of the community. Dissemination of findings within the community and movement toward action are important steps in CBPR and AOCD.

AOCD requires the involvement of both insiders and outsiders to ensure the collection of accurate (defined as reliable and valid) data and the correct interpretation of these data. AOCD might include understanding both the emic and etic perspectives of uninsured families within a cultural and geographic community. This understanding may lead to action and, perhaps, policy changes that reduce barriers or increase access. For example, Latina women may have little access to public health department services if their local health department does not have translation capacity. Coming together during a forum educates providers on the ramification of the deficiency and sparks new ideas and innovative approaches to solving problems. AOCD allows for solutions to emerge based on the compilation of realities that come from various perspectives. No one group or sector is responsible for change; rather, direction and change come from a negotiated process. The exchange of perspectives and ideas allows insiders and outsiders to see community health from fresh perspectives and builds partnerships that are stronger and can move forward in directions that positively affect health.

Often emic and etic perspectives are explored and interpreted through the use of qualitative methods. A research partnership may choose to conduct focus groups, photovoice, or qualitative interviews—methodologies that also are outlined within this chapter and the chapter on qualitative research. More quantitative methods may be less useful during the early stages of AOCD because they may not allow for sufficient flexibility and exploration of perspectives. They may, however, provide important data in less exploratory or developmental research.

FOCUS GROUPS

As a qualitative methodology, focus groups provide the opportunity to investigate more fully participant responses and a reaction related to an issue and allow new areas of inquiry to emerge. The methodology can reveal key nuances and perspectives that clinician researchers may not be able to foresee.[18] In brief, focus groups usually are comprised of six to ten participants who are guided through a set of general predetermined open-ended questions outlined in a *focus group moderator's guide*. The guide may be based in a behavioral theory[18] or may allow for theory to explain phenomena to be developed based on the findings, much like a *grounded theory* approach to research.[19] Either way, the guide should be agreed on by the partners. Not only should the research objectives be mutually agreed on, but in addition the selection of focus groups as a methodology and the line of inquiry delineated in the guide should reflect the most meaningful approach and language as agreed on by the research partners.

After an introduction to the focus group process (once of course informed consent to participate has been obtained) and a review of the ground rules (e.g., speaking one at a time, respecting various opinions, maintaining confidentiality), the participants, who sit in an informal circle, respond to open-ended questions. Group interaction is an explicit component of this methodology. Instead of the clinician researcher asking each person to respond to a question in turn, participants are encouraged to talk to one another, asking questions, exchanging anecdotes, and commenting on one another's experiences and perspectives.[18] The moderator must be skilled and experienced in soliciting discussion from all participants in a group, reminding participants that there are no wrong answers, affirming all opinions, and probing for detail. Probing for detail, whether through examples, clarification, or further exploration, is key to successful qualitative data collection, especially when using focus groups. In most cases, qualitative research requires the clinician researcher to allow the design to emerge more fully during the project's evolution[20]; thus, all potential questions cannot be predicted. The moderator's guide is meant to serve as an outline, but the moderator must facilitate the discussion beyond what is written within the guide. The moderator may need to probe into a perspective to develop and understand it more fully. However, the moderator must be skilled at keeping the discussion on track. If the discussion deviates from the purpose of the focus group, the moderator must be able to bring the discussion back to the purpose of the focus group.

Furthermore, besides a moderator, successful focus groups most often involve at least one *note taker* who documents participant speaking order and body language and facial expression that cannot be captured by audio-recording, but may provide important insight during the data analysis and interpretation phases. Because anonymity may be desired, names of participants are not used. Rather, participants may be assigned numbers that are added to the focus group transcript in order to track which focus group participant is saying what. It may not be important to know the name of a participant; however, it may be important to attribute certain quotations to certain participants. Perhaps only one participant has a certain perspective about a topic that she or he continues to reiterate. When analyzing the transcripts, it may be important to recognize this and "weigh" the findings accordingly.

The note taker also documents nonverbal communication. If a participant is noticeably uncomfortable with a discussion topic or the focus group discussion, but does not assert her or his unease or disagreement, such observations should be noted by the note taker. Overall, the note taker is documenting what is going on during the focus group session that may be missed by the audio-recorder and by the moderator who is leading the session.

When applying a CBPR approach to focus group research, the research question, moderator's guide, and recruitment methods must be developed and agreed on by the research partners. Data analysis and interpretation should be completed in partnership to allow community participation.

PHOTOVOICE

Photovoice is a qualitative method of inquiry that:

1. Enables participants to record and reflect on their personal and community strengths and concerns;
2. Promotes critical dialogue and knowledge about personal and community issues through group discussions and photographs;
3. Provides a forum for the presentation of the lived experience of participants through the images, language, and contexts defined by participants themselves.[21,22]

As a CBPR method, photovoice improves quality and validity of research by drawing on local knowledge, developing local theory, and progressing toward action, hallmarks of CBPR. Photovoice engages participants in the following procedure:

- Attending an informational training session to receive a disposable camera, and determine the topic for their first photo-assignment;
- Recording through photography each photo-assignment;
- Sharing and discussing their photographs from each photo-assignment during photo-discussion sessions; and
- Organizing a forum to present their photographic and thematic data to local policy makers and service providers identified by participants as potential collaborators and advocates for change.

BOX 8–3

SHOWED

SHOWED follows the following discussion outline:

What do you *see* here?

What is really *happening* here?

How does this relate to *our* lives?

Why does this concern, situation, strength exist?

How can we become *empowered* through our new understanding?

What can we *do*?

Photo-discussions typically begin with a review and discussion of themes that emerged from the analysis of previous sessions followed by a "show and tell" activity that allows each participant to share her or his photographs and explains how the photographs relate to the photo-assignment. These discussions follow a Paulo Freirian-based[23] model of root-cause questioning and discussion known by the acronym *SHOWED*.[24] At the conclusion of each photo-discussion, the group develops a new photo-assignment by asking, "Given what we have learned so far, what should we explore next?" (Box 8–3).

The photo-discussion data are analyzed like other qualitative data, through exploring, formulating, and interpreting themes. The participants share these themes with local community leaders, service providers, and policy makers. These photographs serve as the medium through which issues are discussed to raise awareness among a core group of allies, mobilize these allies, and plan for change.

Photovoice transitions from knowledge, or raised consciousness around issues and assets, to direct community action. Although a relatively new methodology, photovoice has been found to be a flexible method both in terms of the issues it has been employed to explore and address and the geographically and culturally diverse groups with which it has been employed. It has been applied in partnership with a number of communities including Latino youth in the rural southeast[21]; Chinese women in the Yunnan Province, China[25,26]; homeless men and women in Michigan, USA[26,27]; youth peer educators in Cape Town, South Africa[28]; urban lay health advisors[4]; and public health department leaders and constituents.[29]

IN-DEPTH INTERVIEWS

Individual in-depth interviews are another common data collection methodology. Simply, these interviews are *unstructured*, *semistructured*, or *structured* depending on the research goals. Unstructured interviews are characterized by questions that emerge during the interview process. The research partners may have general topic areas or categories, but the questions are asked as they are formulated in the natural course of the discussion. There is no predetermined wording of questions. This style is more conversational and increases the salience and relevance of questions. A problem with unstructured interviews is that different information is collected from different individuals based on different questions. Less systematic and comprehensive resulting in data analysis challenges, unstructured interviews may be useful for initial exploration or case studies.

Semistructured interviews by definition provide more structure for the interviewer. Topics and issues to be explored and discussed are specified in advance, often in outline form. Semistructured and structured interviews require an *Interview Guide* that leads the interview process. Leading a semistructured interview, the interviewer decides the order and sequence of the questions during the course of the interview. The interviewer may probe for detail and develop questions and their wording during the interview process. Data collection using this approach is more systematic than an unstructured approach. Because semistructured interviews remain conversational and situational, gaps in data can be explored and closed. However, important and salient topics may be inadvertently omitted as interviews go in directions that jeopardize comparability among interviews and the data collected.

Structured interviews are often well defined prior to the interview. The sequence and exact wording of questions are determined in advance. All interviewees are asked the same basic questions in the same order and manner. Structured interview questions may be *open-ended*, *closed-ended*, or may comprise a combination of question type. Open-ended questions tend to provide more exploratory, developmental, and contextual data. Data from open-ended questions tend to be more descriptive. For example, an open-ended question that was asked of health-care providers who worked in an undocumented Latino community in western North Carolina was: "If you could envision an answer to meeting the health-care needs of the local Latino community, what would that vision be?" Answers were descriptive and complex, providing not only ideas about how to meet health-care needs in the short and long term but also providing further information about what health-care needs existed in this community and root-cause explanations.

Closed-ended questions are characterized by response options that are *fixed*. Participants choose among a list of fixed responses. An example of a closed-ended question from a structured interview that was implemented among Latino men was: "Some men report having sex with other men for a variety of reasons; have you ever heard of a male friend having sex, including oral or anal sex, with another man?" The response options were: "yes," "no," and "refused to answer."

Closed-ended response options simplify data collection and analysis because many questions can be asked in a shorter period of time and responses can be easily aggregated and compared. The disadvantage, however, is that participants must fit their experiences and feelings into predetermined categories. This may distort the true experiences and feelings of the participants by limiting their response choices.

Conventionally, closed-ended interviews collect data on a topic by asking individuals questions to generate statistics on the group or groups within a community or population that those individuals represent. Closed-ended interviews do not tend to be formative or exploratory; rather they ask questions about a variety of factors that influence, measure, or are affected by health. For example, population-based closed-ended interviews may document and follow health status. Or, closed-ended interviews may provide local data and a baseline for evaluation of intervention efforts. Once a local CBPR research project has evolved and developed a research intervention to effect change (e.g., individual behavior change, community change, or policy change), interviews comparing baseline data to intervention implementation or post-intervention follow-up may provide information on how well the intervention is working.

When applying a CBPR approach to research, the research question, measurement method (e.g., interview, questionnaire), and items or questions to be included must be agreed on by the partnership. Furthermore, recruitment and administration must be decided. Questions that the research partnership will want to answer include:

1. How will participants be recruited?

2. What type of compensation will be provided?

3. Who will administer the interview or questionnaire?

4. Will interviewers be used or will the questionnaire be self administered?

Clinician researchers may think she or he knows the best way to recruit interviewees and administer a questionnaire. However, community partners may provide great insight that may increase recruitment and response rates as well as honesty.[30,31] What seems scientifically sound to the researcher (e.g., reducing bias and threats to validity) may inhibit responses.

Qualitative and Quantitative Data Analysis

Analyzing and interpreting any type of dataset, whether qualitative or quantitative, using a CBPR approach is challenging. Ensuring the participation of all partners in the process can be daunting. Clinician researchers may have a variety of data analysis software to choose from that community partners may not have the time or energy to learn and apply. Thus, creative ways to examine data may be necessary. During qualitative data analysis, community partners may review and provide perceptions on potential themes through their detailed reading and rereading of the transcripts separately. The clinician researcher may choose to analyze the data using a software program to code and retrieve non-numeric data (e.g., Nvivo,™ ATLAS.ti,™ Ethnograph,™ NUD*IST™). Coming together, the research partners compare broad categories, resolve discrepancies, and begin the process of interpreting the findings through the development of themes. Themes based in qualitative data are most often directional. Themes can be described as potential assertions that can be tested later through subsequent research. Examples of themes developed using qualitative analysis include: (1) *While participants realized the importance of condoms for disease prevention, attitudes about condoms were negative.* Or, (2) *Undocumented Latinos felt that they have no right to access public health care.* Quotations are usually abstracted from the qualitative transcripts to illustrate the themes.

Quantitative data analysis poses similar challenges. How can community members who lack quantitative data analysis skills or software training participate in this phase? Clinician researchers should communicate and solicit feedback with the partnership throughout the process, keeping the partners up to date on statistical approaches, decisions, and rationales. Furthermore, clinician researchers should not assume that partners do not want to be engaged in the analysis process. After all, CBPR promotes knowledge gain and skill development on all sides. As mutual co-learners, the clinician researcher is learning about the partners, and the partners are learning as well; this learning may include learning data analysis skills.

Because it may be difficult to ensure participation of community partners, getting a commitment from one, two, or three partnership members who are from the community may be key to the data analysis. The whole research partnership may choose not to participate in all phases of the research process, but establishing guidelines that ensures community member representation in each phase of the process is key.

In this section only a few research methods were described. However, it is important to note that a clinician researcher need not give up traditional research methods, but may infuse a CBPR approach into any research method.

How to Get Started with CBPR

Beginning the exciting work of CBPR requires a clear understanding of partnership principles and values, as outlined earlier in this chapter. Below, we outline some pivotal tasks in the clinician researcher's effort to engage in CBPR.

Network, Network, Network

A first task in the CBPR process requires the development of a network with other individuals with a similar health area of interest or concern. A relatively easy and helpful initial contact for a clinician researcher may be a local public health department. Providers and educators within health departments around the country are likely to have connections with community agencies working with those affected by and committed to a variety of health concerns. A clinician, administrator, nutritionist, intern, health educator, and/or epidemiologist within the public heath department might already be working with established local health coalitions or community groups. Dialoguing with these potential partners represents a good solid start in this process well worth the effort. A simple review of a public health department Web site or a telephone call to the health department may offer initial guidance and contacts, and an informational interview with a health department staff member will begin the networking process essential throughout CBPR. As a clinician researcher, "casting a wide net" facilitates networking contacts to identify overlapping health concerns and resources including talent that may support the research process synergistically. Networking also initiates the establishment of trust that is key to success in CBPR.

The clinician researcher must understand the local communities and work in collaboration and not through confrontation with local *stakeholders*. Stakeholders typically are individuals who are affected by the health issue and those who will be part of the research as well as affected by the research and subsequent change. Stakeholders may include community members experiencing the problem, service providers, and community leaders, among others.

In addition to contacting and networking with a local public health department, making connections with those health-care providers in the community who are working with individuals and community members affected by overlapping health and research priorities may provide access to potential partnerships. The clinician researcher benefits from thinking broadly about those individuals providing care, for example, nutritionists, exercise physiologists, physical therapists, mental health providers, and so forth. Furthermore, becoming familiar with other local CBOs, community agencies, and service providers and making contact with representatives from a variety of organizations will yield helpful results. The clinician researcher may find partnerships for CBPR within the local school system, within clinical settings, clubs and service agencies, and/or retirement communities, just to name a few more possibilities.

Build Trust

Once commonalities have been identified, the clinician researcher will begin a process of *trust building.* Trust building is especially important as communities have felt exploited as "living laboratories" for universities and medical centers. Often communities are inundated by research projects that test hypotheses, but do not benefit the community itself. Communities may be apprehensive about committing to a partnership, and the clinician researcher may have to overcome a history of research that had not been initiated and conducted in a respectful manner.[32] A positive relationship is built by working hand-in-hand with community members. A clinical researcher may choose to spend some up front time volunteering with a CBO and serving on local health coalitions. This serves several purposes. First, it advances a genuine and mutually respectful relationship between key community leaders whom the clinician researcher may need and want to have on board as partners in the research. It also may open other doors for the clinician researcher; the clinician researcher may be unfamiliar with all the players and may use the opportunity to identify informal community leaders who may be committed to a health issue and may be interested in the research. Third, it allows the clinician researcher the opportunity to understand community structure, decision-making processes, and levels of influences through their role as a participant observer. Finally, community service allows community members to interact with the clinician researcher in a setting that is not focused on any one agenda. By selecting the right place to volunteer and thus "being seen," the clinical researcher may build community trust by association. If a Latino-serving CBO is well respected by the local Latino community, for example, the clinician researcher will gain more immediate community favor, and thus participation, by spending time there. Such volunteer work

not only builds trust, but also begins to offer emic and etic community perspectives to the researcher.

Building trust includes building relationships. Relationships between community members, CBO representatives, and clinician researchers may involve informal "working" meetings that allow partners to get to know one another. Community events such as street fairs, church gatherings, and forums as well as parties and celebrations are ideal places for community members, CBO representatives, and clinician researchers to come together. These types of opportunities show commitment to the community and allow for community members, CBO representatives, and clinician researchers to know one another better. This improves trust and communication, which improve the research process.

Maintain Relationships

Key to trust building is *relationship maintenance.* While it may be easy to feel that one has built trust, one must remember that partnerships cannot be taken for granted. When things are being done "behind the scenes," gaps in the research process may exist and the clinician researcher must be present within the community. For example, getting a research protocol approved by an Institutional Review Board (IRB) or Ethics Committee may require a delay in the research process, and the clinician researcher will want to touch base with partnership members to provide informal status reports. This is important because the clinician researcher does not want to lose community interest, motivation, or momentum. Community members do not necessarily understand the confusing steps that universities, research institutions, and funders require. Time should be spent in dialogue explaining these steps and their rationales.

Negotiate Partnerships

Subsequent tasks in the CBPR process include bringing key community members and CBO representatives together. This may be easy if an existing community health coalition exists. The coalition can determine whether a health issue is of interest or not. If a health issue is not a focus and yet data suggest that it contributes profoundly to morbidity and morality of the community that the coalition serves or represents, the clinician researcher has to walk the fine line between asserting what she or he perceives to be "important information" and staying true to the priorities of the community. Exploring community priorities and perspectives may yield important insight or even areas of overlap. It may require creatively thinking or thinking "outside of the box." The clinician researcher may provide data and increase awareness affirming her or his agenda or she or he may decide that the community-prioritized agenda is important and an opportunity to build trust and relationships. Nothing can impede or destroy trust between a clinician researcher and the community members and representatives than going into a community to "fix" something without asking community members what they prioritize. After all, community members are not inanimate objects to be "fixed"; they are potential partners. CBPR requires the clinician researcher to be flexible, and no place is this flexibility more evident than in adaptations related to community priorities. A clinician researcher may be required to take on other priorities as identified by the community in the spirit of partnership.

The clinician researcher may begin with a community–health coalition or may need to identify and build a network of community members and CBO representatives. Through this network, the foundation of a partnership may be established. Although growth may occur throughout, this network may evolve into a partnership through the hard work of those involved.

A Case Study: HoMBReS: Hombres Manteniendo Bienestar y Relaciones Saludables

HoMBReS, an acronym for "Hombres Manteniendo Bienestar y Relaciones Saludables" (Men Maintaining Wellness and Healthy Relationships), is an ongoing intervention research project in rural North Carolina that was initiated through a partnership of lay community members; CBO representatives; and university clinicians, practitioners, and researchers. A community health coalition known as Chatham Communities In Action (CCIA) was formed in 1991 as part of the North Carolina Community-Based Public Health Initiative (CBPHI).[33,34] Because of the rapidly growing Latino community in North Carolina and their early success in diabetes prevention within the African American community, CCIA, with expanding Latino membership, chose to explore Latino health concerns within their local community. A subgroup of CCIA members met with university researchers to develop a plan to explore the health-care priorities of the Latino community.

The research partnership, which initially was comprised of current members of CCIA, came together first to determine how to further develop and expand the research partnership to include more Latino representation. Local Latino-serving CBOs and interested individuals who were not involved with CCIA were invited to participate in the process. This inclusion required time to build trust and clarify goals. These added members included representatives from the Liga Hispana de Fútbol de North Carolina (LHFNC; North Carolina Hispanic Soccer League), a local Latino *tienda* (grocery store), and a farm worker advocacy group. LHFNC is a nine-county Latino soccer league of more than 1600 adult men. The League president along with various other interested League members became involved in the research partnership. The research partners continued to build trust among themselves as research partners through personal relationships, genuineness, respect, and "being there." CCIA representatives and the researcher spent many dinners meeting with League representatives. While CCIA had a history of working with the university, these relationships could not be assumed or taken for granted. Building and maintaining trust and communication always play a paramount role in CBPR.

The expanded research partnership gained consensus on the research aims. This process involved answering two equally important questions. First, the research partners had to ask themselves: "What do we want to know?" Second, the partners had to ask themselves: "Why do we want to know it?" This distinction is important because a CBPR approach recognizes that knowledge for knowledge sake (i.e., the accumulation of scientific knowledge) is important, but the immediate application of knowledge to affect the health and well-being of the participating community is equally important. The researchers had many curiosities and theories they wanted to explore, but the research partners kept the focus on the practical use of knowledge gain.

In this study, the research partnership chose to explore health concerns of Latino men primarily because the majority of Latinos newly arrived to the United States are male, especially in rural North Carolina. The research partnership had to come to agreement on the research and recruitment design and the roles and contributions of the partners. They decided to use focus groups to explore health priorities. The partnership created, reviewed, revised, and approved the focus group moderator's guide. The League president recruited focus group participants and two partnership members served as the focus group moderator and the note taker. The note taker was the university researcher who was fluent in Spanish. A Latino-serving CBO hosted the focus groups. Five focus groups were completed.

The first stage of data analysis involved members of a subgroup from the research partnership sorting the focus group transcripts into broad content categories. After the initial sorting process was complete, the analysis team came together to compare broad categories and begin the process of interpreting the findings into conceptual domains. Once themes were created, they were presented to the research partnership and other community members including LHFNC members for *number checking* and interpretation. This was done by writing themes on flip charts, after which they were presented to the research partners and representatives from the soccer league and reviewed, discussed, and revised. Several iterations of this process were completed.

Findings were disseminated through community and national presentations, report writing, and manuscript development. Because action is a key component of CBPR, the findings also were used for funding proposals and intervention design. All partners had equal access to the findings. For example, CBO representatives used findings for grant preparation, and community members used the findings to advocate for Latino men's health. It was through the initial focus groups that sexually transmitted diseases (STDs) and human immunodeficiency virus (HIV) infection were identified as priorities by members of LHFNC as well as the potential use of the social network of the League to develop, implement, and evaluate a lay advisor as an intervention.

The HoMBReS intervention study was funded by the Centers for Disease Control and Prevention (CDC). The goal of this CBPR study is to reduce the risk of STD/HIV infection among Latino men through the development, implementation, and evaluation of a lay health advisor intervention. In brief, HoMBReS is a three-year quasi-experimental research study with five interrelated objectives:

1. Develop and implement a lay health advisor intervention to reduce STD/HIV risk behaviors among members of the soccer league.

2. Evaluate the efficacy of the intervention by comparing soccer league members in the intervention to those in the delayed-intervention comparison group using self-reported sexual risk behaviors and utilization of STD/HIV counseling, testing, and treatment services;

3. Evaluate the changes experienced by the lay health advisors by being trained and serving as lay health advisors;

4. Assess the feasibility of engaging a soccer league in implementing a lay health advisor intervention designed to reduce STD/HIV transmission among Latino men;

5. Assess the feasibility of collecting biomarker data (i.e., urine for chlamydia and gonorrhea testing) from soccer league members, comparing those who have lay health advisors and those who do not.

The lay health advisors, known as *"navegantes"* ("navigators"), are trained to provide STD/HIV prevention education and prevention information and service and resource referral to their teammates. They serve as: (1) sources of STD/HIV information and refer-

ral; (2) opinion leaders to change risky behavioral norms resulting from culturally infused male gender socialization; and (3) community activists to work with organizations such as the local public health department to better address the needs and priorities of Latino men in culturally relevant approaches.

This project has been successful in the recruitment and training of a strong cadre of *navegantes* because of the initial "buy in" of the LHFNC. Without their history of interest, support, and involvement, the idea for STD/HIV primary prevention and the use of team members as lay health advisors would not necessarily have been considered. Had it been considered, the risks would have been higher because buy in would not have been garnered. Less knowledge about whether men would want to participate in a 16-hour, theory-based training and what that training should include would have left more opportunity for misjudgment on the part of the researcher. Instead, the partnership approach has ensured that fewer problems are incurred and when unavoidable roadblocks do occur, creative solutions that have a higher potential for success can be explored because more perspectives and options can be considered.

Discussion

It has been asserted that ensuring the health of the public will require clinicians, researchers, and agencies to join forces with organizations of both community insiders and outsiders to generate new understandings of health status, explore health status predictors and measures, and uncover innovative ways to effect change in the health status within vulnerable communities.[3,35] While this may seem logical, the process of partnership requires time to establish trusted relationships, create a research infrastructure, and develop a history of partnership. The investment of time to build these trusted relationships is essential for successful CBPR; however, this effort is well worth the expense in time, energy, and resources if true changes in health status are to occur.

While no road map exists to conduct CBPR, it is important to note that often individuals, including researchers and community members, who are unfamiliar with CBPR confused *community placed* with *community based*. Community-placed efforts simply imply that clinicians, practitioners, and researchers leave the traditional institutions such as the hospital or medical center and go into the community to do their work. However, community-based efforts are more than going outside physical walls of these traditional institutions. CBPR requires partnering with communities and basing efforts in the reality and structures *preferred* by the community.

Health research through community partnership is a viable mechanism for health promotion and disease prevention[3,6,8,9] because CBPR improves the quality of research, increases community capacity, and advances positive health outcomes by

1. Bringing community members into a study as partners, not just as *subjects*;

2. Using the knowledge of the community to understand health problems and design meaningful interventions;

3. Connecting community members directly with how research is done and how it is used;

4. Providing immediate benefits from the results of the research to the community that participated in the study.

CBPR can be infused into any research design. In this chapter, four methodologies were briefly presented and one case study was described. Clinician researchers who are exploring the use of CBPR in their own research and practice should remember two important issues. First, key to using a CBPR approach is the inclusion of lay community members, CBO representatives, health department and other agency staff, and university personnel, including students and faculty researchers.[4] Together these partners must share control over all phases of the research process, including: community assessment, issue definition, development of research methodology, data collection and analysis, interpretation of data, dissemination of findings, and application of the results to address community concerns. CBPR recognizes that lay community members themselves are the experts in understanding and interpreting their own lives.

Second, CBPR is committed to movement toward action or intervention. This action may be loosely defined, including: community organizing and mobilization; the development of new and authentic community member and agency partnerships with concrete tasks; and measurable plans for action with assigned responsibilities and defined timelines. The actions may be focused on immediate changes to improve health-related conditions, such as changes in a clinical practice protocol that increases adherence to an AIDS medication, policies that increase access to community mental health services, or even improved lighting on an outdoor neighborhood running/walking track to encourage utilization. Furthermore, actions may be focused on long-term changes in social determinants of health, such as improved racial equality in administrative and political representation through community mobilization and organization.

CBPR not only may be an effective tool to addressing the complex health problems facing vulnerable communities but it is also considered to be a just and democratic approach to research; as has been noted by community members, "Nothing about me, without me,"

implies that community members have a *right* to participate in all aspects of the research endeavor. While CBPR is a challenging approach to research, CBPR offers the clinician researcher the opportunity to participate in a co-learning process of sharing resources, knowledge, skills, and attributes to increase the quality and validity of research. Increased quality and validity thus yield more effective interventions and improved health outcomes.

References

1. Centers for Disease Control and Prevention, Agency for Toxic Substances and Disease Registry Committee on Community Engagement. Principles of Community Engagement. Atlanta, GA: US Department of Health and Human Services, 1997.

2. Green LW. From research to "best practices" in other settings and populations. American Journal of Health Behavior 2001;25: 165–178.

3. Institute of Medicine. Unequal Treatment: Confronting Racial and Ethnic Disparities in Health Care. Washington, DC: National Academy Press, 2003.

4. Israel BA, Schulz AJ, Parker EA, Becker AB. Review of community-based research: Assessing partnership approaches to improve public health. Annual Review of Public Health 1998;19: 173–202.

5. Minkler M, Wallerstein N. Introduction to community based participatory research. In Minkler M, Wallerstein N (eds). Community-Based Participatory Research for Health. San Francisco, CA: Jossey-Bass, 2003, pp. 3–26.

6. O'Toole TP, Felix Aaron K, Chin MH, Horowitz C, Tyson F. Community-based participatory research: opportunities, challenges, and the need for a common language. Journal of General Internal Medicine 2003;18:592–594.

7. Viswanathan M, Eng E, Ammerman A, et al. Community-Based Participatory Research: Assessing the Evidence. Rockville, MD: Agency for Healthcare Research and Quality, 2004.

8. Wallerstein N, Duran B. The conceptual, historical, and practice roots of community-based participatory research and related participatory traditions. In Minkler M, Wallerstein N (eds). Community-Based Participatory Research for Health. San Francisco, CA: Jossey-Bass, 2003, pp. 27–52.

9. Wandersman A. Community science: bridging the gap between science and practice with community-centered models. American Journal of Community Psychology 2003;31:227–242.

10. Eng E, Blanchard L. Action-oriented community diagnosis: a health education tool. International Journal of Community Health Education 1991;11:93–110.

11. Eng E, Parker EA. Natural helper models to enhance a community's health and competence. In DiClemente RJ, Crosby RA, Kegler MC (eds). Emerging Theories in Health Promotion Practice and Research: Strategies for Improving Public Health. San Francisco, CA: Jossey-Bass, 2002; 126–156.

12. Lincoln YS, Guba EG. Paradigmatic controversies, contradictions, and emerging confluences. In Denzin NK, Lincoln YS (eds). The Handbook of Qualitative Research. Thousand Oaks: Sage, 2000; 163–188.

13. Habermas J. The Theory of Communicative Action. Cambridge, MA: Polity Press, 1984.

14. Steuart GW. Planning and evaluation in health education. International Journal of Health Education 1969;2:65–76.

15. Cassel JC. The contribution of the social environment to host resistance: The Fourth Wade Hampton Frost Lecture. American Journal of Epidemiology 1976;104:107–123.

16. Kauffman KS. The insider/outsider dilemma: Field experience of a white researcher "getting in" a poor black community. Nursing Research 1994;43:179–183.

17. Steuart GW. Social and behavioral change strategies. In Phillips HT, Gaylord SA (eds). Aging and Public Health. New York: Springer, 1985.

18. Rhodes SD, Hergenrather KC. Exploring hepatitis B vaccination acceptance among young men who have sex with men: facilitators and barriers. Preventive Medicine 2002;35:128–134.

19. Glaser BG, Strauss AL. The Discovery of Grounded Theory: Strategies for Qualitative Research. Chicago: Aldine, 1967.

20. Sandelowski M, Davis DH, Harris BG. Artful design: writing the proposal for research in the naturalist paradigm. Research Nursing and Health 1989;12:77–84.

21. Streng JM, Rhodes SD, Ayala GX, et al. Realidad Latina: Latino adolescents, their school, and a university use photovoice to examine and address the influence of immigration. Journal of Interprofessional Care. 2004;18:403–415.

22. Wang C, Burris MA. Photovoice: Concept, methodology, and use for participatory needs assessment. Health Education and Behavior 1997;24:369–387.

23. Freire P. Pedagogy of the Oppressed. New York: Herder and Herder, 1970.

24. Shaffer R. Beyond the Dispensary. Nairobi, Kenya: Amref, 1983.

25. Wang C, Burris MA, Ping XY. Chinese village women as visual anthropologists: a participatory approach to reaching policymakers. Social Science and Medicine 1996;42:1391–1400.

26. Wang CC, Yi WK, Tao ZW, Carovano K. Photovoice as a participatory health promotion strategy. Health Promotion International 1998;13:75–86.

27. Killion CM, Wang CC. Linking African American mothers across life stage and station through photovoice. Journal of Health Care for the Poor Underserved 2000;11:310–325.

28. Moss T. Youth put their world on view. Children First 1999;3: 3–35.

29. Wang C. Picture this: a snapshot of health in Contra Costa. Unpublished Report, 1988.

30. Angell KL, Kreshka MA, McCoy R, et al. Psychosocial intervention for rural women with breast cancer: The Sierra–Stanford Partnership. Journal of General Internal Medicine 2003;18:499–507.

31. Lauderdale DS, Kuohung V, Chang SL, Chin MH. Identifying older Chinese immigrants at high risk for osteoporosis. Journal of General Internal Medicine 2003;18:508–515.

32. Rhodes SD, Yee LJ, Hergenrather KC. Hepatitis A vaccination among young African American men who have sex with men in the deep south: psychosocial predictors. Journal of the National Medical Association 2003;95:31S–36S.

33. Margolis LH, Stevens R, Laraia B, et al. Educating students for community-based partnerships. Journal of Community Practice 2000;7:21–34.

34. Parker EA, Eng E, Laraia B, et al. Coalition building for prevention: lessons learned from the North Carolina Community-Based Public Health Initiative. Journal of Public Health Management and Practice 1998;4:25–36.

35. Institute of Medicine. The Future of Public Health. Washington, DC: National Academy Press, 1988.

Section Resources

Besides the references cited within this chapter, supplemental resources are listed below.

CBPR

Minkler M, Wallerstein N, eds. Community-Based Participatory Research for Health, 1st ed. San Francisco: John Wiley & Sons, 2003.

Eng E, Moore K, Rhodes SD, Griffith D, Allison L, Shirah K, Mebane E. Insiders and outsiders assess who is "the community": Participant observation, key informant interview, focus group interview, and community forum. In Israel BA, Eng E, Schulz AJ, Parker EA (eds). Methods for Conducting Community-Based Participatory Research for Health, In press.

Agency for Healthcare Research and Quality: *http://www.ahrq.gov/clinic/evrptpdfs.htm]pr*

Campus-Community Partnerships for Health: *http://depts.washington.edu/ccph/*

Preventing Chronic Disease: Public Health Research, Practice and Policy: *http://www.cdc.gov/pcd/issues/2004/jan/03_0024.htm*

Community-Based Participatory Research: Implications for Public Health Funding: *http://www.cprc-chmc.uc.edu/reports/APHA%20article%20on%20CBPR.htm*

Building a Truly Engaged Community Through Participatory Research: *http://www.med.wright.edu/ra/re/2003/tindall.html*

Creating Partnerships, Improving Healththe Role of Community-Based Participatory Research: *http://www.ahrq.gov/research/cbprrole.htm*

Photovoice

Photovoice: *http://www.photovoice.com/*

Moss T. Photovoice. Children First 1999;3(27):28–29.

Wang C. Project: Photovoice involving homeless men and women of Washtenaw County, Michigan. Health Education and Behavior 1998;25(1): 9–10.

Wang C. Photovoice: A participatory action research strategy applied to women's health. Journal of Women's Health 1999;8(2): 185–192.

Wang C. Using photovoice as a participatory assessment and issue selection tool. In Minkler M, Wallerstein N (eds). Community-Based Participatory Research for Health. San Francisco: Jossey-Bass, 2003, pp. 179–196.

Wang C, Burris MA. Empowerment through photo novella: portraits of participation. Health Education Quarterly 1994;21(2):171–186.

Wang C, Cash JL, Powers LS. Who knows the streets as well as the homeless? Promoting personal and community action through photovoice. Health Promotion Practice 2000;1(1):81–89.

Health Disparities

Institute of Medicine. Engaging the Public in the Clinical Research Enterprise: Clinical Research Roundtable Workshop Summary. Washington, DC: The National Academies Press, 2003.

Wallerstein N. Powerless, empowerment, and health: implications for health promotion programs. American Journal of Health Promotion 1992;6:197–205.

Qualitative Research

Patton M. (ed). Qualitative Research and Evaluation Methods, 3rd ed. Thousand Oaks, CA: Sage, 2002.

Miles M, Huberman AM. Qualitative Data Analysis, 2nd ed. Thousand Oaks, CA: Sage , 1994.

Krueger RA, Casey MA. Focus Groups: A Practical Guide for Applied Research, 3rd ed. Thousand Oaks, CA: Sage, 2000.

Morgan DL, Krueger RA. The Focus Group Kit, Volumes 1–6. Thousand Oaks, CA: Sage, 1997.

chapter 9

Data Analysis

Meredith A. Davison, PhD and Bruce R. Niebuhr, PhD

Chapter Overview

This chapter provides a very basic overview of data analysis and statistical tests. It covers some of the common statistical techniques in an effort to provide a first step in the use and understanding of statistics. A large number of books are available on statistics and statistical analysis, and every research and graduate student should have at least one as a reference and guide. A course in statistics should be part of every Master of Science research-based program and, at least, reviewed in professional entry level master's programs. Readers who are truly interested in research should take more than one statistics and research design course above and beyond what is offered as part of their physician assistant (PA) education. Decisions about data analysis must be made prior to data collection and data analysis planning is part of research methodology. Even if you are fairly confident and accomplished in the use and understanding of statistical tests, it is advisable to consult a statistician about the type of analysis that should be used in any investigation. Very careful attention should be paid to the type of research being conducted and the type of data produced by the investigation. Careful selection of the right statistical tests will result in proper data analysis and greater confidence in your conclusions drawn from the results of analysis. If you are a master's or doctoral student, it would be wise to include a statistician on your thesis or dissertation committee. In your career as a practicing PA, an understanding of data analysis is a key part of your interpretation of the medical and research literature

Introduction

Why should PAs use statistics? Although some PAs earn advanced degrees and engage in health-related research, most are, first and foremost, clinicians. All PAs have been exposed to statistical analysis in their education, but many may not see the relevance to their clinical practice. The most basic use of statistics for the PA is to assist in the understanding of research articles that help in the making of important decisions for our patients and practice. A good understanding of the basis for what you do is a key to success. Every day the practicing clinician is called on to make determinations and decisions as to the most cost-efficient, least harmful, or most appropriate types of treatment. These decisions are best made by a careful reading and understanding of the medical literature and, frequently, this understanding requires a basic understanding and appreciation of statistical analysis and inference.

As a PA, you are not expected to be a statistician. Biostatistics is as much a specialty as orthopedic surgery or pediatric oncology. If you conduct a research study, consultation with a biostatistician is essential. However, regardless of whether you ever participate in clinical research, you must be able to critically analyze the results of research studies in order to make decisions regarding clinical diagnosis and treatment. Your primary objectives as a PA engaged in evaluating the data analysis of a research study are to:

1. Become intimately familiar with the types of data produced in the study.
2. Become familiar with the most common statistics. This will allow you to read a journal article and grasp its use of statistics and how the study's conclusions flow from the statistical analyses and results.
3. Understand the rationale behind the selection of statistical analyses and how specific analyses test the study's hypotheses.

In this chapter, we look at descriptive statistics, inferential statistics, styles of results presentation, and statistical reference texts and computer software options. Mathematical and statistical formulas are used sparingly in this chapter. If you are deeply involved in research, you may wish to conduct some data analyses yourself. Further detailed statistical descriptions can be found in the references listed in the bibliography for this chapter and elsewhere in the book.

Levels of Measurement

The first step in deciding on the appropriate type of statistical analysis is to determine the level of measurement that is to be used. As a general rule of thumb, the higher the level of measurement, the more information can be ascertained from the data. The most basic level of measurement is the nominal. With this level of measurement you have divided your responses into named groups or categories; for example, you might have asked your subjects to choose the group to which they belong: surgical PAs, primary care PAs, other PAs. Their choice allows you, the researcher, to group your subjects by category.

The nominal level of measurement limits the researcher in the type and number of statistical and mathematical analyses. Primarily, only descriptive analysis or summary can be used. These are data that let you tell how many subjects fall into each category. In the preceding example, you might find that of the 100 PAs you surveyed, 23 percent reported that they worked in surgery, 61 percent were in primary care, and the remaining 16 percent were in other specialty areas (Table 9–1). Some common nominal data types are gender, race, religion, eye color, year in school, home state, and so forth. Think of nominal data as information that helps you categorize something or someone.

Ordinal measurement provides an ordering (sometimes ranking) between variables. However, the distance between each option is not defined. For example, you may want to allow your subjects to indicate their degree of agreement or disagreement with a series of statements. There is no defined distance between "Agree" and "Strongly Agree" or "Neutral" and "Disagree." One of the most common forms for ordinal measurement is the Likert scale. The traditional use of the Likert scale is to provide the subject with a statement and ask for the level of agreement or disagreement with that statement. The true Likert scale is a five-point scale with the following terms:

| **Strongly Agree** | **Agree** | **Neutral** | **Disagree** | **Strongly Disagree** |

Table 9–1
Definitions of Data Types

Data Type	Definition	Example
Nominal data	Data that categorize	Gender, eye color, race, PA class, practice specialty
Ordinal data	Data defined by an ordering, but the distance between the choices or values is not defined	Likert scales, preference scales, rankings
Continuous data	Data with numeric values. Two types: interval and ratio.	Numbers
A. Interval data	Data with a defined interval between the values, but with by no true zero (0) value	Ambient F° temperature. "0" does not indicate a total lack of temperature. It is a value on a scale. The temperature interval difference between +61° and +62° is the same as the interval difference between −61° and −62°
B. Ratio data	Data with an absolute zero (0) value, where "0" means there is a total absence of what is being measured.	Visual acuity, range of motion, blood pressure, lead level, etc.

While offering more possibilities for deeper analysis than nominal measurement, ordinal measurement still has some limited options for statistical analysis. There are a number of types and ways to use ordinal scales. Ranking is also a form of ordinal scale. Many ordinal scales are referred to as verbal frequency scales. Often numbers are used for the responses to ordinal measurements. There is a real debate on whether these numbers can be analyzed using those statistical tests for ratio or interval data. Again, it is best to consult a statistician.

It is only when you use the two higher levels of measurement, interval and ratio, that you have the possibility of using the most sophisticated statistical analyses. Interval measurement differs from ratio measurement because the ratio measurement has an absolute zero. With both of these measurements, there is an ordering of the points, but the distance between each point on the scale is exactly the same. An example of these measurements would be asking your subjects for the specific number of years since they had graduated. A year is a well defined and understood time interval with the difference between any consecutive points the same. That is, the difference between 4 years and 5 years is the same as between 65 years and 66 years. Also, the presence of a value "0" does not mean total absence of the variable being studied. For example, "0" degrees Fahrenheit does not mean the total absence of heat because you can have negative temperature numbers indicating lesser heat. Thus "0" in this case is just one value on the scale. Continuous data (interval and ratio) offer the researcher the option of the highest level of analytical operations and enable the possibility of using inferential statistics to determine the significance of differences or associations between groups and variables.

The four levels of measurement and the appropriate types of statistical analyses to be used with each level are illustrated in Figure 9–1. Remember, parametric (normal) and nonparametric describe the distribution of the subjects or variables. Continuous data are always considered to have a normal distribution.

Descriptive Statistics

A study may yield a large amount of raw data that are organized and summarized by descriptive statistical methods. Summarizing the data is the essential first step in understanding the results and moving to the inferential methods used to test the hypotheses of the study. Think of description statistics as those processes or analyses that "describe" the sample.

In summarizing data by descriptive methods, the key concepts are measures of central tendency and measures of variability. In common parlance, measures of central tendency are averages; the most commonly used measures are the **mode**, **median**, and **mean**. The mode is the most frequently occurring score. The mode can be found for variables that are nominal, ordinal, interval, or ratio. The median is the midpoint of a sequence of ordered variables or the point at which half the values are above and half are below. Medians can be found for ordinal, interval, or ratio variables. The mean is the sum of the scores divided by the total number of scores. The mean can be found for interval or ratio variables only.

To illustrate the measures of central tendency, look at the following hypothetical data set: The length of stay in the cardiac care unit for seven patients following an acute myocardial infarction was 3, 12, 5, 7, 5, 8, and 9 days, respectively. Calculation of the statistics can best be understood by first sorting the data from lowest to highest numerical value: 3, 5, 5, 7, 8, 9, 12.

The mode, the most frequently occurring score, is 5.

The median, the midpoint of the ordered scores, is 7.

The mean, the sum of the scores divided by the total number of scores, is 7 (3 + 5 + 5 + 7 + 8 + 9 + 12 = 49)/ 7 = 7.

By themselves, measures of central tendency can give a misleading view of the data. For example, suppose that for a second group of five patients the length of stay was 7, 7, 7, 7, and 7 days, respectively. Just as in the first data set, the mean of this data set is 7. What differs, how-

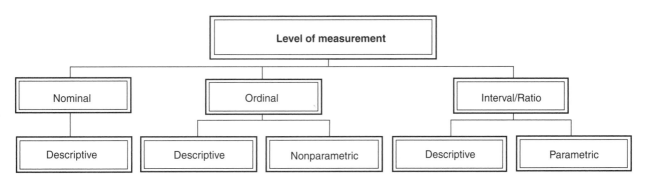

FIG. 9–1. Levels of measurement.

ever, is the variability of the data. In the first group, the length of stay varies from 3 to 12 days, while in the second group everyone had the same length of stay, 7 days.

The three measures of variability most commonly reported in biomedical research are the range, standard deviation, and standard error of the mean. The simplest measure, the range, is the difference between the highest and lowest scores. In the first example, the range is $12 - 3 = 9$. The range gives an easy "rough cut" of the variability, yet it is of limited value because it does not include all of the data in the computation. As a point of interest, the range of the second example is "0" $(7 - 7 = 0)$. This is a statistical anomaly.

The standard deviation (SD) is the key descriptive statistic used to report variability. Mathematically, it is the square root of the variance. The variance is the sum of the squared differences between each score and the mean, divided by the number of scores minus one. The formula is:

$$\sum (X - M)^2 / (n - 1),$$ where X = each score, M = the mean, n = the total number of scores in the sample.

To calculate the SD for the first data set example provided, you would thus need to take the square root of the following equation:

$$[(3 - 7)^2 + (5 - 7)^2 + (5 - 7)^2 + (7 - 7)^2 + (8 - 7)^2 + (9 - 7)^2 + (12 - 7)^2] / (7 - 1)$$

This calculates out to be the square root of 9, or 3. The standard deviation for this sample data set, therefore, is 3 days. The standard deviation is the most commonly reported measure of variability.

The standard error of the mean (SEM) is another descriptive statistic. The SEM is the standard deviation divided by the square root of n, and it represents an estimate of the population standard deviation. In this example, the SEM is 1.1, found by calculating 3 divided by the square root of 7.

Although computation of such basic statistics can be done with a statistical calculator, use of computer software such as Microsoft Excel® or SPSS® is preferred, particularly because the software allows for data management as well as computation. In addition, use of statistical software minimizes the opportunity for computational error.

Inferential Statistics

Following a determination of the level of measurement and a descriptive review of the data, the researcher needs to again ask the original question, "What is the hypothesis?" Most research studies are looking for either a relationship between two or more variables or for a difference between the variables. In the study described earlier, we might be interested in determining whether there is a relationship between a patient's age and the days that he or she spent in the hospital following surgery. In this case, we would probably perform a correlational analysis to determine the potential relationship between these variables. Conversely, if we had hypothesized that the length of stay in the hospital cardiac care unit was shorter in patients who had HMO insurance as compared to patients with PPO insurance, we would analyze for a difference between patients with PPO insurance and patients with HMO insurance. The length of stay in days would be the variables analyzed.

What statistical tests to use is a big question. Literally hundreds of tests are available and we cannot even begin to provide information on all of them or the situations in which they would be used. Decision trees for choosing an appropriate statistical test are provided in Figures 9–2 and 9–3 as a guide for some common statis-

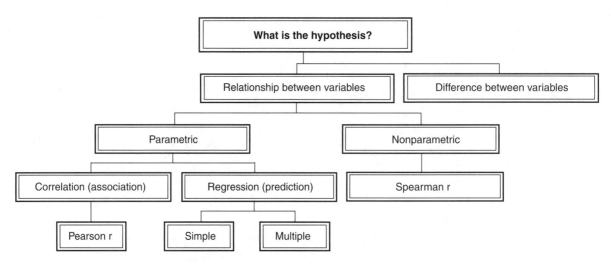

FIG. 9–2. Testing for relationship between variables.

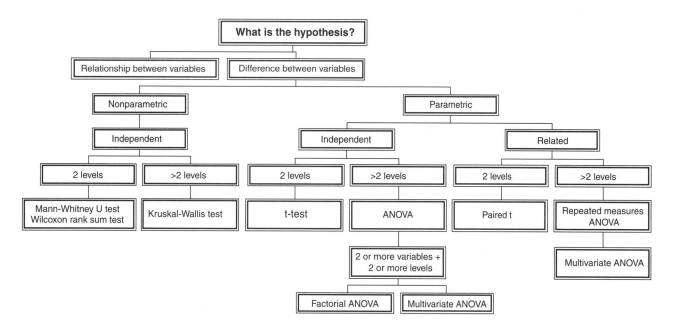

FIG. 9–3. Testing for differences between variables.

tical tests. More information on making a decision is included at the end of the chapter. Again, consulting a statistician is very helpful in making the right decisions.

Inferential statistics are the tools used to draw inferences about the results, particularly to test the hypotheses of a study. A researcher studying a problem usually formulates a hypothesis, such as "Aspirin reduces the incidence of colon cancer" or "Problem-based learning produces better clinicians than conventional instruction." Statistical inference, however, is based on the testing of a null hypothesis. The null forms of the above hypotheses are "Aspirin has no effect on the incidence of colon cancer" and "There is no difference in the effectiveness of clinicians trained/educated by problem-based learning and conventional instruction." So as you develop your investigation, you need to consider how you state your problem(s).

In statistical hypothesis testing, the researcher and statistician select a significance level, called alpha (α). By convention, α level is set at .05 or .01 and reported without a zero in front of the decimal point ($\alpha<.05$). Remember, the alpha level is set by the investigator and can be some other level besides the ones indicated. However, you should have very good reasons for not selecting .05 or .01. When the data are analyzed, the statistical test yields a "p" value. The "p" value is the probability that the observed result could occur by chance if the null hypothesis is true. (The p value is also reported without a zero in front of the decimal point.) If $p < \alpha$, then the researcher rejects the null hypothesis; if $p > \alpha$, then the researcher retains (does not reject) the null hy-

pothesis. If you reject your null hypothesis, you are saying that the opposite of your null hypothesis is true. If you retain your null hypothesis, you are saying that the null hypothesis is true.

Hypothesis Testing: Nominal Data

Much of medical data are nominal, that is, one patient has a diagnosis of breast cancer; another patient has a second myocardial infarction. Epidemiological studies also yield nominal data, that is, a patient did or did not get the disease. In a study about smoking, the null hypothesis might state, "Smokers are not more likely to have asthma." For this study, with smoking or not smoking as the variables, an appropriate statistical test would be the Chi-square (X^2). (We realize that asthma is a multifactorial disease.) The Chi-square test is simply a way to determine whether an event has occurred more frequently than it would be expected to occur by chance alone. The observed X^2 value will be compared to the probability of the event occurring by chance. For example, if the X^2 value was greater than 3, the probability is $< .05$, and the researcher can reject the null hypothesis and conclude that there is sufficient evidence that asthma occurs more commonly in individuals who have a history of smoking cigarettes.

Epidemiological studies use nominal data to produce incidence and prevalence rates. For example, a study is conducted in which it is found that cigarette smokers were seven times as likely as those who never smoked to develop lung cancer or heart disease. In other words, the relative risk for smokers was 7. Is this risk statistically significant? For these data, a confidence interval is used to test the null hypothesis that the relative risk = 1 (no added risk of smoking). If the researchers set α = .05, then they use a confidence interval of 95 percent. Note that confidence intervals are reported as percentages; in this case, the confidence interval was found by calculating [(1 − .05) × 100 percent] to give 95 percent. The 95 percent confidence interval for these results was 3.5. This means that we are 95 percent confident that the actual relative risk is between 3.5 and 10.5 (7 ± 3.5). Because the 95 percent confidence interval does not include the relative risk value of 1, the result is significant at the .05 level. The researchers reject the null hypothesis and conclude that smoking increases the risk of lung cancer or heart disease.

Analysis of Continuous Data: Measures of Association

Determining the association or relationship between two continuous (interval or ratio) variables is a common statistical problem. What is the relationship between a woman's age and hemoglobin level? What is the relationship between blood sugar level and weight in those who are obese? The measures of association most commonly used are subsumed under the general labels of correlation and regression.

Suppose a clinical educator is concerned about the reliability of an examination on interpreting electrocardiogram (ECG) tracings. Ten students were given the test on Monday, and then were given a parallel test on Tuesday. The exam scores are then correlated. Because the student scores are an interval/ratio variable, the

Pearson product-moment correlation technique can be used. The result of the statistical manipulation is an "r" value. This is the correlation coefficient. Values of the correlation coefficient, r, vary between −1 (a perfect negative correlation) and +1 (a perfect positive correlation). An r value of 0 indicates a lack of relationship. The scores on the two days are graphed in Figure 9–4.

An experienced researcher/statistician would view Figure 9–4 and interpret the correlation as moderate to strong (based on the clustering of the points about a straight line) and as positive (as Monday's scores increase, so do Tuesday's). The correlation in this example was computed as r = .88. Is the result statistically significant? The null hypothesis of no relationship between the two tests results (variable) or (r = 0) is tested at the .05 level of significance. The observed p value is less than .05. The researcher rejects the null hypothesis that there is no relationship and concludes that there is a significant correlation between the two administrations of the EKG exam, supporting its overall reliability.

Beyond the simple two-variable correlation are multivariate regression techniques in which relationships among many variables can be examined simultaneously. Regression is based on the concept of predicting one variable from another and assigning a probability to these predictions. Complex multisite clinical trials and epidemiological studies are increasingly being conducted utilizing these methods; including discriminant function analysis, factor analysis, path analysis, and logistic regression. In addition, nonparametric correlational techniques exist for ordinal and ranked data. Discussion of these methods, however, is beyond the scope of this book.

Analysis of Interval/Ratio Data: Comparisons of Groups

The most powerful statistical tests are those that use interval and ratio data from well designed studies. Ordinal data are often treated as if they were interval and then subjected to such tests. A decision as to whether this is acceptable or not is best left to the statistician. Remember, even if an ordinal value is assigned a "number" value, the distance between the ordinal values is not defined. There is a technique, Rasch Analysis, which can be used with ordinal data, but it is beyond the scope of this basic introduction to completely discuss it.

An example of an appropriate use for analyzing the difference between groups would be study of a new antihypertensive drug that is tested against a placebo. Fifty patients are randomized to either treatment or control. After a course of treatment, the diastolic blood

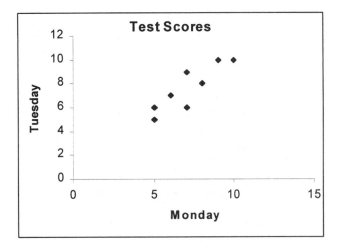

FIG. 9–4. Example of correlation.

pressure (DBP) is measured. The appropriate statistic to test the null hypothesis is the t-test (sometimes referred to as the Student t-test). The researchers set the α level at .05. Statistical analysis produces a t value. In this case, $t = 6.4$. Using t tables, this would yield a p value less than .05, so the researcher could reject the null hypothesis and conclude that the new drug significantly reduced diastolic blood pressure.

The t-test (or Student t-test) is perhaps the most commonly used parametric test. It allows for a comparison of the means of two groups. (A paired t-test allows for comparison of the same group at two different times.) The t-test is actually a special case of a general set of methods collectively known as analysis of variance (ANOVA). Data from complex designs can be analyzed with ANOVA because multiple independent variables, multiple dependent variables, and many subgroups can be tested within a single ANOVA model.

An example, using only one independent variable and one dependent variable will be described. Imagine that you wanted to test the efficacy of over-the-counter pain remedies for nonmigraine headache pain. A total of 25 patients were randomly assigned to one of five drugs in a double-blind manner. The patients were asked to rate their headache pain on a 0–10 scale (where 0 is no pain and 10 is excruciating pain). The null hypothesis was "There is no difference in pain ratings between pain medications." The α level was .05. After one month, the results were compiled and summarized. Then the researcher could perform an ANOVA test that produces an F ratio. The F value is reported with its associated degrees of freedom that are based on the number comparison groups and the number of subjects. If the F yielded a score that had a p value $<.05$ the researcher could reject the null hypothesis that there were no significant differences among the drugs. However, what drugs were different from which others? Several multiple comparison procedures are available, selection of which can be left to the biostatistician. (F values are found in tables produced with most statistical texts.)

Meta-Analysis

Many evidence-based medicine and review studies now rely on the technique of meta-analysis to simultaneously analyze a large number of research studies to determine a conclusion. Meta-analysis can be defined as a process of using statistical integration of the results of several studies to reach an independent conclusion. It is not a singular statistical test or procedure, but rather a general conceptual approach. The steps to completing an overview are:

1. Define the hypothesis.
2. Collect the "units of measurement," the research studies that have been done on the defined topic.
3. Convert the statistics to common values, for example, z scores, r values, and so forth.
4. Compute the measures of central tendency, variability, and prediction from the accumulated data measures.
5. Determine whether the hypothesis is supported.

The advantages of meta-analysis are several: it is precise, rigorous, and quantifies decision-making about a question. It is also more objective than traditional literature reviews because the criteria for the inclusion of studies are explicitly stated for inclusion of multiple related studies, which limits bias. In addition, a meta-analysis is replicable, at least in theory, and any reviewer should reach the same conclusion if the same criteria are applied to the same studies. There are, however, disadvantages to the technique of meta-analysis. Since a variety of studies that have utilized different measures of the same variables and statistical techniques in different settings are combined, there may be a loss of information about individual differences in the various studies. Size effect may be an issue, particularly if some studies are large and some are small. Chapter 6 discusses evidence-based medicine and has additional information on meta-analysis.

Choosing the Right Statistical Tests

Our best advice is to consult a statistician. With that said, here is a general and simple guideline to some statistical testing.

Choosing the right statistical procedures to test your data can be a major challenge. After all, there are people who make their careers dealing with statistical analyses (statisticians or biostatisticians). For most master's level students and for some doctoral students, the math of statistical analysis can be overwhelming. We should all be thankful for calculators, computers, and statistical programs that can do the math for us. With these resources, the math problem is eliminated. Unfortunately, the main problem is still with us: What statistics do I need to make sense of my data?

There are many ways to answer this question. The easiest is to have a statistician do the work for you. This is the thing to do if you are not a student. If you are a student, we suspect that thesis and dissertation committees would take great umbrage at that suggestion. They would be right, of course. For students, learning the process of scientific investigation is what is really important in your thesis or dissertation work. Despite the thoughts of your committee, it probably helps if you can consult with a faculty member with expertise in statistics. We advise having a person with statistical expertise on your committee. Whether you are a student or not, you must still have some understanding for the application of statistical tests and what they mean, even if a statistician does all the work for you. Whether you are a student or not, we hope that the following guidelines and definitions will help you make some decisions about the best statistical analyses for your data.

You analyze your data for a purpose. The statistical tests that you do should be the most appropriate for your purpose. Primarily, we analyze data to summarize, to identify relationships, and to identify significant differences while controlling confounding variables for all three purposes. The results of your analysis will allow you to extrapolate your findings to a population or group within a population. The choice of statistical tests should be optimal for the type of data to be analyzed and meet the purposes of that analysis.

First: Before selecting statistical tests, you must know what kind of data you have. Are your data continuous, ordinal, or nominal? As review, please remember that

1. *Continuous data* are unlimited values that are equally spaced along a continuum. They are numbers or values of some sort that have a defined interval or ratio. Examples of continuous data are blood glucose levels, weight, cholesterol levels, weeks, years, or months, IQ scores, mathematic value, and so forth. These are numbers.

2. *Ordinal data* are those values that have some type of ordering, but with no defined spacing between categories. Examples of ordinal data would be the approximate time of day that a person takes their medications: On arising, before breakfast, before lunch, mid-afternoon, with supper, at bedtime. Likert scale descriptors are ordinal: Strongly Agree, Agree, Neutral, Disagree, Strongly Disagree. There is order, but no defined interval.

3. *Nominal data* are categorical designations. There is no order to the categories. Examples of nominal data are marital status, gender, race, profession, church, year of PA education, and so forth. Many times these are descriptive terms that define a category.

Investigations can involve all three or only one type of data. Your choice of statistical analysis will depend on the type of data and how you want to compare the data.

Second: Once you are clear on the type of data you will use, you must decide whether your data is parametric or nonparametric.

1. Parametric analyses assume that a normal or near-normal distribution exists. For continuous data, one should always assume a normal or near-normal distribution.

2. Nonparametric analyses do not assume a normal distribution exists. Nonparametric analyses can be done on data with a normal distribution, but they are not as powerful as parametric tests. Nonparametric tests are normally used for ordinal data. Continuous data can be converted to nominal or ordinal form. An example of this would be grouping ages into age ranges.

Third: You need to consider the relationships of your data. Are your results "paired" or "matched?"

1. Result data is considered "paired" if you measure the same sample after some intervention (example: a treatment of some type).

2. "Matched" samples are those where the characteristics of the experimental group are "matched" as closely as possible to a control group.

Fourth: Next the number of variables plays a part in your choice of tests. Do you have one, two, or more than two variables (multiple)? Of course, you should know your variable type: independent or dependent. You can have no independent variables, one independent variable, or more independent variables. Remember your tests are for each dependent variable. You may have more than one dependent variable for each independent variable, but multiple measurements are for each dependent variable only.

There are many, many statistical tests. Below are some of the more common tests with brief descriptions of the test. Please remember that many other tests exist that may be more appropriate for your study. Also, be aware that these tests may be used in studies that are not included in the examples. The examples are representative and not inclusive or exclusive.

Fifth: What are you trying to explain?

1. The relationship between variables.

OR

2. The difference between variables

Different tests are used to examine these relationships and differences. (Remember, you can do both in a study.)

Statistical Tests

The following are brief descriptions designed to provide a starting point and basic concept for the reader, so that you can begin to develop an idea of what tests should be used. Many more statistical tests are available and the choice of tests depends on study design and types of data.

Descriptive statistics: the trends of the sample: mean, mode, median, range. They are used to describe a sample and sometimes to demonstrate how a sample may reflect a population, if that population's measures of central tendencies (descriptive statistics) are known.

***t*-Test**: tests the difference between two group's means; can be one-tailed or two-tailed, can be used with paired or unpaired samples. Some times called the "Student's *t*-test."

Analysis of variance (ANOVA): tests the differences among the means of three or more groups for one or more variables.

Analysis of covariance (ANCOVA): a variant of ANOVA that allows adjusting for extraneous, additional, or undesired variables.

Cochran's Q: compares proportions between three or more matched groups

Multiple analysis of variance (MANOVA): a variant of ANOVA that allows for study of multiple dependent variables. If MANOVA results are significant, ANOVA must be done for each variable.

Duncan range test: a test used after ANOVA to identify means that differ significantly from one another.

Kendall's rank-correlation: a test of the linear relationship between two ordinal or continuous variables.

Kruskal–Wallis test: a nonparametric test for significance when using two independent samples. It is comparable to ANOVA, but for rank-ordered data.

Mann–Whitney test: sometimes call Mann–Whitney U test; it is the nonparametric equivalent of a *t*-test. Used with ordinal data for two groups.

Multiple regression analysis: any statistical method that evaluates the results of more than one independent variable on a single dependent variable.

Newman–Keuls test: tests for significance in multiple post hoc comparisons.

Pearson's chi square test: a test of categorical data for goodness of fit or comparisons of observations.

Pearson's product moment test: a test of the strength of linear relationship between two interval or ratio (continuous) variables.

Regression analysis: a method of predicting dependent variable variability by one or more independent variables. Most commonly used are Simple Linear Regression and Multiple Linear Regression.

Spearman rho: a test that demonstrates the degree of relationship between two ordinal variables that may not have normal distribution.

Tukey test: a test to identify significantly different groups after ANOVA.

Wilcoxon rank sum test: a test of significance for two paired ordinal data samples.

Tests that can be used with continuous data:

Descriptive statistics
t-test
ANOVA
ANCOVA
MANOVA
Duncan range test
Kendall's rank correlation
Pearson's product moment test
Regression analysis
Multiple regression analysis
Tukey test

Tests that can be used with ordinal data:

Descriptive statistics
Cochran's Q
Kendall's rank correlation
Kruskal–Wallis test
Mann–Whitney U test
Pearson's chi square test
Spearman's rho
Wilcoxon ranked sum test

What Test to Use?

The choice of the right statistical test can add power to your findings and provide strong support for outcomes and conclusions. There are so many tests (many more than the ones listed here) that for most investigators, particularly novice investigators, confusion reigns. Many investigators will use those tests that are most familiar to them and ones that they have used in the past. Understanding what a statistical test can and cannot do is very valuable, but limiting if one only uses a few tests for all their work.

The number of dependent and independent variables influences your choice of tests, then the category of your data (nominal, ordinal, continuous). Remember you are testing each *dependent variable* separately. Now you must ask one big question: What do I want to do; summarize, explore relationships, or test for significance of difference?

What follows is one way to some useful tests.

To summarize data: Descriptive statistics

To examine the frequency relationship of ONE variable to a theoretical distribution:
          Chi-square test for goodness of fit

To examine the frequency relationship of TWO variables to each other:
          Chi-square test for association

To examine the measured relationship between two variables:

| For ordinal data: | Spearman's rho test |
| For continuous data: | Pearson's correlation coefficient |

To examine the measured relationship of multiple variables:
          Multiple regression test

To examine the significance of difference between groups:

For one group: *t*-test

For two independent groups:

| Ordinal data: | Mann-Whitney U test |
| Continuous data: | Independent samples *t*-test |

For two related groups

| Ordinal data: | Wilcoxon matched pairs test |
| Continuous data: | Paired samples *t*-test |

For multiple independent groups:

| One independent variable: | One-way ANOVA |
| Multiple independent groups: | MANOVA |

For multiple related groups: Repeated measures ANOVA

Presentation of Results

Results of a study are presented in the body of the text, tables, figures, and charts. Examples of these methods have been included in this chapter. A general rule to follow is that extensive results are most easily comprehended when presented in graphical form (e.g., figure or chart) and least comprehended when written into the body of the text. Tables provide the middle ground. A second general rule is that tables and figures do not stand alone and must be referred to and described in the body of the text. See Chapters 10 and 13 for more information.

Summary

In this chapter, we presented an abbreviated and short overview of some of the most common types of statis-

tics used in biomedical and educational research. As a PA participating in a research project, you will wish to understand the rationale behind the biostatistician's selection of statistical analyses and how those analyses test the study's hypotheses. The chapter and bibliography also give you the basis to perform selected data analyses yourself.

Suggested Readings

General References

Bruning JL, Kintz BL. Computational Handbook of Statistics, 4th ed. Glenview, IL: Scott, Foresman, 1997.
Campbell MJ, Machin D. Medical Statistics: A Commonsense Approach, 2nd ed. New York: John Wiley & Sons, 1993.
Lang TA, Secic M. How to Report Statistics in Medicine: Annotated Guidelines for Authors, Editors, and Resources. Philadelphia: American College of Physicians, 1997.
Norman GR, Streiner DL. PDQ Statistics, 3rd ed. Philadelphia: B.C. Decker, 2003.
Dawson B, Trapp R. Basic & Clinical Biostatistics 3rd ed. New York: Lange Medical Books-McGraw-Hill, 2001.

Analysis of Variance and Regression

Cohen P, Cohen J, West SG, Aiken LS. Applied Multiple Regression/Correlation Analysis for the Behavioral Sciences. Mahwah, NJ: Lawrence Erlbaum, 2000.
Glantz SA, Slinker BK. Primer of Applied Regression & Analysis of Variance, 2nd ed. New York: McGraw-Hill, 2000.
Harris R. ANOVA: An Analysis of Variance Primer. Itasca, IL: FE Peacock, 1994.
Winer BJ, Brown DR, Michaels KM. Statistical Principles in Experimental Design, 3rd ed. New York: McGraw-Hill, 1991.
Menard SW. Applied Logistic Regression Analysis. Thousand Oaks, CA: Sage, 1995.

Computer Software

Software for statistical analysis is categorized as (1) general purpose data analysis programs with statistical application; (2) complete statistical packages; and (3) special purpose software for specific applications. All the software listed here are for personal computers running Microsoft Windows 98/2000/XP or Apple Macintosh operating systems.

General Purpose Data Analysis Software

Microsoft Excel. Part of Microsoft Office, general purpose software includes several statistical tools.
Third-party statistical add-ons are available. Web Address: *http://www.microsoft.com*

Complete Statistical Packages

MiniTab. MiniTab, Inc., State College, PA. A very popular package for student use. Web address: *http://www.minitab.com*
SAS. SAS, Inc., Cary, NC. A comprehensive and powerful package. Web address: *http://www.sas.com*
SPSS. SPSS, Inc., Chicago. A comprehensive and powerful package. Web address: *http://www.spss.com*

Specialized Software

Mathcad. Mathcad, Inc., Cambridge, MA. Calculation software, not only for statistics. Web address: *http://www.mathsoft.com*

SigmaPlot. SPSS, Inc., Chicago. Primarily a graphing package, it includes extensive analysis tools. Web address: *http://www.spss.com*

Design-Expert. Stat-Ease. Software set up and analyzes experimental designs. Web address: *http://www.statease.com*

Web Sites Particularly Useful to Faculty and Students in Teaching and Learning Statistics

StatLib. A system for distributing statistical software, data sets, and information. Archives of statistical routines and data sets. Maintained at Carnegie-Mellon University. Web address: *http://lib.stat.cmu.edu/*

Rice Virtual Lab in Statistics. Excellent simulations and demonstrations. Maintained at Rice University. Web address: *http://www.ruf. rice.edu/~lane/rvls.html*

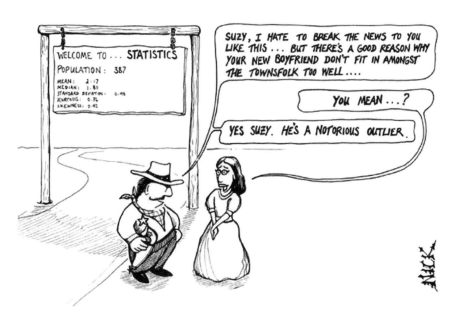

Reprinted by permission of Nick D. Kim.

chapter 10

Results

Anthony A. Miller, MEd, PA-C

Chapter Overview

This chapter discusses the results of data analysis. In most manuscripts, the results section is the shortest and most graphically displayed section. It is important that findings and, particularly, key findings be presented clearly in a logical fashion. The Results section should be the "facts and only the facts" in nature. Your (the author's) opinions, interpretations, and conclusions belong elsewhere. The use of graphs and charts can be useful methods for presenting your results. The "Results" section of a research paper (sometimes referred to as the "Findings" section) is considered one of the more important parts of a research report. It is where key findings and outcomes of the study are reported, and where the author indicates whether or not the hypotheses were supported or rejected. All preceding sections of a research report are designed to build up the reader's anticipation for what is shared in the Results. In addition, it should be consistent and articulate well with the preceding Methods and Data Analysis sections, which describe how the research was conducted, how the data were obtained, and how the data were analyzed. As an author and investigator, you must be careful to keep any interpretation or opinion from the Results section that could bias a reader's interpretation.

The Discussion section, which describes the interpretations of the author and his/her conclusions of the results, is where you get to give your opinions. The Results section should be neutral in every aspect, allowing readers to form their interpretations and conclusions.

Ultimately, the Results section is the "meat" of the research report. The results provide the base for all that follows and, most importantly, for interpretation of meaning. The Results "comprise the new knowledge that you are contributing to the world."[1]

Introduction

The Results section should present only key findings related to the research question, *without* the author's conclusions as to the meaning and importance of the data. That will follow in the next section. The Results section is typically one of the shortest parts of the research report and should be written clearly and succinctly, generally in the past tense for experimental or quasi-experimental studies and in the present tense for descriptive studies. For ethical reasons, all of the key findings should be reported, not just those supporting the hypotheses. Information or descriptions of what was done belong in the preceding Materials and Methods (or

Methodology) section and should not be included in the Results section. Remember you have already presented what you did and how the data was handled.

A common mistake for beginners is to report raw data rather than summarize and present findings. The author's primary task in the Results section is to provide a picture of the data for the reader. The following excerpts provide an example of a poorly written segment in the results section and an improved segment.

Facts Without Interpretation:

"The mean resting pulse rate for the 10 control subjects was 74 $\pm$ 4 (SD) compared to the 12 athletes with a mean resting pulse rate of 66 $\pm$ 5 beats per minute."

Improved:

"The mean resting pulse rate was 11 percent lower in the 12 athletes than in the 10 control subjects [66 $\pm$ 5 (SD) vs. 74 $\pm$ 4 beats per minute, $p < 0.05$)]."

Note that the magnitude of the difference (11 percent) is reported as well as the probability value indicating that the difference was statistically significant. The first example is ambiguous and leaves it to the reader to determine the meaning of the data whereas in the second example, the author informs the reader what is important about the data.

The Results

The Results usually begins with a description or profile of the subjects, and includes relevant demographics so that the reader has a good understanding of how representative your sample was compared to the population. Numbers, percentages, and central tendency statistics should be used to describe the study sample. An example of this section might read: "Fifty-two percent ($n = 78$) of the physician assistants responded to the survey. There were 20 questionnaires returned 'unforwardable.' Of the respondents, 33 were male and 45 were female. The average age was 34 (SD = 6.5)."

After describing the sample used in the study, the researcher should report the results of the statistical analysis with sufficient detail to permit the reader to determine that appropriate analyses were conducted and that the hypotheses were supported or not. For descriptive research, frequencies, ranges, and measures of central tendency should be reported. For experimental or quasi-experimental research, the inferential or associational statistics should include the test statistic, the direction, and the level of probability. Several recent editorials and reports have advocated for the inclusion of confidence intervals (95 percent level) or effect size in results; arguing that statistical significance indicated by a p value is insufficient alone.[2–5]

Authors are cautioned about use of the word "significant" in their discussions of data. "Significant" means "statistically significant" or "clinically significant" when written in the scientific literature. Some authors see events or numbers of subjects affected as significant because of the event or the effect. However, something is significant only if the statistics support that judgment.

Some experts recommend that the rationale for choosing each statistical procedure be included in this section.[6] This may be particularly important if a novel approach to analysis was used or if the procedure is considered controversial. It may be appropriate to include such descriptions in the Methodology section. Always assume that your readers have a working knowledge of statistics and research design. If you are publishing in the medical or scientific literature, don't insult your readers.

Finally, indicate which hypotheses were supported. Indicate clearly whether the reference is to the null hypotheses or research questions or to alternate hypotheses. At this point, do not explain or interpret why the hypotheses were or were not supported; the data should speak for themselves. Your *conclusions* regarding the results should be described in the "Discussion" section of your work.

Tables and Figures

For the sake of clarity and brevity, tables and figures are often used to show research results. Because many researchers use commercially available software for data analysis, the tables and figures are often preliminarily produced through the software program before the author begins writing the text of the Results section. Tables and figures are particularly useful for readers when numerical results are reported. Avoid the temptation of making the topic sentence (first sentence of the paragraph) a reference to a table or figure. For example, "Table 1 presents the means and standard deviations for the control and experimental groups," is an inappropriate topic sentence and provides no useful information. A better example is "The experimental group showed a 10 percent improvement in scores over the control group (Table 1)."

Many commercial programs (Microsoft Excel,® Harvard Graphics,® SPSS®) make it fairly easy to create your own tables and graphs, often without having to reinput your data. Because tables and figures are more expensive to reproduce compared to reporting your results in the body of the text, it is important to use only those graphic elements that are most important to highlight your primary findings. If a large number of numbers, statistics, or other results need to be presented, a well organized table is ideal.

Tables are used to organize, condense, and list numerical data. Examples include those that describe your study sample (Table 10–1), compare groups (Table 10–2), or show correlations (Table 10–3). The types of analyses performed on the research data dictate the format for display in a table. For qualitative or nonexperimental studies, tables are sometimes used to summarize or compare textual information (Table 10–4).

Tables should be clear enough to stand alone without explanation in the text. Although tables can be helpful for the organization and display of your important findings, they can be confusing if not used and constructed appropriately. Be sure to include all the relevant information for the type of statistic you are reporting (e.g., test statistic, degrees of freedom, probability value, direction, and so forth in the case of inferential statistics). Because readers tend to make comparisons first horizontally and from left to right, primary comparisons in tables should be shown horizontally.[7] Box 10–1 lists additional general guidelines for the use and construction of tables and Table 10–5 shows the elements of a typical table.

Graphs, charts, pictures (including radiographs), computer-generated images, diagrams, flowcharts drawings, and so forth are considered figures. There are a variety of types of graphs, including line graphs (Figure 10–1), scatter graphs, histograms (Figure 10–2), bar graphs (Figure 10–3), and pie charts.*

Generally speaking, frequency polygons and histograms are used to plot frequency distributions. Bar graphs are different from histograms in that the columns are separated and are best used to show comparisons for two or more groups when the independent variables are categorical. When developing graphs (particularly bar graphs), care must be taken to ensure that proportions of the width and height provide an accurate display of the data and are not misleading because of dimensions of the graph. Line graphs are used to show the relationship between two quantitative variables.[8] The intersection of the x- and y-axes in the lower left-hand corner is typically zero (0). If there is discontinuity

Table 10–1
Demographic Profile for PA Class of 1999 ($N = 20$)

	Mean	Median	Low–High	SD
Age	28.10	26.50	23–44	5.44
Previous health-care experience (months)	21.95	20.50	12–60	10.97
High school GPA	3.09	3.00	2.25–3.90	0.42
Undergraduate GPA	3.36	3.32	3.00–3.90	0.31

Table 10–2
Comparison of Job Profiles for PA Classes of 1997 and 1999*

Demographic Characteristic	Class of 1997 ($n = 12$)		Class of 1999 ($n = 18$)	
	Frequency	Percent	Frequency	Percentage
Specialty				
Family medicine	6	50	6	33
Pediatrics	1	8	4	22
General internal medicine	1	8	0	0
Emergency medicine	3	25	2	11
General surgery	1	8	3	17
Other	0	0	2	11
Location				
Urban	5	42	8	44
Suburban	5	42	7	39
Rural	2	17	2	11
Practice type				
Solo	1	8	5	28
Group	4	33	7	39
Hospital	5	42	5	28
Other	2	16	0	0
Unknown	0	0	1	5

*Note. Because of rounding, percentages may not all total 100.

---

*Note that all data portrayed in the tables and figures for this chapter are fictitious and are not intended to represent any actual research study or source. Readers should consult the Instructions for Authors section in journals to which they intend to submit manuscripts for specific guidelines and requirements.

Table 10–3
Intercorrelation Between Educational Outcomes for PA Students ($N = 50$)

	HS GPA	College GPA	Basic Science GPA	Clinical GPA	Packrat Exam	PANCE
High school GPA	—	.77**	.54*	.36	.12	.11
College GPA		—	.79*	.23	.34*	.17
Basic science GPA			—	.22	.27	.21
Clinical GPA				—	.56*	.62*
Packrat exam					—	.81**
PANCE						—

Note. GPA = grade point average; * $p < .05$. ** $p < .01$.

Table 10–4
Comparison of Common Cardiac Murmurs

Diagnosis	Location	Timing	Pitch	Quality
Aortic stenosis	Second right inter-costal space, sternal border	Midsystolic	Medium	Coarse
Aortic regurgitation	Base, patient seated and lean-ing forward	Early diastolic	High	Blowing
Mitral stenosis	Apex, patient in left lateral decubitus position	Diastolic	Low	Rumble
Mitral regurgitation	Apex	Holosystolic	High	Blowing

Adapted from Seidel HM, Ball J, Dains J, Benedict G. Mosby's Guide to Physical Examination, 4th ed. St. Louis: Mosby-Year Book, 1999, pp. 467–471.

in an axis, it should be represented by a pair of diagonal lines (-//-) to show the missing portion. The dependent variable is generally plotted on the vertical (y) axis.

Many software programs create graphs using color, but most journals reproduce the graphs in black and white. Therefore it is important to ensure that sufficient contrast exists between adjacent bars. Also keep in mind that, although certain other features (e.g., three-dimensional bar graphs) available with commercial software may enhance the appearance of the report for a PowerPoint® presentation, the graphs may not reproduce well when the size is decreased and they are reproduced in black and white. The American Medical Association recommends a shading contrast of at least 30 percent.[7] In addition to using shading to distinguish bars or pie chart sections, many commercial programs allow different patterns such as cross-hatch marks. A

good rule of thumb is to use the y (vertical) axis for the dependent variable or variable of interest.[8] Pie charts are used to show percentages or proportions of different quantities (e.g., types of students in a cohort) and are used to display results of descriptive research. Box 10–2 provides a quick review of general guidelines for the construction of graphs.

When presenting results in paragraph or graphically, double and triple check your numbers and data for accuracy. Make sure that your graphs present your results accurately and clearly. An inadvertent mistake in one number could make readers cautious about all your results. More than one error will probably make them ignore everything, even if your conclusions and interpretations are correct.

A major advantage in using figures and tables is that a large amount of data can be presented in a relatively

BOX 10–1

Guidelines for the Construction of Tables

1. Choose a clear and specific table title so that there is no confusion about the contents.

2. Number tables consecutively using Arabic numbers from the beginning of the report and label them accordingly.

3. Use subheadings for the columns and rows. Format cells so the data are clear and easy to read; often alignment on decimals is preferred.

4. Limit your information and include only material related to your descriptive title. For example, do not mix sample demographics with inferential statistics.

5. Do not explain your table in the text; it should speak for itself. However, the table first must be identified in the text (e.g., Table 1).

6. Use table formats that are consistent and that conform to the publisher's guidelines. However, table formats should be consistent within the report. Check with the publisher in advance to see if it prefers submission of tables and figures separately or incorporated within the text.

7. Avoid excessive lines. Generally, vertical lines for columns are not needed, but there should be sufficient space between the columns so the table is easy to read. In addition, tables should be limited to one page.

8. Be sure to include appropriate units of measure (e.g., mg/dL).

From Wiersma W. Research Methods in Education: An Introduction, 7th ed. Needham Heights, MA: Allyn and Bacon, 2000, pp. 393-394. Copyright © 2000 by Pearson Education, adapted by permission of the publisher.

Table 10–5
Anatomy of a Table

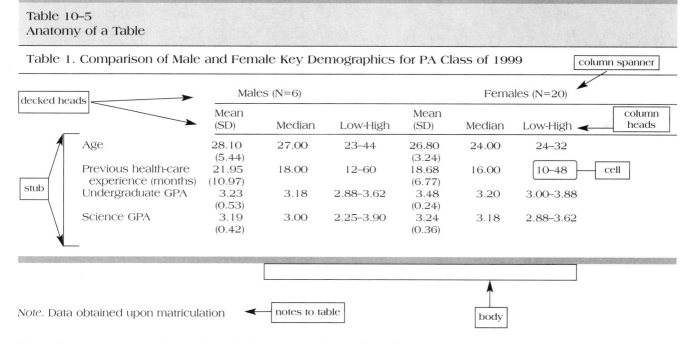

Table 1. Comparison of Male and Female Key Demographics for PA Class of 1999

	Males (N=6)			Females (N=20)		
	Mean (SD)	Median	Low-High	Mean (SD)	Median	Low-High
Age	28.10 (5.44)	27.00	23–44	26.80 (3.24)	24.00	24–32
Previous health-care experience (months)	21.95 (10.97)	18.00	12–60	18.68 (6.77)	16.00	10–48
Undergraduate GPA	3.23 (0.53)	3.18	2.88–3.62	3.48 (0.24)	3.20	3.00–3.88
Science GPA	3.19 (0.42)	3.00	2.25–3.90	3.24 (0.36)	3.18	2.88–3.62

Note. Data obtained upon matriculation

The table example above shows the typical construction for a table with descriptive data and includes identification of the different parts. The title identifies the table numerically and the description informs the reader of the purpose. Notice how decked heads are used in order to show the comparisons between the two groups. The left column identifying the independent variables is called a stub. In some cases, a stub head is included if it is not clear what the column contents consist of. In this table, the stub head could have been labeled "Key Demographics." Table notes can be used to clarify the data or certain cells, provide probability information (see correlation table), or define abbreviations. Publishers (or instructors) may have specific requirements for tables or require that it conform to a particular style manual so it is best to consult with them in advance.

From Wiersma W. Research Methods in Education: An Introduction, 7th ed. Needham Heights, MA: Allyn and Bacon, 2000. Copyright © 2000 by Pearson Education, adapted by permission of the publisher.

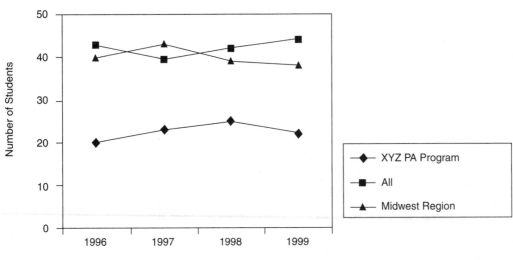

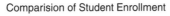

FIG. 10-1. Example of a line graph.

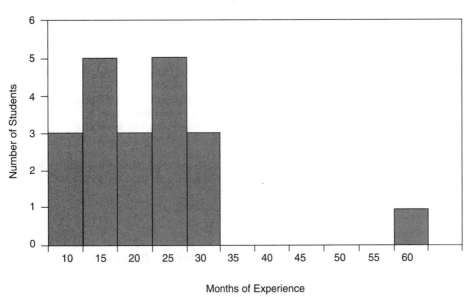

FIG. 10-2. Example of a histogram.

small print space. Number of pages is important to publishers. Well designed figures and tables can provide a large amount of data in a digestible manner and enhance the appearance of a manuscript.

Summary

The Results section of your report is for presenting the results of your statistical analyses. It should be clearly written in a concise, exact format. Tables, graphs, and other figures help present data in a way that makes the results easy to read and readily understood and invites interpretation. The Results is also where you comment on the rejection or retention of null hypotheses or whether research questions were supported or answered. The Results is free of author (or any other) bias. Remember, your interpretations and conclusions do not belong in the Results section. Think of this section as the place for the "facts" of your research results.

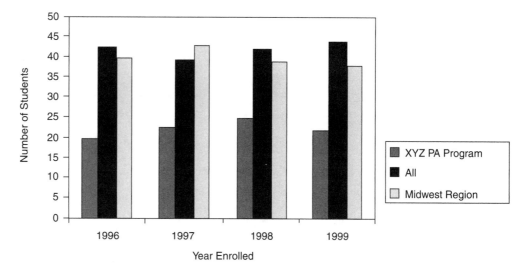

FIG. 10-3. Example of a bar graph.

General Guidelines for Developing Graphs

1. Select the proper type of graph based on the data, statistical analysis, and clearest presentation to the reader.

2. Refer to figures in the text and number consecutively. (Tables and figures are numbered separately.)

3. Be sure there is enough spacing for ease of interpretation and the grid is scaled proportionately.

4. Check spelling (including caption) and ensure data were entered and plotted correctly.

5. Ensure there is sufficient contrast or distinctive patterns to clearly separate segments of pie chart or bars on bar chart. Avoid 3D or other special effects.

6. Check with publisher for guidance on overall size, font size, resolution, and style specifications.

7. Legends should be included if needed and abbreviations explained.

8. Update permission from copyright holder for reproductions or adaptations from other sources.

9. For photographs and other illustrations, be sure to mark "TOP" so the publisher has the proper orientation for typesetting and layout. In addition, be sure they are labeled and identified with your name and article title in case they are separated from the manuscript.

References

1. Day RA. How to Write and Publish a Scientific Paper, 5th ed. New York: Oryx Press, 1998, p. 44.
2. Gehlbach SH. Interpreting the Medical Literature, 4th ed. New York: McGraw-Hill, 2002, pp. 157–158.
3. Sterne JA, Smith GD. "Shifting the evidence – What's wrong with significance tests?" British Medical Journal 2001;322:226–231.
4. Zeiger M. Essentials of Writing Biomedical Research Papers, 2nd ed. New York: McGraw-Hill, 2000, p. 156.
5. Wilkinson L, Task Force on Statistical Inference. Statistical methods in psychology journals: guidelines and explanations. American Psychologist 1999;54(8):594–604.
6. DePoy E, Gitlin LN. Introduction to Research: Multiple Strategies for Health and Human Services. St. Louis: Mosby, 1994, p. 285.
7. American Medical Association. American Medical Association Manual of Style: A Guide for Authors and Editors, 9th ed. Philadelphia: Lippincott Williams & Wilkins, 1998, p. 54.
8. American Psychological Association. Publication Manual of the American Psychological Association, 5th ed. Washington, DC: American Psychological Association, 2001, p. 141.

chapter 11

Discussion

Richard R. Rahr, EdD, PA-C and Virginia A. Rahr, RN-C, EdD

Chapter Overview

The Discussion section of your paper is where you state your interpretations, conclusions, and opinions about your work and the results. This is where you get to answer the questions you posed in the beginning of your manuscript. Of all the sections of a thesis, dissertation, or manuscript for publication, this section most reflects the author and his or her views. There can be a number of subsections in the Discussion section, such as summary, conclusions, implications, interpretations, recommendations, and a closing. The subtitles and sections will depend on the type of work being produced and local and publication requirements. The author also has some discretion on what sections to include in the Discussion section. Discussion should center on the importance of the results and their application in society, patient care, education, or profession. Write the Discussion section of your research report carefully, so that your readers can clearly understand and appreciate the results and outcomes of your study. Be thorough, but concise.

Introduction

The traditional Discussion section of a research report covers the following areas: implications, limitations, discussion, bias considerations, recommendations, and conclusions. A review of several other "how-to" research books would show that similar descriptor terms, such as summary, interpretation, and analysis, are sometimes used in the Discussion section. Even the order of the subsections will vary. This chapter focuses on the terms most commonly used in the research literature, which are the aforementioned six descriptors. However, local requirements or publication requirements may be different.

Implications

In the Implications section the author explores the meaning of the research results. This is the author's opportunity to think critically about the research results and draw or make inferences. For example, what changes are indicated in clinical practice, or in education, based on the research findings? What do the results mean to medicine and society? Even if there were no statistically significant findings related to your research study's hypotheses or questions, there is still meaning to the research effort. One inference from nonstatistically significant results is that current theory or practice is sound or supported by the data. Your recommendations for such studies might well be to make no change in practice and to continue with the current best evidence-based practices. If your investigation found no significance, then you have the opportunity to discuss why and what that means in light of what is known. If you have a significant hypothesis confirmation that has strong clinical implications, however, you might recommend a new approach to the problem or a change in practice.

Remember, major changes in practice are seldom based on a single study unless it was very large, well designed, and carefully controlled investigation. Meta-analysis, which is the integration and evaluation of several or many independent research studies, is now considered one of the highest levels of research sophistication, particularly for evidenced-based practice. Even in evidence-based analysis, questions are often raised that need further investigation.

The implications of your study may point out the potential value of a finding, or the need for replication of the study, or modifications in a subsequent study to strengthen the research results or findings. What you believe your results implicate are important and should be stated in positive terms. Your arguments should be rational if you are contradicting accepted dogma or theory.

An example of an implication: if the use of a new experimental antibiotic called antibiotic X increased the effective cure rate for osteomyelitis by 25 percent over the currently available drug treatment, and if antibiotic X were without any major side effects, then you would certainly recommend the new experimental drug for the treatment of osteomyelitis. If you found that giving antibiotic X with the addition of daily treatments in the hyperbaric chamber made no significant difference in the overall treatment outcomes, however, then you would not recommend that the two treatments be used in tandem. The implications must be in line with the author's working knowledge of the problem that was studied as well as the results.

If the Pearson product moment statistical test is used to measure the variable, and it gives a statistical correlation with a significant r-value of .70, then this would seem to be a good correlation. If you do further testing, however, with a second statistical analysis called the r^2 value (the coefficient of determination), then the r^2 value would be .49 ($r = .70$; $r^2 = .49$). This second statistic would account for only 49 percent of the correlation variance. The fact that 51 percent of the research study variance is not explained should cause you to be conservative in listing implications and recommendations. Your discussion must make sense of your statistical analysis and the results.

The implications subsection of the Discussion section is not the place where you state that the data proved, verified, confirmed, or demonstrated that your hypothesis was right or wrong. You will have written the analysis of data and findings in Results sections of your research report. There you will have used phrases such as "the hypothesis was accepted [or rejected]." In the Implications section, however, you might appropriately state what the research findings suggest (e.g., a change in practice or no change in practice). The implications need to be thought about and written about in relationship to the literature reviewed, current theory, practice, theoretical constructs or framework of the research study, and how your research findings fit into all of these factors. (This is why your methodology is so important.) Your implications should have practical and clinical significance and be clearly supported by the research findings.

Limitations

The limitations section of the Discussion part of the research paper is of utmost importance because it provides a clear picture of the study's defects or weaknesses (or limits). Problems or limitations should be recognized and pointed out by the researcher, so that they can be considered in light of the overall worth of the study. This explanation may allow those weaknesses to be avoided if the study is replicated. The researcher may realize, in retrospect, that there were flaws in the methodology, the sample size was seriously limited by variables that might not have been foreseen, or there may have been other problem areas. All studies have limitations. It is much better to put these limitations in front of the reader because it gives credence to your conclusions and your understanding of your investigation. If you realize your study limitations, then your conclusions were made with those limitations known. Again, when you realize the limitations of your study and reach your conclusions with limitations known, your implications are stronger.

The author needs to state clearly to whom and in what situations the research project's findings or outcomes can be generalized and applied. How well did the sample participants represent the population? The researcher may have inadvertently attracted or recruited only a certain subgroup of the intended population. For example, even though the researcher sought to have a representative sample of both men and women of various age groups, perhaps only women within a certain age range were willing to participate in the study. Your findings and conclusions must take this limitation into consideration. Also, can the data from such a study be generalized to the whole population? For some studies, a pilot study may help discover some of these types of problems (limitations) and help guide your methodology to eliminate or limit such problems. The fewer limitations you have; the better off you are.

The limitations section should also discuss the randomness of the sample selection and potential for error in the sampling and to acknowledge the limitations if the sample was one of convenience (e.g., students in your classroom, all patients attending the clinic on a certain day). Having an experienced researcher as a guide and mentor can assist you in developing a study that is as strong as possible within the ever-present constraints of a practice or educational setting.

Other considerations to address include whether there may have been errors in the data entry, especially if an outside independent person does not audit the data after entry. The level of data quality needs to be discussed, as well as the probability of coding errors. You are responsible for the accuracy of the data, even when someone else enters it.

You should also consider whether an intervening variable or researcher effect (the Hawthorne effect) could be responsible for the results, rather than the independent variable being tested. The level of statistical significance should be discussed as it relates to practical or clinical implications. The amount of variance that is explained is important so that the research outcome impact is not exaggerated. For example, in many educational research studies using learning styles, the learning styles identified have a direct correlation with the learning environment, teaching techniques, and teacher learning style; however, these correlations address only a very small number of total variables responsible for student success. The student's finances, life stresses, living conditions, intelligence, work ethics, study habits, test-taking skills, and social support may be variables that are equally or more important.

The Limitations section must be honest and forthright about all the research study's shortcomings or weaknesses. Such forthrightness gives the researcher, the research project, and its outcomes greater credibility and potential for acceptance. It also assists other researchers to be aware of such limitations and thus try to avoid them as much as possible in future investigations.

Discussion

The discussion subsection of the Discussion section is an informative section that is used to meld together the research report, forming the interpretation of the results, their implications, and the study's limitations into an objective presentation. In previous parts of the research report, such as in the presentation and analysis of data, there was no room for the author's subjective thoughts and insights. The discussion subsection is refreshing in that it allows and encourages authors to give their view of the impact and importance of the research outcomes. This is the author's opportunity to refer to the previous review of literature and the theoretical framework and to discuss how these aspects relate to the current research study's findings. The author can judiciously interject subjectivity based on previous clinical and research experiences and wisdom (expert opinion). How did the data's significance or nonsignificance relate to the conceptual framework of the literature that was reviewed? This is where you get to answer that question in your opinion based on your investigation.

This section is also where we expect to see some practical application of the research findings. For example, does the matching of the teacher's learning style with the student's learning style in the classroom improve the student's performance? If so, then the author would discuss the relationship of the new finding to the old method of putting all learning styles learners with one teacher. The next issue to address would be the implementation of the new learning style research finding. Is it practical to match the student's learning style with the teacher's learning style, or is it more practical to use the "old" way of having one teacher address all the learning styles by using different teaching techniques in one classroom? This is where the author's research, knowledge and wisdom come into play. In a small school it may be impossible to match students with a teacher of the same learning style, but the approach may work well in a larger college or university. A clinical example could be the matching of patients with providers of the same gender. Is the effectiveness of the encounter perceived to be better by patients; by providers? Again there may be a number of other factors that influences these perceptions. The discussion section is the place where all of this could be explored in light of the research findings.

The discussion section is also where the author may want to discuss the characteristics of survey tools, limitations, generalizations, statistical methods, and bias considerations of the research project. Ultimately, this part of your report is your opportunity to critically discuss your evaluation of the research outcomes and their impact. In some formats, the discussion section is the last subsection of the chapter.

Bias Considerations

It is very easy for a researcher to want certain outcomes or results for their research project. A good way to prevent you from becoming biased in this way is to write the study hypothesis using the null hypothesis format. If you force yourself to put the research question into the null hypothesis format ("There is no significant difference between [the independent/influencing variable] and [the dependent/influenced variable]"), then you will be less likely to focus on a desired outcome. This method helps you maintain objectivity. A good researcher should concentrate on the process and methodology of the study and let the results fall where they may. The results are the results. If the process is sound, the results are accurate. That is the basis of research.

If the null hypothesis is rejected, then you have a positive correlation outcome and likely a valuable study. If you were doing a learning style research study and you phrased the null hypothesis: "There is no statistical difference between the concrete-sequential vs. the abstract-random student's grade in a lecture-only format course," then this would keep you from believing that the lecture format is better for the concrete-sequential student. The null hypothesis states that there will be no difference between variables tested, which helps to keep the researcher unbiased and focused on true data outcomes. Most basic science research is null hypothesis based.

A second bias effect can be caused by the extra and close attention a researcher may give to the study group, which can sometimes affect the outcomes of the study. The more attention the researcher gives the subjects, the more the subjects may want to please the researcher and give responses that they believe the researcher is seeking; consequently, the greater effect this intervening variable will have. It may be that an effect occurs simply because the subjects are aware that they are in a research study. This phenomenon, referred to as the "Hawthorne effect," can be likened to a placebo effect. The term Hawthorne effect came from a series of experiments conducted at the Hawthorne plant of the Western Electric Corporation. In this series of studies, it was discovered that the researcher's attention and the workers' knowledge that they were part of an experiment affected their rate of assembly of electric generators, rather than the adjusted variables such as lighting and working hours. Be careful in the collection of data to make sure your attention is not affecting the study's outcomes. You need to control for this potential bias variable in the research study. It is very easy for a researcher to influence a study in the way the investigator wants.

Other ways to prevent bias in a research study are to do a random selection/assignment of the subjects, have control groups for comparison, do a double-blind crossover study of subjects when this is possible and feasible, and have objective outside reviews of the overall design and methodology. All of these efforts should be discussed.

Recommendations

The Recommendations subsection of the Discussion section of a research paper usually states the author's ideas on what future research is needed based on the outcomes of the current study. For example, recommendations could include the suggestion to expand the existing research by adding more subjects to the current research plan or to conduct "next step" studies. Other directions could be to develop a new research design, use a new data collection instrument, or address the gaps or weaknesses in the study. Recommendations may include making the study a double-blind crossover model, adding a control group, or suggesting that an outside independent investigator repeat the same study to determine if the results can be replicated.

The overall purpose of the recommendations subsection is to alert the reader that additional questions need to be asked and answered, or that some variables or inconsistencies were not controlled for or addressed in the research need to be explored. The author should avoid providing so many recommendations that the most important ones become obscured. The author should strive for relevance, clarity, and brevity in his or her recommendations.

Conclusions

This is usually the last section of the paper and it is generally brief. The Conclusions subsection of the Discussion section should begin with a brief restatement of the aim of the study and the major research question(s) or hypotheses. Following that, the author should state the major findings of the study, using a format that can easily be followed such as using bullets or numbers to separate each finding. For example: "This study showed that patients who are treated for chronic severe pain with analgesic medication administered 'around the clock' rather than on a PRN schedule had a higher level of functional status, demonstrated by more time spent out of bed during daytime hours." Based on this finding a major implication might be to change the treatment protocol to regularly scheduled rather than PRN medication administration for patients with chronic severe pain. Clearly stated implications for practice, when backed by sound research findings, help to build evidence-based practice and improve the care of patients.

A good contrast and comparison of the results with relevant underlying literature dogma is expected. For

BOX 11–1

Key Criteria for the Discussion Section

1. Clearly state what your research findings contribute to the understanding of the defined problem or question.
2. Be specific about implications for practice or education or society, based on your research findings.
3. Describe how your findings fit into the present body of knowledge or change it.
4. State how your findings support or enhance prior research findings, OR does your research present a contrasting view of other researchers' findings?
5. If your findings are novel, new, or in contrast to accepted norms, you must have strong support for your interpretations.

BOX 11–2

Pitfalls to Avoid in the Discussion Section

1. Drawing conclusions or formulating implications that cannot be clearly supported by the research findings
2. Providing so many recommendations for further study that the most important recommendations are lost.
3. Having an apologetic tone when describing limitations or study design weaknesses. Be matter of fact.

example, the author can point out that the same or similar research findings have been reported, and the author may here want to refer the reader to a specific section of the Review of Literature section of the paper. The author may wish to restate the strong and weak points of the research study; however, redundancy should be avoided unless a point is restated purposefully. The Conclusions subsection also provides the author the opportunity to share personal opinions and experiences that highlight and emphasize the impact of the research study. This should be done carefully, however, and these comments by the author must be clearly related to the current study and should not merely be the author's "general opinion." The overall practical value is important in the context of educational or health-care practice and this should be stressed in the Conclusions section.

The Conclusions subsection is much like a "closing" abstract, but with a bit more detail than is allowed in an Abstract. It should provide a complete but concise overview of the research study while bringing the Discussion section to a close. In summary, Box 11–1 presents key elements that the Discussion section should ensure, while Box 11–2 provides reminders of pitfalls to avoid in this section.

Suggested Readings

Bailey DM. Research for the Health Professional: A Practical Guide, 2nd ed. Philadelphia: FA Davis, 1991.

Jenkins S, Price CJ, Straker L. The Researching Therapist: A Practical Guide to Planning, Performing and Communicating Research. New York: Churchill Livingston, 1998.

Publication Manual of the American Psychological Association, 5th ed. Washington, DC: American Psychological Association, 2002.

chapter 12

Bibliographies and References

Albert F. Simon, DHSc, PA-C

Chapter Overview

This chapter examines the different documentation styles commonly used when writing research papers. It also looks at the application of documentation for references through footnotes and the proper construction of bibliographies. An understanding of the copyright law and fair use doctrine is discussed to provide a basis for awarding proper credit to sources used in the construction of the research paper. Finally, the chapter looks at how the Internet can assist in finding source material for research projects. Unless otherwise noted, the terms "thesis," "dissertation," and "research paper" are used interchangeably in this chapter.

Choosing a Style for Research Projects

Although there are many styles or formats that one may use when constructing a research paper, most colleges or universities dictate a style that has to be followed for constructing the technical aspects of the paper (the bibliography, citation style, etc.). It is not uncommon for particular departments or schools within universities to have their own requirements regarding which style to use. Added to these challenges is the required style that

journals will want for published articles. A number of style manuals can be used, and before choosing one for your writing, you need to check which one is required by your institution or the potential publisher of your manuscript. Three of the major style manuals commonly (but not exclusively) used for scholarly works are discussed here and form the basis for this guide. These include the *Publication Manual of the American Psychological Association* (APA), *The Chicago Manual of Style,* and *The Modern Language Association (MLA) Handbook for Writers of Research Papers.* These three style manuals are referred to simply as APA, CHI, and MLA, respectively. As pointed out earlier, it is prudent to determine a style choice in conjunction with your mentor, faculty advisor, or department chair before beginning your project. This person will be able to provide the appropriate direction in selecting a style that conforms to the requirements of the institution, university, department, or particular project. Recognize that individual universities or schools within universities may publish their own style manuals that, while based on one of the major style forms (i.e., APA, MLA, or CHI), add particular additional requirements or modifications to which a writer must adhere. Writers must also be aware as they embark on writing an article or book chapter intended for publication that many journals or publishers have specific style requirements. These requirements are generally published in the journal under a section defined as "information for authors" and also contained on their Web sites. Publishers will usually send authors specific guidelines for form and style soon after contracts are issued for contributions.

The APA, CHI, and MLA styles are most often employed for writing undergraduate research papers and theses at the graduate level. Dissertation styles may follow one of these three or other specific institutional or department guidelines. It is not uncommon for research works and dissertations to be published in the style of professional or academic journals germane to that discipline.

Each of these three styles has unique features. The CHI and MLA are the most similar, but there are differences between them, largely related to how the various elements of information (author's name, etc.) are formatted or which elements are used. For example, APA does not generally use content notes, whereas MLA and CHI do. Beyond these comparisons, there are literally thousands of differences in indentations, punctuation, and format among the three styles. The differences may seem trivial to the novice, but publication and departmental requirements are generally very strict in specifying the exact style to be used and used correctly. Your paper could be turned down because you did not follow style recommendations.

Box 12–1 illustrates the differences between the three major styles plus the AMA style, which is used for a number of medical publications. This is the same citation of a source that is a textbook by a single author.

BOX 12–1

Examples of Various Citation Styles

Chicago
Simon, Albert and Miller, Anthony, eds. 2000. *Appleton and Lange's Outline Review for the Physician Assistant Examination*. New York: Appleton and Lange.

APA
Simon, A. and Miller, A. (Eds.). (2000). *Appleton and Lange's Outline Review for the Physician Assistant Examination*. New York: Appleton and Lange.

MLA
Simon, Albert, and Miller, Anthony, eds. *Appleton and Lange's Outline Review for the Physician Assistant Examination*. New York: Appleton and Lange, 2000.

AMA
Simon A, Miller A, eds. *Appleton and Lange's Outline Review for the Physician Assistant Examination*. NY: Appleton and Lange; 2000.

Again it is most important that one follows the style exactly. Writers are advised to consult the complete style guides for the style in use to ensure that proper format is achieved when citing references.

There is no absolute advantage of one style over another. Selection is largely a matter of convention, tradition, preference, or what is dictated in the guidelines for the assignment (e.g., when writing a thesis, dissertation, or paper for coursework or publication).

The APA style is widely used in the social sciences. It offers a "clean" format that encompasses parenthetical citations within the text that contain the author's name, year of publication, and page number (used only for direct quotes). The references are then keyed to an alphabetical list contained at the end of the paper.

The MLA-style format is the one recommended by the Modern Language Association. It is widely used by teachers of English, other languages, and in the humanities. MLA format provides for parenthetical references used directly in the text of the paper. These references are keyed to a list of works cited and found at the end of the paper and in content notes. These three features—parenthetical notes, list of works cited, and content notes—are the key elements of this style.

The Chicago style is most popular for newspapers, magazines, and many scholarly and nonscholarly publications, so it is quite likely that you have already seen numerous examples of writing in this format. For years, many proofreaders, editors, and authors have used *The Chicago Manual of Style* as a guide to proper format and punctuation. This manual is often cited as the definitive authority for accuracy. When following the CHI format, documentation is noted by either a footnote or endnote style. In this style, the notes are placed on a separate sheet at the end of the text (i.e., endnote) or are listed numerically at the bottom of each page of text (i.e., footnote), or notes are placed throughout the text that give either author commentary or list information needed to locate the source.

Each of the three style manuals contains a comprehensive guide to the proper documentation of sources and other technical details of publication (e.g., how an author would properly document a computer bar code as a source). One may purchase these guides in their unabridged form at traditional bookstores or outlets, but many are available either in print or online at university libraries around the world. Each is also available on the World Wide Web at various sites. Depending on the depth of guidance that one needs, abridged handbooks that contain the most common or salient features of each style also may be used. Two excellent examples of these publications are *The Brief Holt Handbook*[1] and *The Thesis Writer's Handbook*.[2] These types of synopses provide a quick reference for general guidance and are helpful in many situations. Their compact size makes for handy reference, but the amount and scope of information they contain is limited.

Although most of the focus of this discussion has been on the three major style guides, it is important to realize that one may be required to use any one of the literally hundreds of styles available. There is no hard and fast rule as to which style to choose; most of the time the style selected for use is decided by mandate of a journal, department, university, or particular professor. Of course it is important, once the appropriate style has been identified, to use that style consistently throughout your manuscript.

Some of these styles may even be proprietary for a specific company, but beyond the three major resources (APA, CHI, and MLA), most are specific to a learned society (e.g., American Institute for Physics or The American Medical Association). Even the U.S. government has a style manual of its own.[3] Fordham University maintains an excellent Web page with a reasonably comprehensive list of links to styles manuals at *http://www.library.fordham.edu/researchguides/guides.html* Remember, it is important to always consult with your faculty mentor, university guidelines or bulletins, your editor, and the author guidelines to determine style requirements prior to writing.

Documenting Sources Using References and Bibliographies

When doing research, one synthesizes opinions, facts, and information from disparate sources. This information is woven together with one's own thoughts to form the basis for a thesis or other publication. Much of the information gleaned in a literature search and used as background material represents others' original work. Whether used as a direct quote or paraphrased, it is appropriate, necessary, and required to acknowledge this work using the proper documentation. Any information that is used and not accepted as "general knowledge" in one's field should be acknowledged (documented, that is, cited) with entries as citations within the text or in a bibliography (or both). The way that you document your citations is determined by the editorial style you are using. Each editorial style has its own specific format for citations and how they are listed. The type of work cited may take varied citation formats.

Documentation is provided in two major ways:

1. Providing specific documentation of facts and the opinions of others, either on each page or at the end of a chapter or section, by the use of citations in the form of footnotes or endnotes.

2. Listing the sources of information used by constructing a bibliography. The bibliography is usually at the end of the manuscript.

The process of documentation involves constructing a list of all the sources of information used in the production of your document. It is also customary to indicate the pages where the information can be found. Be sure to completely and accurately record the facts about your sources from the original publication (e.g., the information following the title page of a book). (See Chapter 4.)

Reference Citations Using Footnotes or Endnotes

In providing acknowledgment, one may use numbered reference citations marked at the end of the appropriate sentence or in the document text followed by bibliographic listings at the end of the chapter or paper. This notation style is known as an endnote. Another popular way to provide documentation is to use a footnote. Footnotes consist of numbered citations that are coupled to documentation notes at the bottom of the page.

Although endnotes and footnotes are popular ways to document sources, there are several other methods to do this. Depending on the style that is chosen (APA, MLA, or CHI), the reference may also be displayed as parenthetical citations or author–date citations. Endnotes and footnotes seem to be giving way to the Bibliography format in many scientific writings.

Bibliographies

Proper documentation also requires that one provide a list of all works used as reference material in the construction of the research paper. The term "bibliography" suggests a list of all works consulted during the background research for the paper, whether they were actually cited in the paper or not. Particularly for dissertation preparation, the meaning of bibliography may encompass all works that would be available on the subject. To properly place the scope of the list in perspective, some academic departments or thesis committees may prefer terms such as "selected bibliography," "references," or "works cited." Consult the guidelines published by your university, editor, or academic advisor to ascertain the correct phrase for your research paper.

The bibliography generally follows the endnotes section of the paper (if an endnotes section is used) and is arranged alphabetically by first-author names or by numbered sequence of occurrence in the paper. There will be slight differences in bibliographic format depending on the style being used. Consult the specific style guidelines to determine the proper format.

By reviewing your bibliography or reference list, the reader of the thesis can obtain a sense of the depth and quality of the research performed as background to the paper. This may be deduced by the types of works one cites, the date of publication, and their appropriateness. The bibliography should contain enough information in each citation for readers to locate the source if they so desire. A reader may want to go to the original source for some fact that you have used to build your research.

There are two variations one might use when preparing a bibliography. The first is an annotated bibliography, which allows authors' comments to be appended to any or all of the entries contained in the list. The second is to group the entries by source type. In this configuration, the list is divided into primary and secondary, then published and unpublished sources. Entries within each category are listed alphabetically. Remember that primary sources are the original works such as a book or video. Secondary sources are derived from primary sources and contain critical comments from others who are knowledgeable about the subject. Secondary sources can be in many forms, such as articles, case studies, or books.

Bibliographies can also be useful in conducting the background research for your thesis. Initial, topic-oriented research will undoubtedly produce articles that contain bibliographies from other authors that relate to your research question. These bibliographies are often useful as leads in completing your subject research. It is acceptable to use these citations as leads, but one must be diligent in locating the sources and doing additional searches to validate the appropriateness of each entry. It is improper to simply copy the citation into your bibliography.

General bibliographies such as *Books in Print* and the *Bibliographic Index* are available in most libraries and can be a start to locate other sources of information. For thesis work at both the graduate and undergraduate levels, general bibliographies may seldom produce sources that are usable because they list works primarily written for the lay public.

Specific bibliographies such as *Index Medicus* are available and direct the reader to more in-depth sources in particular subject areas appropriate to research at the graduate and undergraduate levels, as well as non-education–related research. This is a valuable resource for clinicians in clinical research.

Copyrighted Material, Fair Use Provisions, Public Domain, and Plagiarism

Standards of academic conduct require one to acknowledge all material used in the production of a thesis or other work, whether it was copyrighted or not. Material that falls within the so-called "public domain" can be used without permission, but should be acknowledged as to source. Generally, "public domain" means material that has not been copyrighted or for which the copyright has expired.

Copyrighted material is a different matter and requires that permission of the copyright holder be obtained prior to using the material. One exception to this statement is a provision called "fair use." The 1976 Copyright Act is a comprehensive law that deals with the legalities of using copyrighted material. Under this law, copyrighted material may be used without the permission of the copyright holder for certain specific uses. These uses are referred to collectively as "fair use."

Fair use covers an array of situations that allow one to use copyrighted material without written permission. Unfortunately, fair use is a bit of a shadowy area where general guidelines exist, but there still are many instances where disagreement exists about what constitutes fair use. One realizes after reading the copyright law that it is written to allow for a broad range of interpretation, making "fair use" applications possible. As an author, one wants to respect the integrity of the work of others and, of course, stay away from encounters with the legal system. Make no mistake; the penalty for violation of the copyright laws can be very stiff, up to $150,000 for each willful act of violation. These stiff penalties are intended for willful (intended) violations of the Copyright laws, but even unintentional violations can result in fines being levied against offenders.

The specific outlines of circumstances that constitute fair use are rather vague, but research, teaching, and news reporting are mentioned directly. By popular interpretation, uses that consist of fewer than 150 borrowed words (as long as this does not constitute a major portion of the work) are acceptable, although there are many interpretations. There is a provision of the law referred to as the good faith fair-use defense that can help prevent one from being found guilty of violating copyright laws. But this defense is helpful only if the court believed that the accused violator reasonably thought that the fair use doctrine applied to the material they copied (University of Texas, n.d.). Consistent application of standards of fair use that are reasonable can help protect one from being found guilty of not only plagiarism, but also violation of the copyright laws. A search of the Web will produce several examples of guidelines or tests that can be applied to assist one in correctly identifying fair use practices. One excellent example of such a paradigm and a comprehensive explanation of the fair use doctrine can be found at the following Web site: *http://www.utsystem.edu/ogc/intellectualproperty/copypol2.htm*.

In actuality, the reader will find an entire course on the subject of fair use at this Web site hosted by the University of Texas. This self-tutorial course provides examples from a number of situations and should be considered a must read for those who are interested in keeping to the spirit of the copyright laws.

The public domain rules have also changed dramatically over the past few years. As stated at the beginning of this section, public domain works are those creative works that are not protected by copyright and may be freely used by anyone. With the original law in 1909, authors were required to place copyright notice on their works to prevent them from being categorized in the public domain, but this changed in 1987 when the requirement to include a notice was removed. Currently, all works published before December 31, 1922 are now in the public domain. From this point on it gets very, very complex. There have been numerous changes to the public domain statutes over the course of the 20th century, which are too numerous to recount in this chapter. Fortunately, there is an excellent resource located at *http://www.unc.edu/~unclng/public-d.htm* that details all of the changes and dates that one must keep in mind in making these decisions.

Also, you need to remember that certain works cannot receive the protection of the copyright laws and are always considered pubic domain. This list includes such items as facts and works that lack originality; the most popular example here is the telephone book. Any government publication is also considered public domain. There are other examples as well, which are detailed at the following Web address (and other sites): *http://www.copyright.cornell.edu/training/Hirtle_Public_Do main.htm*. Public domain works still should be cited in the reference list as appropriate to the style of the research paper in which they are contained.

If you are uncertain if a work is in public domain or copyright protected, qualified legal counsel should be sought prior to publication so that infringement of copyright privilege may be avoided. Also remember that if a work you intend to cite is not in public domain and does not qualify for the fair use provision, it will be necessary to obtain permission to use the work from the author and possibly publishing companies. Granting of such use may require that a fee be paid for the right to use that property.

The copyright law states that any literary work (which includes computer software and programs by the way) produced after January 1, 1978 is automatically protected by copyright (*isomedia.com*, n.d.). Some prefer to afford themselves extra protection and actually have their work registered with the United States Copyright office. To register a literary work one must complete a variety of forms and pay a fee to the copyright office. This process provides protection for at least 50 years after the date the copyright application is received by the copyright office. For more information and to obtain forms online visit the United States Copyright office Web site at *http://www.copyright.gov/*

Evaluating Sources

Your research will produce a vast array of sources from which to glean material. For most research questions, the problem is not that one cannot find enough, but rather how to find the appropriate sources. It has already been pointed out that the readers of your paper will be scrutinizing the sources you select for appropriateness and authority. In deciding what sources to reference, one should evaluate several parameters.

You should ask the following questions: Is the source authoritative? Who are the authors of the source, and are they experts in the field? Would the academic community regard the authors as credible? Certainly, it is acceptable to cite dissenting viewpoints from individuals who may be viewed as out of the mainstream of thought or regarded as skeptics. But it is important to put these opinions into context and to construct convincing arguments as to whether these opinions support the conclusions arrived at from your research. Does the article represent current theories or trends? Researchers often attempt to illustrate cutting-edge material in their thesis paper. Currency of references lends credence to the research efforts expended by the author in the construction of the paper. Many departments will have published rules concerning the currency of references. Always check with the style guide published by your department or with your faculty mentor to determine what is appropriate to cite in your paper. When no published rule exists, convention often dictates that references older than three to five years be justified in the text of the treatise. There are occasions when one wishes to cite "classic" works for the particular discipline of one's work. This is an instance where you would have one, or perhaps several, citation(s) that may not be recent.

Other considerations about your sources include where was the article published? Has the reference you are evaluating been through a rigorous peer-reviewed process? Publication in many of the major journals requires that the article receive stringent peer review before publication. This process provides additional confidence that the article contains valid arguments and conclusions that are the results of sound methodology and investigation. In each field of study, certain journals are recognized as prestigious because of their traditional careful scrutiny in selection of articles for publication. Reference articles cited from these sources may carry additional weight when readers review the references-cited list.

In today's world of electronic publishing, one must be careful to evaluate the source of the material when selecting references. Realize that information posted on the Internet may not have received the benefit of peer review and may have simply been put there by an individual to state an opinion. Although this does not imply that the document in question is not valid, one must be careful to evaluate this information for what it is.

Finding References Using Electronic and Internet-Based Sources

Although much of what follows was presented in Chapter 4, it is important to review and consider in light of one construct of references and bibliographies. Just over a decade or so ago, it was uncommon to use anything except print material for conducting research. Now most individuals turn first to the Internet to begin their search for information about a topic. Today most people use the Internet through the World Wide Web. The Web is merely a way to utilize the Internet using a browser. This allows one to access both text and graphics (including movie formats). Although electronic sources have not completely supplanted printed material, no extensive research process would be complete without a search of electronic sources.

Most libraries maintain material on CD-ROMs, DVDs, other digital formats, and other storage devices rather than in print form. Large amounts of printed material can be stored on these devices, facilitating their retrieval.

Most of the time, you will use online searches in conducting your research via the Internet. By connecting computers all over the world, the Internet allows one to access information from anywhere. This also provides a means to enter subject queries, termed "search phrases" or "keywords," into search engines to find material relative to a particular topic.

Search engines are server computers that allow one to search various database files. The extent and breadth of these searches far outreach any that one could perform in a single library collection. Many libraries have placed their entire catalogs and all their holdings online. Almost all of these libraries can be accessed from different locations via queries sent from search engines, so if you are on the Internet, you can access literally hundreds of these search engines.

Various search engines are tailored to specific subjects, such as PubMed for medical topic searches. PubMed can be accessed through the National Library of Medicine Web site at *http://www.ncbi.nlm.nih.gov/entrez*. Indexes of some search engines can be found at *www.search.com*. With some investment of time, one can become familiar with the search engine that fits a particular search need.

When using search engines, it is important to master the skill of phrasing inquiries in a way that produces the most useful results. Each search engine has slightly different rules about how to phrase questions. Most engines have a help section that allows one to modify the search and narrow the results to receive the most helpful responses. Boolean codes or modifiers allow one to be more specific in searches. On most engines, typing the search phrase in quotation marks directs the search engine to search only for those specific words in that specific order. This process helps to narrow the search but requires that one be specific and accurate.

For example, if one wants to find information about John Wayne, but mistakenly types in "John Watne," nothing will be produced about John Wayne, only information about John Watne (although Google and a number of other search engines will detect common misspellings and ask you if you were looking for other terms). Narrowing one's search by proper key phrasing is critical because the volume of information produced from a search can be overwhelming. It is not uncommon to get thousands of "hits" (links to specific data files) from a single search inquiry. Some search engines now categorize results into subject folders to help sort information from your search. The use of search engines on the Internet is free.

Libraries may subscribe to online databases (e.g., DIALOG, Ovid) to provide searches of bibliographic files. These are generally subscription services that charge for each search. Some libraries pay these fees for you, but others pass on the search fee to the user. These commercial search engines often let the user search different databases simultaneously, saving valuable time for the researcher. Some also offer the ability to continually narrow down search terms with progressively more specific search terms, also saving tremendous amounts of time searching through irrelevant "hits." There are a variety of online databases; some cater to the general market, and others are discipline-specific. Searches may be conducted through Google or other search engines available on the Internet for free usage. One must keep in mind that searching this type of engines often does not produce results from professional journals but often more of the "public domain" (nonscholarly) journals and literature. These searches can still be very productive to identify relevant material that complements that which is found in the scholarly literature.

One can also use the Internet to assist in the research process beyond finding published references. E-mail can be used to interview individuals for background material, saving an expensive and time-consuming journey. (This assumes that the person you wish to interview has an e-mail account, almost a sure thing in today's world.)

It is also convenient to conduct research surveys via the Web. A simple search can identify sites that can aid in the production and distribution of online surveys (e.g., *www.supersurvey.com*) which may produce material that would be used and referenced in research work. One can even conduct videoconferences using Internet tools that can save time and money if the computer resources are available.

For all the above, it is important to remember that you must cite your source accurately. Also remember that citing a Web site may not be adequate because the Web site may be importing information from other sources and not be the originator of the work or information.

Summary

Ultimately, one wants the bibliography and reference information to be accurate and attributed properly. Be compulsive in this area. Once a reference style is chosen, follow it throughout your paper. Always cite only original sources that you have checked and read. Good documentation and use of previous works will only strengthen your definition of the problem, literature review, methods, results, and conclusions.

References

1. Kirszner L, Mandell S. The Brief Holt Handbook, 2nd ed. Fort Worth, Harcourt Brace , 1998.
2. Miller J, Taylor P. The Thesis Writer's Handbook. McMinoville, OR: Alcove, 1997.
3. A Manual of Style, 28th ed. Washington, DC: U.S. Government Printing Office, 1993.

Suggested Readings

Isomedia. (n.d.). Protecting your work. Accessed June 1, 2004 from *http://www.isomedia.com/homes/screen/protect.htm*

University of Texas. (n.d.). Fair use of copyrighted materials. Accessed June 1, 2004 from *http://www.utsystem.edu/ogc/intellectualproperty/copypol2.htm*

SECTION III

Research Considerations

chapter 13

Writing and Publishing in the Physician Assistant Profession

James F. Cawley, MPH, PA-C and P. Eugene Jones, PhD, PA-C

A good paper has a definite structure, makes its point, and then shuts up.
Steven Locke, Former Editor, British Medical Journal

"Begin at the beginning," the King said, gravely, "and go on till you come to the end, then stop."
From Alice in Wonderland, by Lewis Carroll

Let thy words be few.
Ecclesiastes 5:2

Chapter Overview

As part of the medical profession, physician assistants (PAs) should share with physicians and biomedical scientists a sense of obligation as clinicians and teachers to contribute to the existing body of research knowledge and the development of the discipline. This applies equally for PA clinical practitioners, PA students, and PA faculty. The development of skills in the dissemination of this knowledge through writing, publishing, and presentation serves as a solid foundation for PAs as they progress through various stages of their careers. Such skills may facilitate expansion of multiple career options.

Skills and techniques in research methods, report writing, and medical publishing have been the subject of much of this book and should be part of the educational preparation of all PAs. An increasingly common graduation requirement for the PA student's professional education is a paper of publishable quality. In this chapter, which builds on material formally presented throughout this book, we review the essential components of a research paper in general and PA-authored research papers in particular. Presentation and posters are also discussed.

There are now more than 90 PA educational programs that award the master's degree. A number of programs require students to write a master's-equivalent thesis paper.

The process by which research papers are transformed into research publications in the biomedical literature is also discussed. In addition, the expansion of clinical investigations and the involvement of more practicing PAs in research require practicing PAs to develop publication and presentation skills.

Style Manuals

Many resources exist for the beginning and experienced writers and researchers. Table 13–1 lists a variety of resources that can enhance your work and help prepare you for submitting and/or publishing your work. Before selecting a particular style manual as a guide, you need to review the journals that offer publishing opportunities for your work. What is the style preferred by the journal or publishing opportunity? If one manual dominates, that is the one you want to obtain first. Ultimately, if publishing is a big part of what you want to do, you will need more than one.

A helpful Web site that includes examples of papers written in four commonly referenced style manual formats can be found at *http://www.dianahacker.com/resdoc/*. In addition, many style manuals now have quick reference links on the Internet, and a useful site to use as a point of departure is published by California State University of Los Angeles at: *http://www.calstatela.edu/library/styleman.htm*

Writing

For the PA student working on a graduate paper, knowledge of the structure and function of the research paper and how to modify it into a published article is an important skill to have. (There is a difference between a thesis or dissertation and a published paper.) This skill is also important to the seasoned PA clinician who has observed an interesting clinical case and seeks to make a contribution to the PA literature by "writing it up" for publication. Finally, such skills are essential for PA faculty and researchers, who not only must guide their students' work but also face the academic career reality of "publish or perish." Thus, given the primacy of writing and publishing in achieving professional success, it is important for PAs to acquire writing skills in the preparation of scientific papers and medical publications.

The proper culmination of any scientific research effort in a formal educational setting, be it a graduate student thesis, a faculty research project, or some other type of academic inquiry, is the production of a written document reflecting the work that was completed. Since time immemorial, recording one's work in formal, writ-

Table 13-1
Style Manuals

Title	Edition	Author/Publisher	Year
American Medical Association Manual of Style	9th	Lippincott Williams & Wilkins, Philadelphia, PA	1998
The Chicago Manual of Style	15th	University of Chicago Press, Chicago, IL	2003
Council of Biology Editors Style Manual	6th	Council of Science Editors, Reston, VA	1994
A Manual of Style	29th	U.S. Government Printing Office, Washington, DC	2000
Modern Language Association Style Manual and Guide to Scholarly Publishing	2nd	Modern Language Association, New York, NY	1998
Publication Manual of the American Psychological Association	5th	American Psychological Association, Washington, DC	2001
Strunk W Jr, White EB: The Elements of Style	4th	Longman, New York, NY	2000
Turabian KL: A Manual for Writers of Term Papers, Theses, and Dissertations	6th	The University of Chicago Press, Chicago, IL	1996
International Committee of Medical Journal Editors: Guide to Uniform Requirements for Manuscripts Submitted to Biomedical Journals		Available at *http://jama.ama-assn.org/info/avinst_req.html*	1997
National Library of Medicine Recommended Format for Bibliographic Citation		US Public Health Service, Department of Health and Human Services	1991
National Library of Medicine Recommended Format for Bibliographic Citation Supplement: Internet Formats		US Public Health Service, Department of Health and Human Services	2001
Scientific Style and Format: The CBE Manual for Authors, Editors, and Publishers	6th	Huth EJ	1994

ten form has been and remains the hallmark of scholarly activities. Since the 1600s, thinking and writing have largely been classified into two types: literary and scientific. The literary style has been associated with fiction, rhetoric, and subjectivity, whereas the scientific style has been steeped in fact, plain language, and objectivity. Through the centuries, this division of style increased as the body of scientific knowledge grew; barbs were increasingly exchanged between the two camps of thinkers and writers. Eighteenth-century Scottish philosopher David Hume thought of poets as "professional liars," and by the mid-1800s literature and science often stood as two distinct domains, particularly in their respective written work. Although dissension and distance still remain between these two broad fields, there are numerous examples of crossovers when talented writers have shed light on scientific truths drawing from both domains. During the 20th century, medical thinking and writing and the expression of medical knowledge have been reflected in the evolution of scientific writing.

Scientific papers are the vital currency of academic endeavors and knowledge dissemination. The quality and timeliness of information and its presentation in scholarly papers are determinants of major decision points in central collegiate activities: assignment of student grades, student advancement and graduation, faculty appointment and advancement, tenure decisions, perceptions of professional leadership, national academic reputations, and more. Publishing in prestigious journals with regularity is the expected and rewarded activity in most academic health centers; however, of all faculty teaching in US colleges and universities, only a small proportion publish regularly.

A health profession's vitality, relevance, and intellectual pedigree are reflected in its literature.[1] If judged by that standard, the PA profession is underachieving. Many believe there is a critical need for the PA profession to improve contributions to both the general biomedical literature and the PA professional literature. For the faculty member or graduate student, writing ability and a familiarity with publishing in the literature of the health professions represent essential professional skills. These skills, which are critical for success, can be learned by students, perfected by faculty, and appreciated by readers, both professional and lay. Beyond the academic setting, this process is also a challenge for the PA clinician. Box 13–1 provides a list of facts and myths about medical writing that are helpful to the PA interested in research.

Research Papers

In medicine, as in most other fields, good scientific research papers are the most common form of expression

---

BOX 13–1

Medical Writing Facts and Myths

Myth: "I'm a physician assistant, not a writer."
Fact: Writing is not a career but a necessary skill for medical professionals.

Myth: "I don't have any talent for writing. I've always been bad at it."
Fact: Writing is a skill, not a talent. Medical professionals should learn to write effectively.

Myth: "Writing has nothing to do with science."
Fact: Effective medical writing requires the same qualities found in scientific thought: logic, clarity, organization, and precision.

Myth: "If a piece of writing gets published, it's a good piece of writing."
Fact: Many published medical papers are badly written.

Myth: "Until I have my ideas clearly organized in my head, I shouldn't start writing."
Fact: The best way to clarify thinking is to start writing. Research shows that the act of writing helps clarify and organize thinking and generate ideas.

Myth: "I'll never be eligible for promotion or tenure unless I get a terminal degree. Why should I bother publishing if it won't help my career?"
Fact: Publishing papers in respected peer-reviewed journals has substantial academic value and generates far more career-enhancing opportunities than having a terminal degree and not publishing.

Adapted from St. James D. Writing and Speaking for Excellence: A Brief Guide for the Medical Professional. Boston: Jones and Bartlett, 1997, p. 13.

---

of a scientific finding. Research papers have a clear, well-defined structure. The logical sequence of the research paper's sections—Introduction (or Problem), Review of the Literature, Methods, Results, and Discussion—is generally accepted as the gold standard of the classic research paper structure. This format requires the author(s) to address a given topic answering five basic questions:

1. What is the issue?
2. What is known about the issue?
3. What methods have been used to investigate the issue?
4. What was found?
5. What are the implications of the findings?

Research papers take several forms, but generally the best form is to begin the paper by posing a question or identifying a problem. The question may address the need for further research on an issue, propose a new hypothesis, or justify further analysis. The conventional format and approach used in research papers is derived from what Huth calls the concept of critical argument.[3] This idea holds that research papers must convey information in such a way that the reader is convinced that the research paper's findings are well thought through and ultimately valid. Critical argument describes text that is coherent and consists of a series of reasons, statements, or facts intended to support or establish a point of view. This tone is "critical" in the sense that it carefully scrutinizes the source of the text's assertions. The "critical argument" is the heart of research writing.

Elements of the Research Paper

Tables

Tables are an essential component, really the hallmark, of the Results section. As ideal vehicles for summaries of numerical and categorical data, tables are often far better than text for conveying this type of information. A table typically includes columns, rows, fields, titles, footnotes, and display trends. A table should stand alone and be readily understood without referring to the text, and each table should present at least one key result. Collectively, tables contain the vital findings of the investigation or study and represent the essence of an original research paper.

Effective tables should be constructed with a purpose in mind. Use of mutually exclusive categories is desirable, and the number of rows and columns should be kept to the minimum needed to convey the results. The use of several small tables is more effective than one large, complex table. Tables should be referred to in the text of your manuscript and placed within the text at a point approximate to that reference.

Illustrations and Figures

Illustrations or figures provide features central to the research paper: evidence, efficiency, and emphasis. The quality typically required for publication suggests that illustrations are best when prepared by professional graphic artists. Illustration examples include radiographs, electrocardiograph (ECG) strips, and photomicrographs. Illustrations must have a descriptive legend. As with tables, figures and illustrations should be referred to in the text at the appropriate point.

Titles

The title of your paper is important, particularly when your work is published. The title may be the reason people are attracted to your work and why they read what you have published. Basically, there are two types of titles. The two types of titles are indicative (what the paper addresses) or informative (describes briefly the paper's specific message). The title should be accurate, succinct, and effective. As clinicians must triage through a voluminous and growing number of biomedical journal articles to determine which ones should be read, the first (and usually only) part read by most readers is the title. Word selection for the title is, perhaps, one of the most critical parts of the paper because it is the principal determining factor in the reader's decision to read the paper. The title should arouse enough curiosity on the part of the reader that your article will be read.

In the review/editing process, authors should not be disappointed or defensive if the title submitted with the manuscript is changed (and it is often changed substantially). Editors are experienced at determining what title would best catch the readership's eye for their particular journal.

Prose Revision

Research articles published in the biomedical literature typically present new and original information on topics relevant to the primary readership. The accepted scientific standard is that the investigators have applied reasonable standards of methodological rigor and have presented their findings in an accurate, concise, and clearly stated fashion. A big part of the accurate, concise, and clearly stated fashion is review and revision of the manuscript. What you think you have stated in your prose may not be what the reader reads. It would be very rare for any author to submit his or her first draft of a paper. Once you have written your paper, you have to review, revise, and reread a number of times. A first step when approaching the revision of a manuscript is to revise for larger segments of content, such as missing or unnecessary information or erroneous/misplaced content or sequence. The next step is to focus on prose, including sentence length, paragraph length, clauses, phrases, modifiers, and word choices. In revising prose, a seasoned writer seeks to develop fluency. Fluent prose runs along as the reader expects it to run. The reader is not jarred by defects that interrupt the line of thought. Short, simple sentences and structure are best. We suggest that once you have gone through your own revisions have two people review your manuscript. One person should be knowledgeable of your subject and scientific writing. The other person should be ignorant of the specific subject and a general reader. Get suggestions for revisions from both and then revise your manuscript again.

References

It is critical for any author to properly cite sources of information used in the paper as references. Two reference citation styles are commonly used in academic and biomedical circles. The so-called Vancouver style is a distinctive academic reference citation method in which the authors and year of publication are cited in the text as they are used. At the end of the paper, these references are listed alphabetically by first author's last name. The Vancouver style cites the author(s) and year as they appear in text, followed by an alphabetized list of full references. This format is typical for graduate school research papers.

The reference citation style used in most medical and health professions journals is the style of the "Uniform Requirements for Manuscripts Submitted to the Biomedical Journals," as developed by the International Committee of Medical Journal Editors.[4] This reference format takes the following form:

Author(s). Title. Journal. Year;Volume:Pages.

An example:

Hanson RL, Pettitt DJ, Bennett PH, et al. Familial relationships between obesity and NIDDM. Diabetes 1995;44:418–422.

One of the most important rules to follow in citing references in an academic paper is to be consistent. Reference citation style and policies are typically included in the "Information for Authors" section published in journals. References cited should include only those documents that are readily available, and the first author should have access to every reference. A good rule to remember is the dictum that "if you can't put your hands on it, don't cite it." Special formats/requirements exist for monographs, government publications, informal documents, Internet sources, and personal communications.

References drawn from Internet sources to be used in an academic paper represent an issue on the frontier of scientific communication. Internet sources are becoming a leading category of reference information used by authors in presenting a paper or defending a thesis. Using Internet sources allows an author to obtain information that should be not only accurate but also current. For instance, if one were writing a paper on the topic of PAs in surgery, an essential "factoid" to be included in the first paragraph of this paper would be the current number of PAs working in surgery. To obtain that information, in the past one may have consulted published information, which would be, by its very nature, dated. Consulting an Internet source, however, would instantly give the author the most current and accurate number available.

Citation of Internet Sources

The value of Internet references applies to many, but not all, online sources. Some Internet sources are unreliable and have questionable credibility. There is, nonetheless, an increasing acceptance and inclusion in the peer-reviewed medical literature (e.g., *JAMA* and the *Annals of Internal Medicine*) of Internet reference sources. The authors believe that Internet reference sources can and should be permitted with the following ground rules:

1. The Internet source is not a personal Internet site (e.g., an individual home page).

2. Any person can readily access the Internet site and obtain the same information cited by the author.

3. The citation contains as much specific information as possible.

4. Always include the date you accessed the information on the Internet.

The following examples of Internet citations are from the *American Medical Association's Manual of Style: A Guide for Authors and Editors*, 9th ed., p. 45.

1. Rosenthal S, Chen R, Hadler S. The safety of acellular pertussis vaccine [abstract]. Arch Pediatr Adoles Med [serial online]. 1996;150:457–460. Available at: *http://www.ama-assn. org/sci-pubs/journals/archive/ajdc/vol_150/no_5/abstract/htm.* Accessed *November 10, 1996.*

2. Gostin LO. Drug use and HIV/AIDS [JAMA HIV/AIDS Web site]. June 1, 1996. Available at: *http://www.ama-assn.org/ special/hiv/ethics.* Accessed June 26, 1997.

Additional care must be taken to ensure that information or texts acquired from Internet sources are properly acknowledged. According to Glass and Flanagin,[5] there are four types of plagiarism:

1. *Direct plagiarism*: Verbatim lifting of passages without enclosing the borrowed material in quotation marks and crediting the original author.

2. *Mosaic:* Borrowing the ideas and opinions from an original source and a few verbatim words or phrases without crediting the original author. In this case, the plagiarist intertwines his or her own ideas and opinions with those of the original author, creating a "confused, plagiarized mass."

3. *Paraphrase:* Restating a phrase or passage, providing the same meaning but in a different form without attribution to the original author.

4. *Insufficient acknowledgment*: Noting the original source of only part of what is borrowed or failing to cite the source material in such a way that a reader will know what is original and what is borrowed.

A key rule to remember is to provide any and all information that is needed to allow the reader to go to the same Internet site and review the same information cited by the author. This is the cardinal rule that also applies to published reference sources. The second rule is completeness; follow a sequence of author(s) (individual[s] or organization), work title, site, latest date, Web address, pages (if applicable), and any other specifics that allow the reader to access the site. If a reader is unable to verify your work, it may create doubts about the validity of your efforts.

Electronic Journals

The number of electronic journals in the medical literature is increasing. There are three forms of e-journals:

Type 1 e-journals are completely electronic with no regular print version.

Type 2 e-journals are titled the same both in the print and electronic versions, but each publishes some unique content.

Type 3 e-journals have both the print and electronic versions publish the same content (Weller, 2002).[6]

A number of e-journals are listed among MEDLINE titles. Although editor's statements on editorial peer review are similar, there are differences in number and type of materials included in the three different types of e-journals.

Approaches to Publication

A potential writer, such as a new PA graduate, experienced PA clinician, or PA faculty member, may take a wide range of approaches to enter the world of the published. For many PAs, the first effort at publication may be somewhat easier and have a greater chance at success in a format other than publication of an original research article or manuscript. As you plan your publication efforts, you may want to consider one of the following options. Something other than an original research manuscript publication will give you experience in dealing with journals, editors, and the review process. A good thing to do before you put a lot of effort into a project or writing effort is to send a query letter to the publishing editor of a journal.

A query letter is an appropriate method for determining interest in a research paper, commentary, or opinion article that might exist among the biomedical editors. The one-page query letter intends to gauge the interest of a particular journal in publishing an article on your topic. Addressed to the editor of one or more journals that might be interested in publishing your paper, a query letter should pique the editor's interest by asking, "Would you consider a submission on [your topic here]?" Avoid forcing the editor to make an immediate decision; recognize that no editor will commit to a publication decision before seeing the final manuscript and obtaining at least one other review. However, if they are not interested in your topic, you and the journal can save a great deal of time and effort by knowing this up front. Send your query letter to a number of journals. But remember, you should submit a manuscript to only one journal at a time. If a manuscript is turned down for publication, then you can submit it to another journal.

Original Articles

In terms of academic currency, original articles typically achieve more value when considering importance of content, relevance for promotion and tenure, and establishing one's reputation within a profession. Original articles are not required to be data-driven clinical projects of "bench science" or laboratory origin. They may instead reflect policy analysis, utilization patterns, cost–benefit analyses, and a host of other relevant topics that contribute to advancing the knowledge base of the profession. The key is that they are original pieces of work that represent original investigation or approach in some manner.

Clinical Review Articles

The clinical review is the most common type of paper appearing in the current PA literature. This reflects, in large part, the need for practicing PA clinicians to obtain an easy-to-read, concise summary of a particular health condition or disease. Review articles cite current theory and clinical practice for specific diseases and conditions, but they do not consist of original research on the disease or condition conducted by the author(s). Typical section headings of a clinical review article include Introduction, Etiology, Pathophysiology, Clinical Manifestations, Diagnostic Imaging/Laboratory Findings, Diagnosis, Treatment, Prognosis, and Health Promotion/Disease Prevention, and recommendations.[3] (See Chapter 6, Section 3.)

Case Reports

Case reports, once a "staple of the menu of clinical literature," and for that matter the format of many academic teaching exercises and presentations, remain an important type of paper appearing in biomedical journals.[3] Case reports are typically detailed, illustrated clinical descriptions of individual occurrences of disease. Over the past 20 years, however, case reports have become less frequent forms of contributions in the biomedical literature and tend to carry little new information. Biomedical journals usually publish clinical research trials, but case reports may provide important information. Those that merit publication include case histories that are unique, or nearly unique, and cases of a new disease or an unexpected association (such as an outlier case or one with unexpected therapeutic events). They may represent notable early clinical observations that herald new diseases. Case studies are frequent in the PA literature and offer the practicing clinician an opportunity to share interesting and informative cases.

Editorials

The editorial section of journals is often the most revealing and, occasionally, the most controversial section of the journal. At times, an editorial in a major biomedical journal is an invited comment on a paper appearing in the same issue. Editors may choose to invite subject matter experts to compare and contrast their opinions with the paper and other known related studies. Articles that have the potential for substantial impact on a disease or society are often complemented with an invited editorial, as are articles that endorse a significant departure from the traditional method of treating a disease or condition. Editorials can be personal opinion pieces that address issues and controversy in society, medicine, and the profession. Editorials sometimes present minority opinions on professional trends and directions. Editorials can be submitted by anyone, but journals may have policies that govern what can be addressed in an editorial. Generally, the editor of the journal makes the decision on whether or not to publish an editorial or not.

Position Papers: A Variant of the Editorial

Many highly respected journals are owned by professional societies, and these often contain official statements and position papers produced by the organization. Some journals choose to publish occasional "point-counterpoint" position papers on controversial topics. Although such articles typically do not contribute new data to an issue, the questions they pose often result in the development of new studies or new ways to approach an ill-defined issue. Position papers may attempt to influence readers, members, or those outside of the profession or professional society. Position papers sometimes will deal with therapeutic or clinical issues. These are usually the result of reviews by experts who then recommend a course of action. It is not uncommon for standards of care to come from such positions or expert opinion.

Book Reviews

Book reviews are common departmental features of biomedical journals. An effective and engaging book review begins when the reviewer, ideally an individual well versed in the field that the book addresses, begins by asking the following questions: Is this book needed? Does it add a new perspective to the topic? Is it a helpful addition to the clinician's library? Reviews of books are commissioned by the editor or the department editor and are thus usually an invited publication. Book reviews may or may not count as "significant publications" by institutional promotion and tenure committees. However, the opportunity to do a book review is a publishing opportunity.

Letter to the Editor

For readers, the well-written, informed, pointed response to a previously appearing article can be among the most interesting sections. Letters to the Editor often include frank challenges to published findings. The real and personal risk of publishing any work in a peer-reviewed journal is that writers open themselves to public and professional criticism and occasionally humiliation when their work is challenged or refuted by experts on the topic. For other writers such as aspiring authors, however, a letter to the editor may represent an entry channel to publication and further contributions. If appearing in a major medical journal, letters to the editor count as a "major publication" and are indexed in *Index Medicus*. Letters to the editor should directly address a recently published paper or provide new information. Letters are usually limited to 500 words or fewer, and journals typically restrict the number of times letters to the editor by a given author can be published. Typically, if a published work is challenged or commented on in some way, the original author is allowed a response.

Abstracts and Posters

An excellent opportunity to present your work in a peer-reviewed forum includes abstract and poster presentations. For PAs, professional meetings such as the American Academy of Physician Assistants (AAPA) and the Association of Physician Assistant Programs (APAP) offer an excellent opportunity for poster and abstract presentation. AAPA's Clinical and Professional Poster Session is conducted every year at the annual PA conference. AAPA's Clinical and Scientific Affairs Council sponsors the session and coordinates the submission and peer-review process. The following section is from the AAPA Web site (*http://www.aapa.org/clinissues/PosterSession.htm*, used by permission), and is an excellent resource for abstract and poster development and presentation:

Frequently Asked Questions

Q. What is a poster?

A. A poster is a common method used to present research in the biomedical sciences. It is actually a bulletin board that displays one or several large pieces of paper. It provides an opportunity to publish a very short article and discuss it with your peers. It is a static, visual medium that you use to communicate ideas and messages. In presenting your research with a poster, you should aim to use the poster as a means for generating active discussion of the research. A great poster is readable, legible, well organized, and succinct. The Science and Engineering Library at the State University of New York at Buffalo has excellent Web resources to help you create an effective poster (*http://ublib.buffalo.edu/libraries/units/sel/bio/posters.html*).

Q. Does it have to be original research?

A. No, although original research is the sine qua non for poster presentations other types of research or scholarly activity are welcome. Appropriate research may be results of a survey, an interventional study, a secondary data analysis, an epidemiologic study, cost–benefit analysis, an evaluation of a diagnostic test, or something else. Interesting case studies, patient vignettes, and innovative practice techniques are also welcome. Posters that have been presented at other professional meetings within the past 12 months are also eligible for submission. Students are strongly encouraged to present research done in the program. Faculty are encouraged to present their educational research, innovative curricular designs, or case studies.

Q. Is the process very competitive?

A. There is no competition to get your abstracts approved per se. In most cases, if you follow the guidelines and present quality work, your abstract will be accepted. In general, originality of work, adequacy of data, and clarity of expression are the determining factors for selection. Specific selection criteria vary for each category as listed below.

- Original research
  - Is the purpose or the objective clearly stated? Is the scope of topic too broad or too narrow?
  - Is the description of the materials and methods understandable? Are the data collection and experimental technique adequate for the study?
  - Are the analytical procedures used adequately described? Is the research design appropriate for the data collected and the subject of the study?
  - Are the results presented in sufficient detail to support the conclusions? Do they follow from the data and analysis?
  - Is the conclusion clear and the interpretation sound?
  - Is the information presented important? Are there

practical implications of the information? Is the information new? Is the research original?

- Clinical report or case study
  - Is the information presented clearly and understandably?
  - Is the information presented applicable to PAs?
  - Is the information clinically important, relevant, and significant?
- Previously presented poster
  - Is the information appropriate for PAs?
  - Does it satisfy the criteria above for original research?
- Educational research or interventions
  - Is the abstract thoughtful, organized, and clear?
  - Is an innovative method presented which is original and effective?
  - Are measurable outcomes presented?
  - Does the project impact special populations?
  - Does the project have value to other PA educators and the PA profession?

Q. Do you have an example of what a poster looks like?

A. The Clinical Affairs and Education Staff created a poster demonstrating the principles of poster design and summarizing the abstract review process. (Link available on Web site.)

Posters

The poster display board is 8 feet wide by 4 feet tall with a 1 inch metal border. The background material is a neutral color cloth. Figure 13–1 demonstrates the look of the classic original research poster. The top banner should include the title, author names, and author affiliations. The poster should read from top left to bottom right. The title should be legible from 8 feet away, the remaining words from 4 or 5 feet away. See the poster guidelines for more information.

Look at Figure 13–1 for examples. Keep in mind these important tips:

- Keep it simple.
  - Present only enough information to support your conclusions.
  - About eight poster panels is the maximum for effective presentation.
- Use graphs, charts, and figures to make your points; less text is better.
  - A good ratio is 20 percent text, 40 percent graphics and 40 percent open space
  - Don't use all capital letters; they are much harder to read.
- Above all be clear, concise, and organized.

Q. Are there any resources to help me prepare my poster?

A. Look for these in your local library:

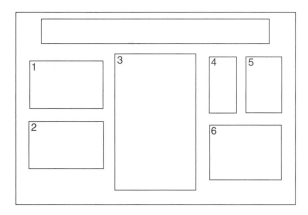
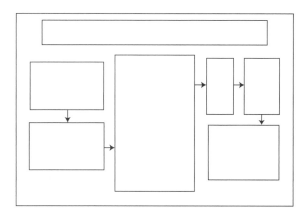

FIG. 13–1. Example of a poster presentation.

Salisbury FB. Appendices—presenting scientific data: "Some suggestions about scientific writing." In Salisbury FB (ed): Units, Symbols, and Terminology for Plant Physiology: A Reference for Presentation of Research Results in the Plant Sciences. New York: Oxford University Press, 1996, pp. 163–187.

Loning RE. Standards for effective presentations (includes section on Poster Presentations, pp. 195–197). In Salisbury FB (ed): Units, Symbols, and Terminology for Plant Physiology: A Reference for Presentation of Research Results in the Plant Sciences. New York: Oxford University Press, 1996, pp. 188–201.

Block SM. 1996. Do's and Don'ts of Poster Presentation. Biophysical Journal 71(6):3527–3529.

Brown BS. 1997. Poster design: six points to ponder. Biochemical Education 1997;25(3):136–137.

Schowen KB. Communicating in other formats: posters, letters to the editor, and press releases—tips for effective poster presentations. In Dodd JS (ed): The ACS Style Guide: A Manual for Authors and Editors, 2nd ed., 1997, Chapter 2.

Hartman KJ. Designing effective poster presentations. Fisheries 21(7):22.

Day RA. How to prepare a poster. In Day RA (ed): How to Write & Publish a Scientific Paper, 4th ed. Phoenix: Oryx Press, 1994, pp. 148–151.

Hailman JP, Strier KB. meetings. Planning, Proposing and Presenting Science effectively: A Guide for Graduate Students and Researchers in the Behavioral Sciences and Biology. New York: Cambridge University Press, pp. 112–115.

Briscoe MH. Posters. In Preparing Scientific Illustrations: A Guide to Better Posters, Presentations, and Publications, 2nd ed. New York: Springer-Verlag, 1996, pp. 131–149.

Pechenik JA. Writing a poster presentation. In A Short Guide to Writing About Biology, 3rd ed. Upper Saddle River, NJ: Pearson Longman, 1997, pp. 258–265.

Davis M. Poster presentations. In Scientific Papers and Presentations. San Diego: Academic Press, 1997, pp. 258–265.

Gosling PJ. Scientist's Guide to Poster Presentations New York: Kluwer Academic/Plenum Press, 1999, 139 pp.

Many other helpful sites exist to offer guidance on poster presentations. A Google™ entry of "poster presentation tips" results in more than 1,000,000 hits. One site with a number of excellent examples of poster compositions is *http://www.aas.duke.edu/trinity/research/vt/postertips.html*. Another helpful site that includes things to avoid when making PowerPoint© presentations is *http://www.anandnatrajan.com/FAQs/powerpoint.html*

Oral Presentations

Many professional meetings provide opportunities for participants to orally present their research. A common method is a 10-minute presentation followed by a 5-minute question and answer session. This is an excellent opportunity to present work in progress or the results of a finished project or study. The most frequently used product for digital presentation of data is Microsoft's PowerPoint.© Numerous self-paced PowerPoint© training courses are available online at *http://office.microsoft.com*. In addition, entering "PowerPoint presentations" on Internet search engines will result in more than a million hits on sites to visit for additional instruction or assistance. A number of excellent sites with general hints for effective oral presentations can be found on the Internet.

Becoming a good speaker and presenter requires experience, effort, and practice. A beginning speaker has only effort and practice at hand. The experience comes from making oral presentations. The first time speaker or presenter also feels nervousness and anxiety, which increase as the size of the audience size grows. These are normal responses and feelings, and even veteran speakers get "butterflies" from time to time. Two key ways to overcome initial fears are to: (1) know your material and (2) practice, practice, and practice some more. There are two common traps that you need to avoid. The first is "Don't read your visual presentation." Too many presenters just read their overheads, PowerPoints, or slides. If all you do is read your visual presentation, there is no need for an oral presentation. There will be very few audiences that cannot read. Use notes or keywords to help you deliver your material and to keep you on course. The second common trap that many first time speakers fall into is that they have practiced to the point where they sound like they are reciting a memorized piece of work. You need some spontaneity and emotion in your voice. Don't recite your presentation. It will be boring. Talk to your audience. Don't try to be funny unless you are good at it. Humor can add much to a presentation, but it must be appropriate for the audience, material, and you, the speaker.

The last key element to being a good speaker and presenter is to stay in the time frame allowed for your presentation. Be aware of your time. Practice will help you frame a time period, but it is never the same as being in front of an audience. It is probably better to end a presentation a bit early than to run over your allotted time. One way to avoid running over is to allow some time for questions at the end of a presentation. In some venues, there will be directions to allow for a set time period for questions. The authors believe that, generally, 5 minutes is a reasonable time for questions. Much depends on the length and subject matter of your presentation. A plus point for always allowing time for questions is that if you run a few minutes long in presentation, the only thing lost is the question period. If you are short of your allowed time, it gives you a longer period to field questions.

Work at being a good presenter. The more experience you gain as a presenter, the less effort and practice you will need to do the presentation itself and the more time you will have to concentrate on your subject. As you begin your presentation and speaking experiences, you may want to look for formats and venues that have short 10- to 15-minute periods or consider panels and co-presentations. Going this way will keep you from being put "under the gun" for an extended time. You may also want to look for small audience opportunities as a way to gain experience.

Physician Assistant Papers

As more PA educational programs during the 1990s either began as, or converted to, awarding the master's degree, theses or master's papers became more com-

mon. A final graduate paper typically requires extensive modification, usually specifically tailored reduction in length in order to be a suitable candidate for peer-reviewed publication. The usual academic format needs to be modified to fit the format required by a specific journal. Be aware that the editor and editorial board members are expert at determining if a master's thesis has been reworked to fit the specifications of a specific journal. Having early publications on one's resume is likely to enhance employment opportunities and professional advancement. Some PA publications have a policy of not accepting manuscripts from PA students owing to the high overall rejection rate of unsolicited manuscripts. If you feel your graduate project is worthy of consideration for publication then send a query letter to either a member of the editorial board or the editor. Acquiring their guidance in advance can increase your chances for publication.

Writing the Paper

Huth (1994) proposed a writing system utilizing a process in which one writes a first draft, places it aside for a couple of days, rereads it, and then begins the second draft (rewrite). This iterative–reiterative process is continued until the paper is finished. Authors should consider sharing the paper with a friend who has critical writing and editing skills. Colleagues with content expertise should also be consulted. Please understand that it may take as many as 10 or more drafts and rewrites until you achieve a final product.[3] Your aim is quality, and this level of effort is the effort that quality requires.

Working with Editors

Writers and editors have historically shared an uneasy alliance. According to Arthur Plotnik (*The Elements of Editing*),[7] editors are foot soldiers in the eternal war between raw talent and the people who process that talent. As long as writers write primarily to advance themselves, and editors edit to satisfy readers, there will never be a lasting peace. Writers know their particular subject; editors know their audience. A well-known truism is that knowledge of the subject does not necessarily translate to good writing, and good writing does not necessarily correlate with good editing. The editor may determine that a writer's style does not correlate with the journal's requirements or quality standards.

When conflicts of interest arise in the editing process, the readership, not the writer, receives first consideration. This is where the writer must have thick skin.

Realize that some of your work and words will be changed in the editorial process. Resist the temptation to think that it's no longer your work when the text is modified to fit the format and preference of the journal that accepted it for publication. Manuscript content is the writer's province, but the form is the editor's specialty. Do not be frustrated if a manuscript has to be revised a number of times. Each revision is reviewed and your changes to meet required or recommended improvements may need further work. Like other biomedical journals, journals in the PA profession are typically expensive to operate, and editors are required to make the most efficient use of their pages. Figure 13–2 shows the stages of publication.

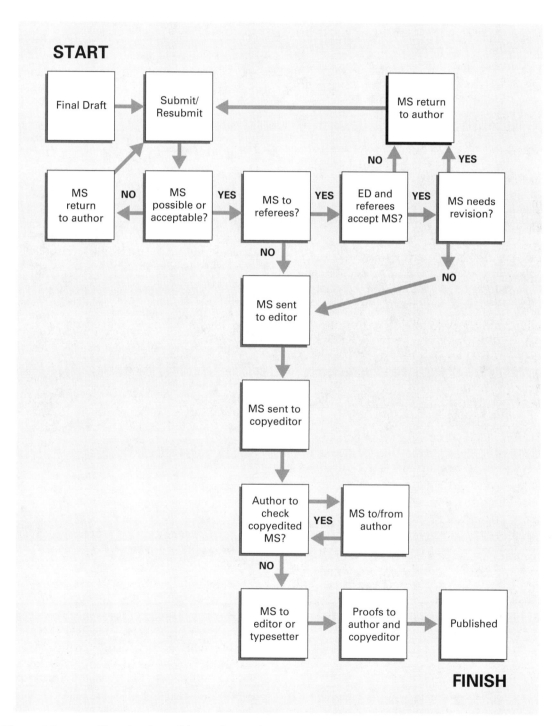

FIG. 13–2. Manuscript process. The refereeing, editing, and copyediting stages in the publication pathway. (Adapted from O'Conner M: How to Copyedit Scientific Books and Journals. Philadelphia: ISI Press, 1986, p. 16.)

Basic Steps in Publication

What is the right journal for your manuscript? Different journals feature different types of formats: Original Reports, Special Articles, Short Papers, Editorials (usually invited), Clinical Notes, and Letters to the Editor. Decide which format you want your paper to have. If you are unsure, contact one of the journal editors or editorial board members for clarification. Is the topic of your proposed paper within the journal's scope? Is the topic represented frequently or only rarely? Would the journal offer the best match of audience with your topic? What formats does the journal accept? Who is the audience? Determine who cares about the message of your paper. Is it best suited for a clinical specialty journal or a general medical journal? Is it best suited for clinicians, educators, researchers, or all of these groups?

Duties of a Potential Author

Based on the topic of the paper, several journals may be publishing candidates. Begin with the most recently published issue of a target journal, and work back for at least 1 year, reading each issue carefully. Review the last few years' publications. Ensure that an article on the same topic you are considering for submission has not recently been published. If it has, determine if your paper merely rehashes existing information or adds new information. In assessing the suitability of your paper for a particular journal, you should also do the following:

1. Read the journal's Statement of Editorial Purpose.
2. Review the journal's editorial board membership.
3. Consult the annually published list of peer reviewers.
4. Read the journal's most recent Information for Authors statement.
5. Evaluate the journal's publishing style regarding article format and requirements for tables, charts, abstracts, footnotes, citations, and references.

In doing these tasks, the author can determine in advance if the project fits a specific journal or if it needs to be modified in differing ways. Have you reviewed and cited the relevant work of leaders, members of the journal's editorial board, and peer reviewers? This is referred to as "chanting the names of the ancestors." Realize that at least one editorial board member and one or more peer reviewers will review your work. If you fail to cite their relevant work, your paper may be deemed incomplete.

Communicate with the Connected

Establish dialog with editors, editorial board members, peer reviewers, or subject matter experts on your topic.

If you have a specific journal in mind, send a proposed outline of your manuscript to determine preliminary interest. Try to get from the "unsolicited" to the "solicited" side of the journal's editors. These are the "connected" people for your publishing attempt.

Request Reprints of Previously Published Articles

Every peer-reviewed journal lists the contact person (usually the first author) for article reprints. Write this person a letter stating how much you enjoyed his or her work. This individual may end up reviewing your manuscript, or you may eventually cultivate a collaborative relationship with him or her. Request a reprint of his or her work.

Requirements and Resources for Writers

An important characteristic of writers is that they possess (or develop) thick skin when working with the paper's revision, rejection, and publishing process. Basic requirements include access to medical literature databases, preferably accessible electronically via online Internet service providers. Writers must be meticulous in their work.

PA students attempting to meet master's degree paper requirements must have access to biomedical literature databases (such as the National Library of Medicine's "Grateful Med" at *http://www.Igm.nlm.nih.gov*). If you have access to academic-based reference librarians, befriend them; they can help you make the literature review and reference retrieval process much less intimidating. Writing also requires uninterrupted time, with ready access to reference and resource material, including your reference documents, a personal computer, and your favorite writing aids. You must schedule time to write on a regular and predictable basis. Close your door if you need to, or write from home, if that option exists.

The Peer Review Process

To evaluate the accuracy of submitted manuscripts, most reputable biomedical journals employ the peer review process. This process typically involves sending the manuscripts to two or three individuals, selected by the editor, who are in a position to judge the value of the work. In the more selective journals, only a few submissions ever make it just to the peer review process. These journals often have full-time editorial positions that are filled by health professionals (e.g., physicians and midlevel providers) who have developed skills in medical writing and editing. This is the case at journals such as the *New England Journal of Medicine*, the *Journal of the American Medical Association*, the *Annals of Surgery,* and the *Annals of Internal Medicine.*

On receipt, most reputable journals conduct an initial internal review of the manuscript. The editor or an associate editor reads the manuscript and determines its eligibility for peer review. If determined to be a possibility, the manuscript is then sent to peer reviewers from various related fields. Often, peer reviewers may be editorial board members and/or editorial consultants who perform these services for the journal on a regular basis.

The peer-review process is regarded as an extension of the basic principles of science and scholarship. Peer review has existed for more than 200 years and has achieved near universal application for assessing research reports before publication. Peer review is considered a critical quality control. Yet despite this widespread utilization, the process has been shown to have flaws and relatively little is known with regard to the quality and utility of the information that is eventually published.[8,9]

Blinded Review

Journals vary in their policies with regard to "masking" the names and affiliations of authors. Most, but not all, biomedical journals mask the identities of authors. A question regarding the value of the peer review process is the potential of a reviewer being familiar with the author's identity, which would create bias. In several disciplines, only a few investigators are involved in a particular field of research, and the identities of authors may be easily recognized by peers. This is the "Achilles' heel" of the peer review process that has led some journals to adopt the policy of unblinded review.

The Publishing Decision

Outcomes of the peer review process may include:

1. Acceptance
2. Minor revisions required
3. Major revisions required
4. Outright rejection

The response from the editor typically consists of a cover letter summarizing the reviewers' comments, recommendations, and the blinded reviewers' evaluation sheets. Always pay close attention to recommended suggestions, changes, or critiques. Address all concerns expressed by the reviewers, including data inconsistencies and errors, even if you disagree with them. (It is not unusual for authors to disagree with peer reviewers.) If you can make your case, the section of the manuscript in question may remain unchanged. Review and save

rejection letters with a copy of the submitted manuscript. Some rejection letters are carefully worded invitations to resubmit. Rejection is part of the process. All successful authors have a history of rejection. Don't take it personally. Resubmit the manuscript with all of the required revisions completed, addressing all of the concerns of the editor and reviewers. As stated earlier, be prepared for a rejection letter. Learn from the experience; everyone has been rejected at some point.

Submitting the Final Manuscript

Assuming that the final version of the manuscript meets all publishing requirements, the packet is then sent to the journal, including the requisite number of manuscript copies. Be aware that journal requirements may vary on specific format of the title page—for instance, whether or not an abstract is required as part of the manuscript. The final packet should also be accompanied by a cover letter that summarizes the basic rationale for the paper. The cover letter must also include an author attestation statement that "the paper, nor its essential substance" is not presently under consideration by another journal and has not appeared elsewhere (e.g., in another journal). This statement must be fully acknowledged and signed by all authors indicating that the work is their own and has not been published or submitted elsewhere.

Authors must follow precisely the Instructions to Authors requirements of the particular journal to which they are submitting. The final draft submission should be flawless. This becomes very important when work is submitted to a journal that has significant competition for space. If an editor must choose between two manuscripts of relatively equal importance, then the one that requires the least amount of corrective action from the editorial staff is more likely to be accepted.

The next step is the receipt of the galley proofs. Be prepared for a rapid turnaround requirement—as little as 24 hours is not unusual. This requires you to drop what you're doing to address the proofs and return them for final typesetting.

Realize that you assign copyright protection to the journal that accepts your work; in reality, it is no longer your paper. If you eventually need to include some of the data again in another manuscript (a published table, for example), you must secure permission from the publisher, even though it was your work to begin with.

Authorship

The author must carefully select co-authors as the research or project ideas are developed. Adding colleagues or friends who contribute little to the work is inappropriate and serves to alienate the co-authors who did perform the work. A co-author should have generated at least part of the intellectual content of the paper and had a part in writing the paper, including reviewing it for possible revision or revising its intellectual content. A co-author should be able to publicly defend all of the content of the paper in the scientific community.

Before you agree to collaborate, know the work habits, reliability, and temperaments of potential co-authors. Are they committed to deadlines? Do they return calls and provide information in a timely manner? Do they do what they say they will do? All of these issues matter when it comes to co-authoring manuscripts. A good rule of thumb is that the more co-authors you have, the more difficult it becomes in getting the paper to everyone's point of agreement and satisfaction. It is important to agree up front about work responsibilities and authorship order. The overall responsibility of the manuscript always rests with the first author.

Assignment and determination of authorship on papers submitted to biomedical journals has undergone significant evolution in recent years. There is now a greater sense of accountability for the intellectual contributions of authors and what types of contributions merit authorship.

Authorship of a paper submitted to a biomedical journal indicates that the individual has invested substantial intellectual effort in the conceptualization and writing of the manuscript.

To qualify as an author, an individual should fulfill the following criteria:

- Participated in the work sufficiently to take public responsibility for all or part of the content
- Made substantial contributions to the intellectual content of the paper in one or more of the following categories:
  - conception and design
  - acquisition of data
  - analysis and interpretation of data
  - drafting of the manuscript
  - critical revision of the manuscript for substantive intellectual content
  - statistical analysis
  - obtaining funding
  - administrative, technical, or material support

Source: Journal of the American Medical Association Authorship Responsibility, Financial Disclosure, Copyright Transfer and Acknowledgment Statement.

Today, most reputable medical journals will require authors to sign a form attesting to their input into the paper and verifying their qualification for authorship designation.

Group authorship sometimes presents problems, particularly with citation. Group authorship is the listing of the name of a group in place of the names of individual authors. Modified group authorship, in which individual names are listed followed by the name of the group, is also used. Group authorship is most often used by investigators associated with studies involving many investigators (e.g., multicenter clinical trials or genomics) because it allows investigators to share credit equally. PubMed is the National Library of Medicine's (NLM's) bibliographic database, with citations dating back to 1966. The NLM has not included group authors in the MEDLINE author field; rather, the group name has been included as an add-on to the title. NLM will now list group authors under a separate "collective name" field. Science Citation Index (SCI) is a scientific and biomedical bibliographic database used to track citations to individual articles. Instead of listing the research group in the author field in its source listing, SCI lists either all individual names in the group or the writing committee members' names in the order they are listed in the article.

Publishing in the PA Profession

Become familiar with the characteristics and orientation of the journals you want to target as potential publishers of your research paper. PA-specific literature is still somewhat limited when compared to that for medicine and nursing.

The PA Literature

The first official journal of the American Academy of Physician Assistants (AAPA) was launched in 1970. Initially, the title was *Physician Associate*, reflecting the then-current name of the American Academy of Physician's Associates. Later, when the name changed to the American Academy of Physician Assistants, the title *PA Journal* was placed on the journal cover. Journals of the PA profession indexed in the Cumulative Index on Nursing and Allied Health Literature (CINAHL) are the *Journal of the American Academy of Physician Assistants* (JAAPA) and *Perspective on Physician Assistant Education*. Nonclinical articles appearing in JAAPA are indexed in *Index Medicus*.

JAAPA, the official journal of the AAPA, is a peer-reviewed journal published by Avanstar and indexed on CINAHL. *JAAPA* publishes original clinical and research articles, clinical reviews, articles on professional issues and workforce policy topics, book reviews, editorials, letters to the editor, opinion pieces, and AAPA professional news and organizational events. *JAAPA* has an editorial board appointed by the AAPA, and the editor-in-chief is a PA.

Perspective on Physician Assistant Education is the official journal of the Association of Physician Assistant Programs. "*Perspective*" is intended primarily for PA educators and features peer-reviewed articles. Edited by a senior PA academician/clinician, it includes papers addressing educational methodology and research issues, and issues of concern to PA educators.

Clinician Reviews is a journal directed toward both PAs and NPs (nurse practitioners). It publishes clinical articles as well as letters, review articles, professional news, and conference summaries. *Clinician Reviews* and *Clinician News* are publications of the Clinician Publishing Group, formed in 1989 by two PAs, David Mittman and Tom Yackeren. By targeting both PAs and NPs, these publications are directed toward a wider audience of midlevel practitioners.

Physician Assistant, a clinical journal published by Springhouse Corporation and edited by a senior physician assistant educator, folded in 2003.

Clinical Advisor is a journal that entered the field in 2001. It contains clinical review articles, advice for clinicians, and editorials by leading PA commentators.

Surgical Physician Assistant is the official publication of the American Association of Surgical Physician Assistants and is a specialty journal for PAs working in surgery.

Advance for PAs is among the latest publications to seek a niche in the growing PA market. This publication is targeted for health professions by Merion Publications, and it emphasizes clinical articles but also covers professional news and nonclinical subjects.

Some Challenges for PA Publications

Over the past 40 years the PA profession has seen journals come and go and, in the main, have had difficulty in gaining recognition beyond their PA readership. Part of the problem is the very specialized interest of PAs for, primarily, clinical review type articles. Part of the problem is the relatively small number of PAs. Part of the problem is that outside of the AAPA, journal publication by PA professional societies is almost nonexistent, except for AASPA, as noted earlier. Part of the problem is that journal publication is a competitive business for the publishers. This circumstance was illustrated in 2003 with the passing of the journal *Physician Assistant*, an event that confirms the realities of the competitive nature of the medical periodical publishing business. Most PAs are full-time clinicians and therefore do not have the time nor direct incentive to write and publish medical articles. Those PAs who do, primarily PA educators, are relatively small in number and tend to write on educational and curricular topics and not on clinical matters. The primary audience for PA journals is PA clinicians who seek material of a clinical nature that will help them to keep current on medical care advancements and make them more effective in serving their patients. To do this, rather than depend primarily on their own literature as is done in many other professions, PAs tend to seek and utilize resources that are available to physicians. After all, PAs share the discipline of medicine with physicians. This literature includes the standard medical journals, both the general journals like *JAMA*, *The Lancet*, and the *New England Journal of Medicine*, as well specialty and subspecialty journals. These publications tend to feature papers reporting original clinical and epidemiological research findings and recommendations for optimal management practices. Many PAs read these journals and, like physicians, depend on these sources to keep current with medical advances.

Thus many PAs who might otherwise seek to write and publish are forced to compete with physicians and biomedical scientists in the medical world who are academics, clinical researchers, or basic science researchers, and have the resources and incentives to write and publish. PAs are not trained to be writers/scholars, but instead are prepared to be clinicians, and most are in no position to produce original biomedical studies and research products sought by journals. As a result the PA literature has tended to focus primarily on concise and current clinical review articles, that is, papers that summarize a specific clinical problem and outlines recommended management. While this focus tends to serve the needs of the primary audience, it does not contain original research material. As a consequence, PA specific journals fail to have a readership beyond PAs. This may change as more students gain research experience as a component of their education, as more PA educators become involved with research, and as more and more clinically practicing PAs have research as part of their practice.[10,11]

Medical Journals

Over the past few decades, many PAs have published papers in biomedical journals.[8,9] These journals are aimed primarily toward physician audiences. They include the major general medical journals such as the *New England Journal of Medicine*, the *Journal of the American Medical Association*, *The Lancet*, and the *British Medical Journal*, as well as leading specialty journals such as the *Annals of Internal Medicine*, *American Family Physician*, and *Annals of Surgery*. These are options for PAs, but are limited in some ways.

It goes without saying that the modern medical publishing business is an intensely competitive enterprise. Virtually all biomedical journals are basically dependent on their sponsors (professional societies and commercial publishers) for their viability. The business operations of these ventures in turn depend, most of the time, exclusively on advertising revenue. This fact of life (that biomedical publications depend on revenues from advertisers) requires editors and editorial boards to balance scientific direction and standards and journal content with the requirements of those who are "paying the freight" in the operation of the publication.

The vast numbers of publications in biomedicine are essentially businesses. Publishing medical journals is an expensive venture. Publishers of various biomedical journals comprise:

1. Professional organizations that sponsor and produce a journal identified as their official journal

2. Proprietary publishing firms

3. Philanthropic organizations, including journals such as *Health Affairs*, a health policy resource subsidized by Project Hope, or the Milbank Memorial Fund Quarterly

Manuscript Flaws that Prevent Publication

Authors fall prey to several pitfalls in the preparation and submission of manuscripts to biomedical journals (Box 13–2). Editors and reviewers are always looking for reasons to be skeptical regarding the worthiness of a manuscript for publication. Although the reasons for rejections are extensive, the author should bear in mind the following common scenarios:

BOX 13–2

Reasons for Manuscript Rejection

Excessive use of philosophy

Loose organizational style

Material not sufficiently important

Information not easily generalized

Methods used unclear

Results described unclear

Statistics used incorrectly

Sample size inadequate

Conclusions unwarranted

Results not compared with similar studies

Inadequate period of observation, use, or evaluation of method

Inadequate review of the literature

Adapted from Geyman JP, Bass MJ. Communication of results of research. Journal of Family Practice 1978;7(1):120.

---

1. The topic is inappropriate for a specific journal. The manuscript is a sound piece of investigation, description, or opinion and is presented in a suitable format, but the topic is not quite appropriate for the particular journal. In some cases, these papers may represent previously rejected or recycled manuscripts that the author(s) didn't bother to reconfigure in the required format for that journal.

2. The use of imperfect style and "crazy-quilt" fonts. A manuscript containing imperfect style that has differing sections with differing fonts and font sizes indicates that it may be a "cut-and-paste" effort, one that is basically recycling the work of others or an uncoordinated collaboration among authors that has not been properly edited. Manuscripts with these types of sloppy narrative reveal inattention to detail and a nonsystematic structure. Editors regard such papers as a waste of time if it appears that the authors have not put forth the proper effort to prepare the manuscript to specifications.

3. "Cut-and-paste" citations were used. Cut-and-paste citations lifted verbatim from reference sources are ill advised. If you are not able to put your hands on a citation in your paper, then do not quote it. Do not be surprised if editors or reviewers ask for verification, particularly if the citation looks suspicious. If you can't provide this verification, it raises questions of plagiarism, and the paper will be summarily rejected.

4. Tables and/or text were used without permission. Give credit where credit is due. If you copy or modify a table from someone else's work, acknowledge the source. You may be required to present permission to your publisher.

5. Errors in mathematical calculations occurred (bad math). Be aware that the journal will calculate any math included in the manuscript, such as percentages in a table. It is always recommended that authors double-check their data, including the math included in tables in the manuscript.

6. The same material was used to publish several articles. Editors are well acquainted with the tendency of authors to partition their work into "least publishable units," a phenomenon also known as "salami science." This is the splitting of one's data set into smaller subsets, each with a narrow focus, in an effort to publish as many papers as possible from one core data set. Examples include submitting single-center reports from multicenter studies, and short-duration reports from long-duration studies. The dangers of repetitive publication of the same material are many. An old or recycled paper must be sufficiently updated or have new data added to justify publication.

7. Citation or reference inaccuracies were found. You are obligated to double-check the accuracy of all citations within your work. Citation error is a serious problem in biomedical publications. One study of peer-reviewed surgical journals found a 48 percent citation error rate, casting doubt in many cases that original reference sources were reviewed by the authors.[12]

On Writing and Publishing

Writing is hard and time-consuming work. Authors must fundamentally calculate the questions of "Why write a paper if it does not stand a reasonable chance of being published?" and "What do I have to say?" Dr. John Billings, founder of the National Library of Medicine, espoused four primary rules for the aspiring author:

1. Have something to say.
2. Say it.
3. Stop as soon as you have said it.
4. Give the paper a proper title.

Strive to Write Clearly

Think clearly and you will write clearly. George Orwell said, "Good prose is like a window pane; that is, what you have to say should not be obscured by how you say it." Prose is bad when readers need to stop and look at it again to understand its message. The central message of a book written by a long-time editor of *JAMA*[13] was embodied in its title, "Why Not Say It Clearly?" Interestingly, this book appeared during a time when biomedical writing was criticized by, among others, Michael Crichton (a well-known author and film and television producer), who was then a recent medical school graduate, as being deliberately "obfuscatory." Writing clearly means using words with the greatest degree of accuracy in transmitting what you wish to communicate to others.

A Step-by-Step Approach to Publishing Your Manuscript

The essential steps in the process of publishing a paper in the biomedical literature are as follows:

1. Determine the central message of the paper.
2. Decide if the paper is worth writing.
3. Identify the appropriate audience for the paper.
4. Select the journal for which you will prepare the paper.
5. Search the literature.
6. Determine authorship and an expected timetable.
7. Assemble the sources and materials needed to write the paper.
8. Develop a structure for the paper; make a detailed outline.
9. Write the first draft conforming it to the journal's requirements for manuscripts.
10. Revise the first draft and cycle through several more drafts; add appropriate tables, graphs, and illustrations.
11. Finalize the manuscript; complete all sections.
12. Obtain comments and critiques from selected "personal consultants."
13. Submit the article to the selected journal in the required format; include a formal cover letter with the appropriate disclaimer.
14. Promptly respond and revise the manuscript as indicated in the editor's communication; respond to all authors' queries.
15. Resubmit the corrected manuscript; proof the final typescript; assign copyright.

Summary

After deciding to attempt to publish your work, one should consider several key steps. These include making sure that your work is a quality effort and your writing is clear and concise. You need to make a careful selection of the journal or journals that may be interested in the type of work you have produced. You may want to contact the editor about his or her interests. Follow the "Instructions to the Author" explicitly. If the journal is interested, work with them on revisions and suggestions for your paper. Be patient because the process takes time, sometimes up to 1 year. If your submission is rejected, it can be for many reasons. It is not personal. In fact, for those who seek to publish often, rejection is part of life. Remember that your work has value to you in the experience you gained in the process of scientific inquiry. If research is a part of your professional life, publication success will eventually occur.

References

1. Kole LA, Currey R. Writing to be published— Why and how (and when). Journal of the American Academy of Physician Assistants 1999;12(3):92, 93, 96.
2. Benson CV. A roadmap for better writing: a guide to writing for JAAPA. Journal of the American Academy of Physician Assistants 1994;7:53.

3. Huth EJ. How to Write and Publish Papers in the Medical Sciences, 2nd ed. Baltimore: Williams & Wilkins 1990.

4. International Committee of Medical Journal Editors: Guide to Uniform Requirements for Manuscripts Submitted to Biomedical Journals. JAMA 1997;277:927-934.

5. Glass RM, Flanigan A. Communication, biomedical II. Scientific publication. In Reich WT (ed): Encyclopedia of Bioethics, 2nd ed. New York: Macmillan, 1995.

6. Weller AC. Qualitative and quantitative measures of indexed health sciences electronic journals. JAMA 2002;287:2865–2866.

7. Plotnick A. The Elements of Editing: A Modern Guide for Editors and Journalists. New York: Macmillan, 1982.

8. Jefferson T, Wagner E, Davidoff F. Measuring the quality of editorial peer review. JAMA 2002;287:2786–2790.

9. Wagner E, Jefferson T. The shortcomings of peer review. Learned Publishing 2001;14:257–263.

10. Hooker RS, Cawley JF. Physician Assistants in American Medicine, 2nd ed. New York: Churchill Livingstone, 2003.

11. Ballweg R, Stolberg S, Sullivan E (eds): Physician Assistant Guide to Clinical Practice, 2nd ed. Philadelphia: WB Saunders, 1999.

12. Evans JT, Nadjari HI, Burchell SA. Quotational and reference accuracy in surgical journals. JAMA 1990;263;1353..

13. King L. Why Not Say It Clearly? Boston: Little, Brown, 1978.

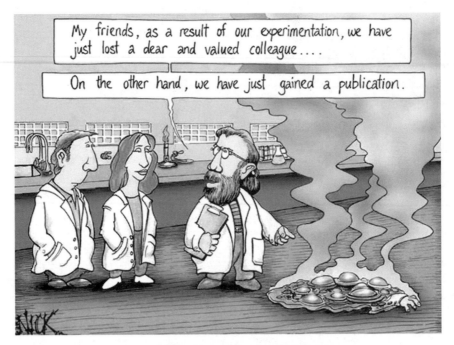

Reprinted by permission of Nick D. Kim.

chapter 14

Ethics in Research

Suzanne M. Peloquin, PhD, OTR, FAOTA

Even if we cannot, strictly speaking, teach people to act properly, we can prepare minds to think about action and to see the uses in experience of acting one way rather than another.

J. Allen (1987, p. 53)

Chapter Overview

This chapter discusses a sampling of the ethical considerations involved in research. Largely because of the notorious medical experiments conducted during World War II, it is clear to most individuals that ethical behaviors are important when human subjects participate in studies. The research process taps many more ethical behaviors than the very clear demand to do no harm and to respect human rights, however. Research in health care is a multifaceted and interpersonal process that scarcely resembles the science that happens in a laboratory. Many occasions for ethical deliberation present themselves to health-care practitioners on a regular basis. Such occasions, though not as dramatic in nature or outcome as the experiments conducted by Nazi doctors, require that physician assistants (PAs) choose the best ethical action from among many actions that are possible.

Scientific inquiry is one aspect of healthcare practice that demands that PAs consider value systems, make critical decisions, and interact responsibly with others. It is the aim of this chapter to provoke you to think more deeply about what it means to be ethical in the practice of research. It is my hope to prepare your minds in the way described in the citation that launches this introduction, so that you might be ready to "think about action and to see the uses in experience of acting one way rather than another."[1]

Thinking About Ethics in Research

In keeping with the aim of this chapter to provoke you to think more deeply, I begin with a fable entitled *The Glass in the Field*.[2] Remember, a fable is a story about animals that is designed to teach lessons about persons. This fable features several large birds—a goldfinch, sea gull, hawk, eagle—and one small swallow. As the title of the fable suggests, the story turns around a large piece of plate glass left standing upright in a field by a construction crew. The first bird to encounter the glass was a goldfinch, knocked cold as he flew into it. When asked by a sea gull what had happened, the goldfinch considered the question and said that the air had crystallized. The sea gull, eagle, and hawk all laughed. They offered other hypotheses: that the goldfinch was struck by a hailstone, that he had had a stroke. They asked the swallow his opinion because he had remained silent on the matter; he said, rather meekly, that perhaps the air *had* crystallized.

The large birds then took wagers from the goldfinch who, annoyed at their laughter, said that they would hit the hardened air if they flew the same course. They took his bet of a dozen worms each and invited the swallow to join them. He declined. The large birds together flew the course described by the finch and were knocked unconscious. The swallow watched. The moral that James Thurber attached to his fable was this: "He who hesitates is sometimes saved."

The moral is a whimsical twist on the old adage, "He who hesitates is lost." The fable tells much about research functions such as experiencing reality, asking questions, formulating hypotheses, and testing in the field. It tells of precision and observation. It exemplifies the kinds of speculations that lead to experimentation in the first place. It illustrates the manner in which researchers can sometimes be at odds with one another about whether and how hypotheses should be tested. It highlights the risks that some investigators take in either formulating or testing their hypotheses and the prudence that others exercise when the risk of harm is present. It shows how incentives to investigate a reality can grow when funding is thrown into the mix.

I use this fable to introduce a discussion of ethics in research because its strong moral theme about hesitation also targets the work of this chapter. Most of the other chapters in this book point to the cognitive and technical demands of research, and these are vital discussions. But many affective challenges, both intrapersonal (within an individual) and interpersonal (between or among individuals), also characterize the quest for knowledge, and these must not be taken lightly or dismissed as peripheral. The fable about *The Glass in the Field* supports the necessity for reflection, an action that is vital to ethical practice. Often, in moments of critical decision making, little time is available to hesitate while pondering the best choice. Time spent beforehand, with a chapter such as this, is a proactive way to prepare for such moments.

The Nature of Ethics and Research

When a person habitually, or even regularly, thinks about the ends and means of an action and accordingly acts to achieve the best ends, that person can be said to

have learned virtue, or grace.[1] Allen's words show his broad understanding of ethics as a deliberation that keeps these thoughts in mind simultaneously: the best outcomes of any action, the goodness of any means or methods used, and the call to honor virtue throughout the process. Allen's understanding characterizes the good researcher who would have to agree that any responsible discussion of the *ethics of research* must occur within discussion of the broader disciplines of both ethics and science. I propose that to set out to discuss the ethics of research is to consider the affective dimension of science alongside its intellectual rigor. Let me elaborate.

As an investigator, it is important that as you develop your project, you also develop and explore the ethical considerations that will be part of your study. Ethics as a discipline seeks to understand the moral duties and obligations that associate with any action. Ethics relies heavily on personal thought, value systems, and the interpersonal responsibilities of those who live their lives and practice their professions in communities. Science has a different focus. Science as a discipline is a search for knowledge. Although the practice of science is best known for its intellectual or cognitive rigor, science also warrants and taps the affective or emotional side of human nature. If one agrees that the affective dimension of human nature includes creativity, imagination, motivation, will, and courage, the link between science and the affective performance of scientists becomes clear. Research is but one of many of the methods of science, alongside other forms of scientific inquiry, such as philosophical and historical work. Scholars in history, philosophy, or the humanities would be the first to agree that their work taps both their intellectual and affective competence. But even the practice of highly focused medical research is commonly understood to have affective demands such as those for personal integrity, interpersonal accountability, and collaborative teamwork.

There is much to consider, then, when the two terms *ethics* and *research* are juxtaposed and the call becomes that of considering moral action as one is searching for knowledge. The challenge to prepare to be ethical in research is far greater than can be met through memorization of any guidelines for research that can be found in ethical codes published by professional groups. The scope of the phrase *the ethics of research* includes any issues that may emerge when the practice of seeking moral duties and obligation (ethics) intersects with the practice of discovering new knowledge (research). Such issues may include the affective energy that it takes to prompt and sustain scientific inquiry, the principles and values that drive a personal or professional quest for knowledge, and the intrapersonal and interpersonal challenges that structure the investigatory process. The values that surface as important to researchers include honesty, beneficence, integrity, altruism, respect, prudence, justice, equality, and fidelity. Because each of these values is known in psychology as either an intrapersonal or interpersonal aspect of personal functioning, I suggest that this chapter on the ethics of research is really very much about the affective dimension of science.

The Affective Dimension of Science

In an essay some years ago about the art of science, I noted that science, as a human practice, taps personal characteristics such as passion, imagination, and intuition, each thought to be affective.[3] Science demands these personal characteristics, alongside its rigor. Bruner[4] noted that science builds on wild and artful metaphors that also rise from the affective domain:

> Let me say now what Niels Bohr told me. The idea of complementarity in quantum theory, he said to me, came to him as he thought of the impossibility of considering his son simultaneously in the light of love and in the light of justice, the son having just voluntarily confessed that he had stolen a pipe from a local shop. His brooding set him to thinking about the vases and the faces in the trick figure-ground pictures: you can see only one at a time. And then the impossibility of thinking simultaneously about the position and the velocity of a particle occurred to him. (p. 49)

How little known is the fact that *quantum theory* sprang from a father's emotional musings about how to love his son!

Perhaps because such stories are not widespread, there is a sad tendency to dichotomize affect and cognition in ways that resemble the longstanding and more popular *art-from-science* split. This splitting makes distinctions that name science as the worthier source of knowledge and thought more valuable than emotion. In this same scheme, adjectives such as *soft* or *fuzzy* or *subjective* attach to affective and interpersonal realms. But science is a human endeavor and as such both requires and reflects the thinking–feeling natures of persons. Just because one is engaged in a *scientific* endeavor does not mean that one is free from having to make affective or ethical considerations.

Years ago, scientist–physician Bernard[5] argued against such dichotomies. He said, "discovery inheres in a feeling about things." He supported engagement in intuitive feelings. Affect, in his view, makes science happen. Most will agree that the forces behind science—curiosity, motivation, a desire to know—seem as much affective as intellectual. Philosopher Goodman[6] reiterated this point as he spoke of the tools and talk in science:

> To suppose that science is flatfootedly linguistic, literal, and denotational, would be to overlook the analog instruments often used... and the talk in current physics and astronomy of charm and strangeness and black holes. Even if the ultimate artifact of science, unlike that of art, is literal, verbal, or mathematical denotational theory, science and art proceed in much the same way with their searching and building. (p. 107)

Simply said, my point is this: Science, as a human enterprise, demands affect *and* cognition from its practitioners, often in equal measures.

Affective Concerns in Research Scenarios

It seems important to consider a few examples that show the practice of science as affective in the sense that it challenges researchers to use their intrapersonal strengths. More specifically, it may help to see the manner in which the work of research often involves value conflicts. A brief overview of what we typically mean by values may be a helpful point at which to start.

The fable that introduced this chapter gave a few examples of strongly held values: The workers who left the plate glass standing upright in the field must have held trust as a personal value in that they left something so costly out in the open. Besides being trusting, they perhaps also valued risk-taking; much could have happened to damage that glass. We might also assume from the fact that they were involved in construction that the workers valued physical activity. We deduce that the swallow, having declined to risk flying over the course that had knocked the goldfinch cold, valued caution. He also valued independent thought, choosing to stay behind even as the large birds ridiculed him. The sea gull, having challenged both the goldfinch and the swallow, seemed to value boldness of idea and action. He clearly valued risk and adventure and perhaps also the leadership role in that he rallied the larger birds to join him in both wager and flight.

Knowing one's personal values requires reflection. The process is a matter of first asking what one's likes and preferences as well as dislikes are, then thinking more deeply about what it is within oneself that draws one to make those judgments. Most often, some value is foundational to our choices and decisions, preferences or dislikes.

Examples of situations that may involve value conflicts are presented next in the form of research scenarios. Some of the scenarios may feel quite familiar to you. Others may cause you to make an imaginative leap into a future within which you will assume a more advanced role related to research. For each of the scenarios, ask yourself:

1. What feelings might surface within the individuals in the case?
2. What personal values might lead the individuals to experience conflict?
3. Which values might make peace or compromise possible?
4. What actions might be taken that could be perceived as good or virtuous?

Scenario 1: You are a PA student. As part of a larger class project, you have been invited to participate in a research project conducted by one of your faculty members. You have been told that your participation is voluntary and anonymous, but you know that if you leave the room it will be apparent that you have chosen to abstain. You prefer not to complete the required personal questionnaires. You worry that your nonparticipation in this project will suggest to your faculty that you lack a commitment to the research agenda of the department and may engender some ill will and recrimination.

Scenario 2: You are a senior faculty member with a reputation for qualitative research in your profession. You have thought yourself a historical scholar for years, and your profession values your scholarship. Your university president has announced that funded grants will be prized as the most prestigious form of scholarship, and all of the schools within your university are revising their salary merit systems to reward such work. You know that merit raises will be hard to come by if you do historical work, but you do not want to abandon your passion. You resent this apparent dismissal of historical research.

Scenario 3: You have practiced in your town for 20 years, and you are known as a master clinician. You receive a phone call from a faculty member who teaches in a local university and who has a strong research background. He tells you that he has a research idea on which he hopes that you might collaborate. He asks if he may send you his proposal. You later read the proposal and realize that the research agenda would mean your doing much more work than you think possible or reasonable. You also see that it reflects a lack of understanding of your patients and the constraints within your practice. You realize that this faculty member is naïve about your clinical practice. You are scheduled to meet with him to discuss the proposal.

Scenario 4: You are a junior faculty member with a master's degree. You teach an innovative course that you think is a good fit for submission to a well-known state agency as a project for grant funding. The chair of your department has a doctoral degree and says that the grant would stand a much better chance of funding if her name were listed as the primary investigator with yours listed in the lesser role of project coordinator. You know that you would earn less credit and hold less sta-tus within your setting as a project coordinator, but you believe that your chair has a valid suggestion.

Scenario 5: You are in your first year of practice and have developed a documentation form to gather numerical data on the progress of patients with chronic diseases. You have monitored its use for the past 4 months and are pleased that your supervising physician seems so responsive to its use. You have heard from a reliable friend that this same physician supervisor recently gave a presentation to staff at a hospital out-of-state. She presented "her" documentation form without mentioning your role in either developing or piloting it.

Scenario 6: You are among several who have worked on a committee that decides to write a publication about the results of a recently completed project immunizing children in the community. You come from different disciplines. In your group are two administrators who launched the project, both very invested in their status and their leadership roles. You are meeting as a group to decide who shall be first author and in which order the rest of the names shall appear in the journal. You have been the strongest and primary writer for the group thus far, and you anticipate that you will also do most of the work on this article. You predict that the two administrators will want to be first or primary authors.

Scenario 7: You are a departmental chair working on an interdisciplinary health-care team. You conceived of a research project with your brother's firm that the team thinks is worth pursuing. Your administrator says to you, in the meeting, that it seems best that you disengage yourself from the project because of your close relationship with your brother. You see no conflict of interest because the nature of the research is such that your being related to a co-researcher will not matter. You want to be part of the team; this was your original idea.

Scenario 8: You are a first-year PA in a rehabilitation setting for individuals with head injury, a population unfamiliar to you. Your supervisor asked you a week ago to invite each client to give consent to participating in an ongoing research project. Not quite sure that you know how to do this with individuals who have significant cognitive impairments, you have been asking them, "Do you want to help us with our research?" You hope that this request will suffice. You feel rather awkward asking your supervisor if this approach is sufficient, because the question would suggest the extent to which you feel a novice with this population and with research.

Scenario 9: You walk into the main office of an outpatient clinic in psychiatry on a Monday morning. A new member of the clerical staff, seated among several other workers, looks up and says to you, "Well, Mr. F. certainly has little emotional sensitivity, according to his answers on the scale you're using! He dropped the research form onto my desk and I've rated it for you. I thought I'd just keep up with them as they come in." This staff member was *supposed* to have followed your instructions to have each participant place an anonymous code number on his or her completed scale, drop it into a large box with a slot, and rate all accumulated forms at the same time in 2 weeks.

Scenario 10: In your study of child abuse, you understand that your responsibility in obtaining informed consent includes initiating a dialogue with each participant regarding the possible consequences of participating in your research. Your project requires that participants review their early childhood histories of abuse and neglect. Your task is to discuss fully with each individual the possibly difficult thoughts and emotions that may surface as they remember their past histories. You are really hoping to recruit participants for your project and don't want to scare them off. How will you proceed?

Within each scenario is a research issue. Within each scenario is also an intrapersonal or interpersonal challenge that invites attention, reflection, and virtuous action. Think about the intrapersonal issues in each scenario. Think particularly about any possible differences in personal values, using the questions posed at the start of this section. Some of the challenges that surface within each scenario may seem trivial at first glance, but the manner in which they are handled can have a significant impact on the researcher, the research process, or its outcome. You will perhaps derive more meaning from your engagement with these scenarios if you discuss them with others after having given them some personal thought.

Values that Shape Good Practice

Beyond the individual values held by any one practitioner, several *professional* values relate to good practice in research. Some professions have articulated the core values that should guide their practice. Both nursing and occupational therapy uphold the following values[7]:

Altruism in scientific inquiry is the unselfish concern of a researcher for the well-being of others.
Equality in scientific inquiry requires that the researcher perceive individuals as having the same fundamental human rights and opportunities.
Freedom in scientific inquiry presses the researcher to allow individuals to exercise choice and to demonstrate self-direction.
Justice in scientific inquiry mandates that the researcher act with fairness, equity, truthfulness, and objectivity.
Dignity in scientific inquiry requires that the researcher emphasize the importance of valuing the inherent worth of each person.

Truth in scientific inquiry requires that the researcher be faithful to facts and reality.
Prudence in scientific inquiry is the researcher's ability to discipline the self through the use of reason.[8]

Now, revisit the research scenarios to determine which of the above values might prompt better interpersonal outcomes as well as virtuous actions in each. Let's say, for example, that you embrace altruism (the unselfish concern of a researcher for the well-being of others) as a dominant value. How would that value shape your communications with the individuals in *Scenario 10* who have a history of child abuse? In all likelihood, with altruism *foremost* in mind, you would convey real concern for each candidate. You would openly acknowledge that although the research project is important to you, at least equally important is the fact that participation could be emotionally painful. You would make every effort to ensure that study participants could easily secure help from counselors made accessible to them. You would communicate your concern and this resource to your participants. Spend some time now looking at the list of values and considering how these might help direct a virtuous course of action in each scenario.

Although a list of professional values with accompanying dictionary definitions seems a helpful enough tool, it takes little stretch of the imagination to understand that dilemmas in research—like those in the clinic—often press one to choose one highly important value over another, hence the dilemma. Matters are sometimes not as straightforward as was my application of the value of altruism to Scenario 10.

For example, Scenario 4 involves a junior faculty member's dilemma over whether to accept the chair's suggestion to yield the leadership role to her on a research grant. Let's say that the junior faculty member ultimately chose to exercise *prudence* by yielding to the chair's suggestion. Given her personal lack of a higher educational status that promised a better review by experts, she abandoned the thought of being a principal investigator. In deliberations over what to do in this dilemma, she had had to reflect on several points. She believed that she would end up doing the most work and that *justice* would be compromised if documents indicated otherwise. And although having *equality* of status with the chair relative to this project, the faculty member reasoned that prudent reliance on the chair's educational status and experience in research would result in funding that would get this project off the ground. She considered several values—prudence, justice, and equality—and their meanings and consequences to her and her project. And so it is, in practice, that no listing of professional values can remove from a practitioner the responsibility to reflect about the broader context within which moral action occurs. In this case, the novice researcher, feeling admittedly a bit torn when it came to upholding her sense of equality and justice, chose to value prudence most.

Communication Competence and Ethical Research

The research scenarios that you have considered also call up this question: What interpersonal challenges are present in research and how might these be met? It's a very appropriate question. Any prior knowledge that you have about assertiveness, setting limits, active listening, and negative inquiry will help you to answer it. Many challenges in the practice of research call for competencies in communicating. The hope is for the best possible outcome: that a PA will interact professionally and effectively. To reinforce that hope, I offer a brief review of foundational communication competencies.

One important capacity is that of communicating desires and needs assertively. To assert a personal opinion or position is not to dominate or to be aggressive but to calmly state one's view. "I statements" often characterize assertive communications. Examples of self-assertions that might work in some of the research scenarios within this chapter are these:

"Although I appreciate the opportunity to be involved in this project, I don't feel comfortable filling out this questionnaire." (Scenario 1)

"I understand that grant work is considered of utmost importance on this campus, but I believe that merit raises should follow the execution of quality historical work as well." (Scenario 2)

"I think that you have a very exciting idea, but I can't assume the level of responsibility that you have assigned to me in this proposal." (Scenario 3)

"If you have time, I'd like to discuss something that's bothering me. I have heard from a reliable source that you are making presentations and using the form that I developed while referring to it as your own." (Scenario 5)

"I don't agree with you on that point. I believe that, as originator of the idea for this project, I should be on the team." (Scenario 7)

"I really do appreciate the work that you have done. As soon as you get a chance, I'd like to speak with you privately about the aims of this project." (Scenario 9)

Another related communication capacity helpful in the ethical practice of research is that of setting limits. An individual can set limits effectively with members of a research team in a number of ways that include the offering of alternatives, compromise, empathic refusal, and broken record. Let's again consider Scenario 3 because it lends itself to illustrations of each of these methods. In this scenario, remember, the master clinician has been asked by a local university faculty member to participate in an enormous way in a research project that has little personal appeal for many reasons. The clinician might set limits in these ways:

Offer alternatives: "I can't do all that you have allotted to me in your proposal, but I *would* be willing to take the lead in gathering some data for you."

Compromise: "If you would be willing to take over a few of my clinical responsibilities, I might be able to help you more."

Empathic refusal: "I understand that you need my involvement, but I can't help you in all of the ways that you've specified."

Broken record: In response to several overtures initiated in rapid sequence by the academic researcher, the PA clinician might respond to each, in turn, in this way: "I'm not comfortable with the level of responsibility that you've assigned me……"No, I can't do that"….."I'm sorry, I'm not able to do that"…."There are too many responsibilities for me to handle."

In setting limits through acceptable ways, a practitioner communicates important values and personal intentions as part of virtuous action.

The capacity to actively listen is also an important aspect of ethical research. Both research colleagues and participants need to be heard, particularly when they are sharing strongly felt ideas or opinions; this need makes active listening an important skill to master. The process of active listening consists of a series of exchanges with a person that convey a desire to really hear and understand.[9] The active listener will:

Focus complete attention on the individual who is speaking and communicate interest through eye contact, posture, facial expression, movement, or gestures.

Reflect back what was said through a paraphrase, including the feeling and content of the communication, by using variations of the formula for the understanding response: "You feel _____ because _____."

Seek confirmation and clarification. Sometimes this step can be incorporated into the previous one.

Offer empathy and support.

Explore events and feelings further.

Facilitate problem solving.

As an example, consider Scenario 8. Let's say that the first-year PA, hearing that the MD supervisor had the reputation for being understanding, approached him to share his lack of knowledge in discussing research protocols with patients who are cognitively challenged. Using active listening, the supervisor might say: "You're feeling a bit awkward about how to approach some patients, and that is totally understandable (variation on the how you feel—because—formula). I felt the same way when I started to explain protocols (offer of support). Tell me how you have been trying to do this so far, and maybe we can figure out ways that will work for you." (exploration of the situation and movement toward problem solving).

Another communication competence that is closely related to active listening is that of negative inquiry. Negative inquiry consists of listening fully, without interruptions or defensive responses, to a complaint that someone wants to air. Instead of either responding defensively or prematurely justifying the offensive behavior, the person first *hears* the complaint, or evidence of listening occurs through paraphrasing. Negative inquiry invites the feelings of another so that the air can be cleared, the problem addressed, and better relations resumed.

In Scenario 5, for example, the PA has a significant complaint about the physician's use of a documentation form. Note here how the physician supervisor, using negative inquiry, might respond to the PA's complaint:

PA: "I'm really upset that you have been using the documentation form that I developed when you do presentations at conferences."

MD: "I've angered you by using the form?"

PA: "Yes. I have heard that you are not acknowledging me for having developed it."

MD: "The problem is that you think that I have not declared your prior work on it?"

PA: "Yes, and it looks to others as if you developed it yourself."

MD: "Is there anything else about this situation that troubles you?"

PA: "No, it just seems unfair to me that you have been doing this."

MD: "So if I were to use the form but somehow acknowledge your efforts, that would be acceptable to you?"

PA: "Yes."

MD: "May I tell you what I have been doing? On the bottom of the form, I have listed you as its primary developer. I'm sorry that I failed to share this with you beforehand. Maybe I should also point that out to my audiences in the future."

The Hazards of Plagiarism

This last dialogue between a PA and MD highlighted ethical concerns about ownership in research. In this case, it was ownership of a documentation form that was useful in gathering research data. In some of the other scenarios, ownership questions emerged relative to ideas and projects (Scenarios 6 and 7). Ownership clashes can occur around use of the titles of *primary* or first author of an article or *primary investigator* on a grant. Often the discussion turns on who should get credit for the work and how fair that determination

seems in light of who did either the most work or most important parts of the work.

One aspect of ownership in research that is familiar to PAs who are still in a student role is that of plagiarism. Commonly understood as taking the idea or work of another and passing it off as one's own, plagiarism is a growing concern today because so many resources are so readily available. The guidelines established in the American Medical Association's *Manual of Style*[10] in a section entitled "scientific misconduct" are helpful in clarifying various forms of plagiarism.

The first definition of scientific misconduct was released by the US Public Health Service in 1989 as "fabrication, falsification, plagiarism, or other practices that seriously deviate from those that are commonly accepted within the scientific community for proposing, conducting, or reporting research" (1989). This definition, known as FFP because of its reference to fabrication, falsification, and plagiarism, remains the official one. In 1993 the Commission on Research Integrity[11] defined scientific misconduct further at the request of the US Public Health Service. The new definition, known as MMI for its substitution of the terms misappropriation, misrepresentation, and interference, has not replaced the old because it does not apply as well as the old one does to all governmental departments.[10]

Iverson et al.[10] described four common kinds of plagiarism:

1. Direct plagiarism: Lifting of passages word for word without placing the lifted material in quotation marks or crediting the author.

2. Mosaic: Borrowing ideas from an original source by using a few word-for-word phrases woven into one's own work, without crediting the original author.

3. Paraphrase: Restating a phrase or paragraph so that although the words differ, the meaning is the same and the author is not credited.

4. Insufficient acknowledgment: Noting only a small part of what is borrowed so that a reader cannot know exactly what is original and what is not.[10]

Within the discussion that follows their descriptions, Iverson et al.[10] said that plagiarism often occurs because of careless note-taking. For example, consider this: A PA student sits in the library or at a computer and records good ideas to include in a paper. The student does not, near each idea, either note the precise source or insert quotation marks. Prompted by these good ideas of other authors, the student then jots down personal thoughts alongside ideas from his or her other sources. Days later, the student begins writing a paper from his or her notes, forgetting or confusing which ideas were original and which came from the resources being used, mixing them in a way that constitutes plagiarism. Careless in his original method of note-taking, the student produces a paper that is plagiarized.

Even if it is inadvertent, plagiarism can be a violation of copyright law and a breach of honesty. Should the holders of the original copyright discover the breach of ethics and law and file suit, penalties could be imposed by the courts. And in many academic centers, violations of academic integrity policies in place can result in serious consequences such as expulsion, suspension, or community service.

Principles and Guidelines for Ethical Research

In addition to intrapersonal and interpersonal approaches that guide research, ethical principles merit consideration. Typically, most individuals understand the phrase *ethics of research* to mean an adherence to sets of principles that are part of institutional policy, ethics committee protocols, professional codes of ethics, or grant funding guidelines. Although this understanding is sound, it is restrictive in light of the broad affective competence required for successful research, as seen in discussion of the research scenarios. Although the PA profession's Code of Ethics does not specify conduct related to research, certainly there are general guidelines within the code that shape research directives for the PA. Examples of statements that apply to research as much as they apply to clinical practice are[12]:

"… providing competent medical care …"

"… to the full measure of their ability …"

"… adhere to … laws governing informed consent …"

"… uphold the doctrine of confidentiality …"

"… place service before material gain …"

Codes of ethics from other professions mandate more specific behaviors for the professional who engages in research. A sampling of such behaviors may be helpful: researchers must attend to and deal with these.

Obtain informed consent from subjects.

Respect the individual's right to refuse involvement in research.

Protect the confidential nature of research gained from investigational activities.

Be honest in receiving and disseminating information.

Give credit and recognition when using the work of others.

Do not fabricate data, falsify information, or plagiarize.

The Code of Ethics for the PA profession implies ethical responsibilities for research. Ultimately, PAs should always be guided by the mandate to "first, do no harm." That mandate prohibits physical, mental, and social harm and includes the honoring of patient confidentiality. In a broad sense, PA conduct must be beyond reproach and actually transcend guidelines articulated in the ethical code. The call to follow the major tenets of honesty, sound communication, ensuring the common good, competence, and confidentiality extends to practice in research. The admonition against conflicts of interest, sexual relationships, and impaired practice generalizes to research as well.

To illustrate the manner in which research issues require the kind of thinking that this chapter encourages, it might be instructive for you to consider a couple of research scenarios while holding ethical guidelines from the Code of Ethics in mind. Eight of the scenarios in this chapter relate in some way to the six principles listed above that come from various professional codes. Take a moment or two to consider how these principles might guide you to virtuous action.

Summary

Research holds many affective challenges. In fact, the research enterprise is enhanced when affective standards are integrated alongside intellectual and technical rigors. You must recognize that what you do—even in the realm of research—has intrapersonal, interpersonal, and ethical dimensions. Medical research lacking such recognition can deteriorate into the experiments done in Nazi war camps. Ethical science is a virtuous quest for knowledge. Ethical research aims to add to the knowledge base of the PA without causing undue harm. Most importantly, research must support the dignity and the values of persons. It must reflect a desire to do the right thing and a persistence in that course in spite of obstacles. It must be characterized by communication practices within which respect, honesty, and confidentiality are key. If, from the start of your research plan, you consider what it means to be ethical in research, you may increase quality health care. And in doing so, you will be manifesting evidence of having learned virtue or grace.[1]

Some Opportunities for Reflection

1. Movies that depict challenges associated with values and research:
   Awakenings, Brainstorm, Charlie, Contact, Dr. Jekyll and Mr. Hyde, Duplicates, ET, Frankenstein, Good Will Hunting, The Fly, The Insiders, Lorenzo's Oil, Nell, Schindler's List

2. Historical events of this century that reveal conflicts with human values and research:

Tuskegee Syphilis Study, Nazi Medical Experiments, early governmental and medical responses to the AIDS epidemic, artificial insemination, the human genome project, cloning, the life-threatening separation of conjoined twins.

3. Books (fictional or phenomenological) that portray the conflict:
   Awakenings, Faggots, Flowers for Algernon, Geek Love, Regeneration

Acknowledgment

This chapter derives from a larger work prepared by the author for the American Occupational Therapy Foundation. J. Dennis Blessing consulted on applications related to the physician assistant.

References

1. Allen J. The use and abuse of humanistic education. In Christensen CR. Teaching and the Case Method. Boston: Harvard Business School, 1987, pp. 50–53.

2. Thurber J. Fables for Our Times. New York: Harper and Brothers, 1940, p. 59.

3. Peloquin SM. Occupational therapy as an art and science: Should the older definition be reclaimed? American Journal of Occupational Therapy 1994;48:1093–1096.

4. Bruner J. Actual Minds, Possible Worlds. Cambridge: Harvard University Press, 1986, p. 49.

5. Bernard C. An Introduction to the Study of Experimental Medicine (Greene HC, trans.). New York: Dover, 1957 (Original work published in 1927), p. 34.

6. Goodman N. Languages of Art: An Approach to a Theory of Symbols. Indianapolis: Hackett, 1976, p. 107.

7. American Occupational Therapy Association. Core values and attitudes in occupational therapy practice. American Journal of Occupational Therapy 1993;47:1085–1087.

8. Webster's New Collegiate Dictionary. Springfield, MA: G. & C. Merriam, 1981.

9. Davidson DA, Peloquin SM. Making Connection with Others. Bethesda, MD: The American Occupational Therapy Association, 1998.

10. Iverson C, Flanagin A, Fontanarosa PB, et al. American Medical Association Manual of Style. A Guide for Authors and Editors. Philadelphia: Lippincott Williams & Wilkins, 1998.

11. Commission on Research Integrity. Integrity and misconduct in research. Washington, DC: Office of Research Integrity, 1993.

12. American Academy of Physician Assistants. Code of Ethics. Alexandria, VA: American Academy of Physician Assistants, 1999.

chapter 15

Regulatory Protection of Human Subjects in Research

Bruce R. Niebuhr, PhD and Raylene Lawrence, PA

Chapter Overview

In Chapter 14, you were introduced to ethical principles and exposed to ethical aspects of health-care research. Practicing physician assistants (PAs) and PA students, no doubt, recognize the ethical principles discussed in that chapter and the need to apply those principles in everything we do. In addition, it should be clear that autonomy, beneficence, nonmaleficence, and justice are essential for clinical practice as well as research.[1] The purpose of this chapter is to describe the manner in which the ethical conduct of research with human subjects has been codified and regulated in the United States.

Specific objectives for the reader are:

- Identify key historical events that shaped the present regulatory climate.
- Review the ethical principles applied to research with human subjects.
- Identify the applicable federal laws and regulations.
- Determine if a research study requires human subject protection.
- Identify and discuss issues of subject selection.

- Discuss privacy and confidentiality of subject information, including use of protected health information.
- Define informed consent to participate in research and the elements needed to document informed consent.
- Discuss the determination of capacity to consent, particularly with vulnerable populations.
- Describe the institutional review board (IRB), its membership, and responsibilities.
- List the criteria for research protocol to obtain IRB approval.
- Describe the ways of providing continuing protection of human subjects over the course of a study.
- Discuss emerging issues in the protection of human subjects in research.

To assist the reader in applying the concepts, short case studies for analysis are included.

Introduction

The modern history of human subject protection is generally considered to have begun with the post–World War II Nuremberg trials of German physicians implicated in crimes against prisoners of war and concentration camp inmates.[2] The revelations that came from these trials were horrific. Under the guise of research, human beings were subjected to inhuman torture, mutilations, and unbelievable atrocities. Part of the judgment of those who had been involved included the *Nuremberg Code* (see Box 15–1). The first principle of that code is that "The voluntary consent of the human subject is absolutely essential"[3] in research. It is clear that consent of the subjects was never a consideration in the research conducted during World War II.

The next major step in world recognition of the rights of human subjects was the World Health Organization's *Declaration of Helsinki*, adopted by the World Medical Society in 1964. This "declaration" provided guidelines for medical doctors in research involving human subjects. These guidelines, in widespread use around the world, have been revised several times.[2] In the United States, at about the same time, the Kefauver–Harris Amendments to Food and Drug Administration (FDA) regulations were adopted to protect people from unknowingly being given non–FDA-approved drugs.

We in the United States have not been innocent of violations of human rights in the name of "research." Among our transgressions are the Tuskegee syphilis study (discussed later), the exposure of people to radiation during the Cold War, retarded school children exposed to hepatitis, people given thalidomide and lysergic acid diethylamide (LSD) without their knowledge, and the list could go on. So even in a country where we consider ourselves to be moral, just, and fair, people have been submitted to research without their consent or understanding of what will happen and what the consequences could be. We must be ever diligent in our protection of people and ever vigilant in our efforts in research that involve people.

A specific stimulus in the United States to regulatory protection was the "Tuskegee Syphilis Experiment" of 1932 to 1972 in which several hundred African-American men were enrolled in a study of the natural history of syphilis without their consent. This "study" was conducted under the auspices of the federal government. The men were not informed of their disease, of what would happen to them, and of the purposes of the tests done to them (some tests and procedures were not beneficial or indicated); in addition, the men were not informed that treatment with penicillin was possible, even after the antibiotic came into common use in the 1940s.[4] Racism certainly played a part in this "research." While the horror of such an experiment can never be explained away or forgiven, one positive result of the Tuskegee Syphilis Experiment and other revelations was the National Research Act of 1974[5] establishing the National Commission for the Protection of Human Subjects of Biomedical and Behavioral Research, which functioned between 1974 and 1978.[6] The Commission's report, known as the *Belmont Report*,[7] provides the ethical basis for federal regulation of research with human subjects (Box 15–2).

The most recent federal legislation impacting human subject research (and clinical practice), the Health Insurance Portability and Accountability Act of 1996 (HIPAA),[8] governs the use of protected health information (PHI) for many purposes, including research. Federal regulations undergo revision at any time, even the recently implemented HIPAA. The reader can keep up with recent regulatory changes at the NIH Regulations and Guidelines Web site.[9] There is no doubt that keeping abreast of regulations of protected health information and human subjects research will continue to evolve in the future.

Ethical Principles

The *Belmont Report* established the basic ethical principles for acceptable conduct of research with human

---

BOX 15–1

Principles of the Nuremberg Code

1. Informed consent of volunteers must be obtained without coercion in any form.
2. Human experiments should be based on prior animal experimentation.
3. Anticipated scientific results should justify the experiment.
4. Only qualified scientists should conduct medical research.
5. Physical and mental suffering and injury should be avoided.
6. There should be no expectation of death or disabling injury from the experiment.

Adapted from Dunn CM, Chadwick G. *Protecting Study Volunteers in Research.* Boston Center Watch, 1999, p. 4.

BOX 15–2

Overview of Protective Federal Regulations

1. Review of research by an Institutional Review Board
2. Informed consent of research subjects.
3. Institutional assurances of compliance.

Basic Principles of the Belmont Report

1. Respect for persons
   a. Individual autonomy
   b. Protection of vulnerable subjects
2. Beneficence
   a. Do not harm.
   b. Maximize benefits.
   c. Minimize risks.
3. Justice
   a. Fairness in distribution
   b. Fairness in selection

subjects: *Respect for Persons, Beneficence* and *Justice* (Box 15-3).

- *Respect for persons* involves, first, that individuals should be treated as autonomous agents, and second, that persons with diminished autonomy are entitled to special protection. Informed consent is the key way to demonstrate respect for the individual's autonomy.

- *Beneficence* requires that persons be protected from harm by maximizing potential benefits and minimizing risks. This principle incorporates both beneficence and nonmaleficence as described in the *Guidelines for Ethical Conduct for the Physician Assistant Profession.*[1]

- *Justice* requires that the potential benefits and risks of the research be distributed fairly among populations.

Case 1: A clinical trial protocol is submitted to an academic health center's IRB. In the proposed trial, a new investigational drug for treating obsessive–compulsive disorder will be compared to a currently approved drug. The researchers plan a "double-blind" study in which neither the subjects nor the health-care professionals (teams consisting of physicians, PAs, and nurse practitioners) treating them are aware of which medication the subjects are receiving. A new member of the board from the community, not a health-care professional, expresses concern that the study as planned cannot be conducted ethically. Her concern is that the principle of *respect for persons* is not met, as the subjects cannot give true informed consent because they will not know which medication they will be receiving.

Do you agree with the board member's interpretation? If not, under what conditions can a "double-blind" study not violate the principle of informed consent? The case analysis is found at the end of the chapter.

When Does a Study Require Human Subject Protection?

Human subjects are living individuals whose physiological or behavioral characteristics or responses are studied in a research project. Data may be obtained through observation or intervention or identifiable private information.[2] In addition to a traditional understanding of subject participation in research, researchers are obliged to consider protection of subjects if a study uses

- Bodily materials collected invasively or noninvasively such as hair, saliva, or urine.

- Material from routine clinical care that would normally be discarded, such as blood.

- Private information such as protected health information (PHI), including cell lines or DNA in which individuals can be identified.

The researcher must decide if a given study includes human subjects. The researcher's decision is guided by the rules of the researcher's institution, including those of the Institutional Review Board (IRB) and the appropriate federal regulations.[5,10]

Subject Selection

Selection of subjects for research must be equitable and meet the principle of justice. The NIH has specific guidelines for inclusion of women and minorities in clinical research.[9] The objective is to maximize potential benefits to all persons at risk for the disease or condition to be studied. A study in which the population of interest excludes subpopulations, particularly women or minorities, requires a compelling societal or scientific rationale. For example, in a study on improving screening tests for prostate cancer, exclusion of women in the sample would clearly be justified. There must also be sound rationale for excluding non–English-speaking subjects. Careful review of local requirements (such as the IRB at your institution) should be done as you design the inclusion and exclusion of your study subjects.

Privacy and Confidentiality of Subject Information

Privacy is defined as "control over the extent, timing, and circumstances of sharing oneself (physically, behaviorally, or intellectually) with others."[2] Research subjects expect that information about them is to be shared only as necessary and will be protected from unauthorized access. PAs and PA students are well aware of the importance of maintaining confidentiality of patient information and this level of confidentiality is extended to research subjects. In some ways, the protection of research subjects and the level of confidentiality exceeds that of patient–provider confidentiality.

The Health Insurance Portability and Accountability Act of 1996[8] governs the use of PHI for many healthcare operations, reimbursement, clinical, and research purposes. Confidentiality of PHI and other private subject information can be protected by

- Using codes to replace identifiers and/or encrypting information
- Separating cover sheets from questionnaires containing data
- Properly disposing paper records and deleting computer files
- Limiting access to authorized individuals with training in protection of subject information
- Storing paper records in locked cabinets or computer files behind password protection

Figure 15–1 provides an example of the language used for the PHI section of a research consent form.

Informed Consent

The key method whereby the autonomy of subjects in research is ensured is by *informed consent. Informed consent* is defined as "a person's voluntary agreement to participate, based on adequate knowledge and understanding of relevant information about the research process, intents, and those diagnostic, therapeutic, intervention or preventive procedures that will be done as part of the study."[2] Figure 15–2 is an example of consent form elements. For consent to be valid[11]:

- The subject must be competent (special provisions described below apply if the subject is not competent because of age, mental status, or incapacity).
- The researchers must disclose all relevant information as to the potential risks and benefits of the research.
- The subject must understand the information. Thus, the researchers must be able to assess the subject's ability to understand the procedures of the study.
- The subject's agreement must be voluntary and free from coercion or other undue influence

Consent with Vulnerable Populations

Vulnerable research subjects are people who are relatively or absolutely incapable of protecting their own interests. The researchers must be aware of the special issues in research involving vulnerable populations, justify the need to involve these populations, and provide additional safeguards as required. These populations include:

- Children
- Individuals who may lack decision-making capacity, including comatose patients
- Prisoners
- Fetuses, neonates, and pregnant women
- Students or employees of the institution conducting the research

CHILDREN

Special procedures are in place in the federal regulations that provide additional safeguards for the protection of children involved in research activities. The regulations require that children **assent** to participation in research and that a child's parents also give **permission** for their child to participate. Assent is a positive affirmation of a willingness to participate. Failure to object is not assent, that is, if the child does not voice his or her assent, this does not mean that he or she agrees to be in the study. Following the child's positive affirmation, the parents must also be approached for their permission. Researchers should consider the age, maturity, and psychological state of each child that is approached for enrollment in a research study. A common general policy is to obtain the assent of all children (ages 7 to 17 years). Nevertheless, each particular IRB may establish its own criteria. Under special circumstances, the requirement to obtain the assent of a child can be waived by the IRB.

OTHER VULNERABLE POPULATIONS

PAs involved in clinical research are likely to interact with vulnerable populations in which the potential for real or perceived coercion or undue influence on subjects to enroll in the study is present or in which the subjects may be incapable of fully understanding the potential risks of the research. Examples of these populations include economically or educationally disadvantaged persons, persons enrolled in emergent care settings, students, employees, and critically or terminally ill patients. Incarcerated individuals are also considered vulnerable. In all cases, the IRB must consider the possibility and justification for including these subjects in the proposed research and safeguards to protect their rights and welfare. If your research protocol includes vulnerable subjects, you must ensure their protection, particularly to prevent them being coerced into participation.

WHAT IS PROTECTED HEALTH INFORMATION (PHI)?

Protected Health Information is information about a person's health that includes information that would make it possible to figure out whose it is. According to the law, you have the right to decide who can see your protected health information. If you choose to take part in this study, you will be giving your permission to the investigators and the research study staff (individuals carrying out the study) to see and use your health information for this research study. In carrying out this research, the health information we will see and use about you will include: *[a specific list of information involved in the study is listed here, such as: your medical history and blood work, information that we get from your medical record, information you give us during your participation in the study such as during interviews or from questionnaires, results of blood tests, and pill counts; demographic information like your age, marital status, the type of work you do and the years of education you have completed.]*

We will get this information by *[ways that PHI will be gathered is placed here, for example: by asking you, asking your doctor, by looking at your chart at the _____(name of health care facility)]*.

HOW WILL YOUR PHI BE SHARED?

Because this is a research study, we will be unable keep your PHI completely confidential. We may share your health information with people and groups involved in overseeing this research study including:

- the sponsor of the study *[name of the sponsor]*
- the company *[name the company]* that makes *[name the study drug]*,
- *[name the collaborators at other institutions that may be involved with the study and their institutional affiliations, such as:]* Drs. John Doe and Mary Smith who are also working on this study at the _____ _____ University *[specify]*.
- the committee that checks the study data on an ongoing basis, to determine if the study should be stopped for any reason,
- the investigators at the *[name of local study sites]*
- The Institutional Review Board and the Compliance Office of the *[study institution]*, and other groups that oversee how research studies are carried out.
- Research office at the *[name of study site(s)]* and
- *[if the study involves a drug or device regulated by the FDA, add:]* the Food and Drug Administration (FDA)

Parts of your PHI may be photocopied and sent to a central location or it may be transmitted electronically, such as by e-mail or fax.

The groups receiving your health information may not be obligated to keep it private. They may pass information on to other groups or individuals not named here.

If you decide to participate in this study, you will be giving your permission for the groups named above, to see and share your health information. If you choose not to let these groups see and share your health information as explained above, you will *not* be able to participate in the research study.

HOW WILL YOUR PHI BE PROTECTED?

In an effort to protect your privacy, the study staff will use code numbers instead of your name, to identify your health information. Initials and numbers will be used on any photocopies of your study records, *[if applicable add: and on any blood or tissue samples that are sent outside of the (name the study site or sites) for review or testing]*. If the results of this study are reported in medical journals or at meetings, you will not be identified.

DO YOU HAVE TO BE IN THIS STUDY?

Being in the study is voluntary. You are free to choose not to be in this study or to stop being in this study at any time. You are also free to not let the researchers and other groups see and share your health information. If you choose not to be in the study or not to let the researchers and other groups use your health information, there will be no penalties. In other words, you will still be able to get medical treatments without being in the study and it will not affect your eligibility for any health plan or any health plan benefits or payments you may be eligible for.

WHAT IF YOU CHANGE YOUR MIND?

You may ask the researchers to stop using your health information at any time. However, you need to say this in writing and send your letter to *[give the name and full mailing address of the person to whom a request to revoke must be sent]*. If you tell the researchers to stop using your health information, your participation in the study will end and the study staff will stop collecting medical information from you and about you. However, the study staff will continue to use the health information collected up to the time they receive your letter asking them to stop.

FIG. 15–1 Example of PHI language for research subject consent form. *Italics* indicate language provided by the investigator or directions for completion. (From The University of Texas Health Science Center at San Antonio IRB at *http://www.uthscsa.edu/irb/_*). Accessed May 18, 2005.

(Figure continued on following page)

CAN YOU ASK TO SEE THE PHI THAT IS COLLECTED ABOUT YOU FOR THIS STUDY?

The federal rules say that you can see the health information that we collect about you and use in this study. *[Explain any limitations that might affect the subjects' access to their PHI, for example: You will only have access to your PHI until _____. If there are no limitations, add: Contact the study staff if you have a need to review your PHI collected for this study. If the nature of the study makes it necessary or preferable to temporarily suspend access, explain this by adding: Because of the type of research, you can only access your PHI when the study is done. At that time, you have the right to see and copy the medical information we collect about you during the study, for as long as that information is kept by the study staff and other groups involved.]*

HOW LONG WILL YOUR PHI BE USED?

[Indicate if the authorization to use PHI expires and if so state when. This element is required to be in an authorization. If there will be no expiration date, you must state that is the case. The following is an example of how that may be stated:] By signing this form, you agree to let us use and disclose your health information for purposes of the study at any time in the future. There is no expiration date because we do not know how long it will take us to finish doing all of the analyses and we will need to use your health information for as long as it takes. *[If there is an expiration date, be sure to make the date far enough in the future that you will not have to go back to the subjects to get a new authorization signed in order to permit all of the analyses and inspections to be completed.]*

[The following text must appear immediately before the signature lines. This text and the signature lines must appear on a single page. DO NOT permit a page break after this point in the consent, unless something additional appears after the signature lines.]

You will be given a signed copy of this form to keep. *[Researchers please note: the HIPAA rules require that the research subject be given a SIGNED copy of the authorization. You must give the subject a signed copy of the consent whether they want it or not, because it contains the authorization.]*

SIGN THIS FORM ONLY IF ALL OF THE FOLLOWING ARE TRUE:

- You have voluntarily decided to take part in this research study.

- You authorize the collection, uses and sharing of your protected health information as described in this form.

- You have read the above information.

- Your questions have been answered to your satisfaction and you believe you understand all of the information given about this study and about the use and disclosure of your health information.

*The University of Texas Health Science Center at San Antonio IRB @ http://www.uthscsa.edu/irb/

FIG. 15–1 *(Continued)*

Case 2: A PA faculty member is studying the development of empathy with patients among PA students. She teaches the program's "Introduction to the PA Profession" course to beginning, first-year students. At the end of the first class period, she describes her study and asks the students to complete a short questionnaire. She informs the students that completion of the questionnaire is voluntary and that if they do not wish to participate, they may leave.

What ethical principles are involved and how do they apply to this situation? Do you have any difficulties with the manner in which the faculty member is recruiting subjects? What changes, if any, would you make in the recruitment procedures? How would you approach the class about their participation?

Function of the Institutional Review Board (IRB)

Each institution engaged in research involving human subjects conducted, supported, or otherwise subject to regulation by any federal department must establish an IRB. Although large, research-oriented institutions such as universities, academic medical centers, or hospitals establish their own IRBs, smaller institutions, or private medical practices, may utilize the services of an independent IRB. Typically, the institutions will assign responsibility for all human-subjects research, not just federally supported, to their IRBs.

CHECK LIST FOR ELEMENTS OF INFORMED CONSENT

YES   NO

—   —   1.   We are asking you to take part in a research study of (*state what is being studied*).

—   —   2.   We want to learn (*state what the study is designed to discover or establish*).

—   —   3.   We are asking you to take part in this study because (*state why the subject was invited*).

—   —   4.   If you decide to take part, we will (*describe in lay language all procedures, their purposes, how long they will take, and their frequency*).

—   —   5.   (*Describe total time over which the subject will be studied.*)

—   —   6.   (*Describe the discomforts, inconveniences, and other risks to be reasonably expected and indicate incidence of occurrence.*)

—   —   7.   (*Describe any benefits reasonably expected. If benefits are mentioned, add:*) We do not guarantee you will benefit from taking part in this study.

—   —   8.   (*If subjects are patients, description of alternative procedures that might be advantageous and disclose any standard treatment being withheld.*)

—   —   9.   (*If the subject will receive any compensation, describe the amount or nature, and how it will be pro-rated if the subject does not complete the study. If being paid by a state voucher, add*): Please note that if you are on record as owing money to the State of Texas, such as for back child support or a delinquent student loan, the compensation will be applied to that debt and you will not receive a check. (*If amount exceeds $600 in calendar year, explain that the income must be reported to the IRS and that subject will receive a form 1099*)

—   —   10.   (*Describe the possibility of costs to the subject because of participation. VA consent forms must include the following [exception: studies being done strictly at the GCRC]:*) If you are a veteran, your only cost for treatment as a subject in a research study at any South Texas Veterans Healthcare System facility would be the copayment that may be required based on your category of eligibility for medical care.

—   —   11.   (*Injury/compensation statement*): If you are injured as a result of the research procedures, your injury will be treated. You will be responsible for any charges. We have no plans to give you money if you are injured.

—   —   12.   (*Confidentiality statement*): (*If Protected Health Information [PHI] is being used, a valid authorization must be incorporated. Information is available on the IRB website: www.uthscsa.edu/irb/hipaa.html If no PHI is involved, include:*) Everything we learn about you in the study will be confidential. If we publish the results of the study in a scientific journal or book, we will not identify you in any way. The Institutional Review Board and other groups that have the responsibility of monitoring research, may want to see your records *which identify you as a subject in this study.*

—   —   13.   (*Right to withdraw*): (*A valid authorization covers this element, however if no authorization to use PHI will be included, add:*) Your decision to take part in the study is voluntary. You are free to choose not to take part in the study or to stop taking part at any time.

—   —   14.   (*Without prejudice statement*): (*A valid authorization covers this element, however if no authorization to use PHI will be included, add:*) If you choose not to take part or to stop at any time, it will not affect your future medical care at the University of Texas Health Science Center at San Antonio or (name of institution/s at which study is being conducted).

—   —   15.   (*Principal investigator's full name and phone number (and after-hours phone number – if digital pager gives instructions how to use); full names of co-investigators who will enroll/perform procedures*): If you have questions now, feel free to ask us. If you have additional questions later *or you wish to report a medical problem which may be related to this study*, (full name and degrees) can be reached at (work and home phone/after-hours numbers with area code). (*Note: If >minimal risk, provide names & number of at least 2 MDs or otherwise clinically appropriate people.*)

FIG. 15–2 Elements of a consent form. (Adapted from The University of Texas Health Science Center at San Antonio @ *http://www.uthscsa.edu/irb/elements03–04july.doc*). Accessed May 18, 2005.

(Figure continued on following page)

CHECK LIST FOR ELEMENTS OF INFORMED CONSENT *(Continued)*

YES   NO

—   —   16.   The University of Texas Health Science Center committee that reviews research on human subjects (Institutional Review Board) will answer any questions about your rights as a research subject (210-567-2351).

—   —   17.   We will give you a signed copy of this form to keep.

—   —   18.   (*Statement of understanding and agreement to participate*): (*A valid authorization covers this element, however if no authorization to use PHI will be included, add:*) YOUR SIGNATURE INDICATES THAT YOU HAVE DECIDED TO TAKE PART IN THIS RESEARCH STUDY AND THAT YOU HAVE READ AND YOU UNDERSTAND THE INFORMATION GIVEN ABOVE AND EXPLAINED TO YOU.

—   —   21.   Information about issues like lactation, pregnancy, contraception and concerns about fathering a child (contact IRB for samples of language)

—   —   22.   If minors involved, the form must address parent throughout: We are asking you to allow your child to take part...

—   —   23.   If minors involved, include lines for Signature of Parent/Guardian; specifying relationship to subject and minor's assent (if age 7 or older)

—   —   24.   Persons obtaining consent must sign *and* print name. (persons obtaining consent must be designated in protocol)

—   —   25.   (*If applicable*): We will tell you about any significant new findings which develop during the course of this research which may relate to your willingness to continue taking part.

—   —   26.   Anticipated circumstances when study may be terminated by sponsor or principal investigator

—   —   27.   If the study involves GENETICS, USE OF DNA, ESTABLISHMENT OF PERMANENT CELL LINES, BANKING OF SAMPLES FOR FUTURE STUDY, HIV TESTING, OR DEVELOPMENT OF MARKETABLE PRODUCTS MADE FROM HUMAN SAMPLES, contact the IRB office for additional guidelines and sample consent form wording.

FORMAT REQUIREMENTS

—   —   28.   Title of study on top of all pages (must be same, word-for-word, as protocol), UTHSCSA and study sites listed under the title on p. 1 (except VA), page numbers on all pages (page 1 of 2, page 2 of 2), except p. 1 of VA consent. VA uses form 10–1086.

—   —   29.   Lines for the signatures of the subject, a witness, the person obtaining consent, printed name & title of person obtaining consent and to record the date & time. VA consent requires a signature line for the subject at the bottom of all pages.

*adapted from the University of Texas Health Science Center at San Antonio
@ http://www.uthscsa.edu/irb/elements03-04july.doc*

FIG. 15–2 *(Continued)* (There are no items 19 and 20 in the consent form, as presented.)

Each IRB must have at least five members, with varying backgrounds to allow for comprehensive review of research activities commonly conducted by the institution. The membership of the IRB is well defined and certain conditions must be met. Membership must include individuals who are qualified through research experience and expertise. The membership must be diverse with respect to ethnicity, gender, and cultural background. One member must not be affiliated with the institution and one member must be concerned primarily with nonscientific issues. Community interests (noninstitutional) must be represented. All members must be concerned with the protection of human subjects. In addition, members must possess the professional competence necessary to review specific research activities; the IRB must be able to ascertain the acceptability of proposed research in terms of institutional commitments and regulations, applicable law, and standards of professional conduct and practice. The IRB must therefore include individuals knowledgeable in these areas. If an IRB regularly reviews research that involves a vulnerable category of subjects, such as children, prisoners, pregnant women, or handicapped or mentally disabled persons, consideration must be given to the inclusion of one or more individuals who are knowledgeable about and experienced in working with these subjects. The IRB may not have a member participate in the initial or continuing review of any project in which the member has a conflict of interest, except to provide information requested by the IRB.

Specific responsibilities of the IRB are to:

- Determine the acceptability of proposed research in terms of institutional policy and regulations, applicable laws, and ethical standards of professional conduct and practice.

- Conduct an initial and continuing review of all research activities to ensure compliance with international standards of ethical practice regarding the use of human subjects in research, in order to ascertain their welfare and safety.

- Approve, deny approval to, or require modifications for the purpose of approval in research activities proposing the use of human subjects.

- Recommend the suspension of an ongoing research activity in case of deviation from the existing guidelines for the use of human subjects in research.

Types of IRB Review

Depending on the level of risk of the research protocol and subject population, the IRB may conduct either an expedited review or full board review.

EXPEDITED REVIEW

For certain kinds of research involving no more than minimal risk, and for minor changes in approved research, the IRB chair or a designated voting member or group of voting members review the proposed research rather than the entire IRB. It cannot be assumed that research that involves only interview or survey data collection poses minimal risk. Sensitive questions may lead to distress that exposes participants to greater than minimal risk. Loss of confidentiality can cause harm to participants, their relatives, and others.

EXEMPT REVIEW

Some types of research projects may be exempt from review. Even if exempt, these protocols may still need to be approved as exempt. This is usually done by the IRB chair or a designee. You will need to check with your local IRB to learn what type of forms or information needs to be submitted for exempt status. Records reviews and surveys are examples of types of studies that may be exempt. There can be absolutely no risk to the subjects.

FULL BOARD REVIEW

When *full board review* is necessary, the research proposal is presented and discussed at a meeting at which a quorum of IRB members is present. Typically, there is a pre-review of the IRB applications by members of the board (at the editor's institution, two members do the pre-review). The investigator then responds to the pre-review and the application is submitted for full IRB review. The application is presented to the full IRB, discussed, and voted on for approval, disapproval, or tabled. The IRB may request additional information, clarification, or set stipulations before final approval is granted. The IRB may require full member approval on resubmission, review of stipulations or requests by a subgroup of the IRB, or allow the chair or chair designee to review further stipulations. Ultimately for the research application to be approved, it must receive the approval of a majority of those voting members present.

Research Exempt from IRB Review

Under federal regulations [45 CFR 46.101 (b)], certain categories of activity are considered research, but may be declared exempt from review by the IRB. This determination should be made by someone other than the principal investigator, and may need confirmation by the IRB.

Exempt types of research include:

- Research on instructional strategies, techniques, curricula, or classroom management methods

- Research involving the use of educational tests, survey or interview procedures, or observation of public behavior

- Research involving the collection or study of existing data, documents, records, or specimens

- Taste and food quality evaluation and consumer acceptance studies

These exemptions do not generally apply to research involving vulnerable populations such as prisoners, fetuses, pregnant women, newborns, or children. Situations in which the information is recorded or

BOX 15–4

Overview of the Responsibilities of the IRB

The primary purpose of the IRB is to protect the rights and welfare of human research subjects. Activities that support that purpose are

1. To ensure that risks to subjects are minimized. For example, the IRB evaluates whether procedures to be performed on subjects (a) are consistent with sound research design and do not unnecessarily expose subjects to risk and (b) whether they are already being performed for diagnostic or treatment purposes.

2. To ensure that risks to subjects are reasonable in relation to any benefits that might be expected from taking part in a research study and to the importance of the knowledge that may result.

3. To ensure that selection of subjects is fair and equitable. For example, the IRB seeks to determine that no eligible individuals are denied the opportunity to take part in any study, particularly those from which they may benefit, based on an arbitrary criterion such as gender or because they do not speak English.

4. To ensure participation is voluntary and informed consent is obtained from each prospective subject or where appropriate, from the subject's legally authorized representative.

5. To ensure that the research plan provides for monitoring the data collected to ensure the safety of subjects.

6. To ensure that there are adequate provisions to protect the privacy of subjects and to maintain the confidentiality of data.

Adapted from The University of Texas Health Science Center at San Antonio IRB at *http://www.uthscsa.edu/irb/*. Accessed May 18, 2005.

obtained by the investigator in such a manner that subjects can be identified, directly or through identifiers linked to the subjects, may not be exempt. Because the decision whether or not a research study is exempt is often a difficult one, many institutions elect, as a matter of policy, not to exempt any or all of the above categories of research from IRB review (Box 15–4).

Case 3: In a surgical group practice, the surgeons use one of two standard techniques for hernia repair. One surgeon proposes to the group that they conduct a systematic study to compare the two techniques. Each surgeon is qualified to perform either technique. The proposal is to randomly assign patients to either technique. Furthermore, since both techniques are approved, and are of equal cost, consent of patients to be included in the study is not necessary (of course, patients will complete the normal consent form for treatment). A PA in the practice expresses ethical concerns about the study and suggests that an outside review would be of value. Another surgeon says that since they are a private practice, not a university or academic health center with an IRB, they are not required to undergo a review or obtain special consent from their patients. If you were the PA, what would you recommend?

Ongoing Protections

Ultimately, the researchers and investigators are responsible for protection of subjects throughout the study. Such protection is accomplished by

- An ongoing process of informed consent
- Reporting of adverse events
- Ongoing data and safety monitoring
- Continuing review by the IRB

A key concept is that informed consent is not a static document (the consent form), but an ongoing process. The researcher is obligated to notify subjects of changes in the protocol or new information (e.g., new information on side effects) that may alter the risks of participation. The researcher must report unanticipated adverse events to the IRB. For multicenter clinical trials, adverse events are also reported to the central coordinating site.

The principal investigator is responsible for the ongoing monitoring of the research project with respect to subject safety and protection of the confidentiality of the data. It is frequently valuable to have an autonomous group evaluate trial data to ensure participant safety and study integrity. This data monitoring may be performed by the IRB or a Data Safety Monitoring Board (DSMB) may be appointed. The role of DSMBs is to provide a multidisciplinary and objective perspective as an independent group of experts to advise the institution and the study investigators. The primary responsibility of the DSMB is to periodically review and evaluate the accumulated study data for timeliness, completeness, and accuracy. This enables the DSMB to assess the safety and welfare of study participants. Items the DSMB may review include but are not limited to:

- Evidence of study-related adverse events
- Evidence of efficacy based on preestablished statistical guidelines
- Data quality, completeness, and timeliness
- Performance of individual centers
- Compliance with recruitment and retention goals of the participants
- Adherence to protocols
- Factors impacting confidentiality

A DSMB may recommend early termination of a study based on safety considerations. An example was withdrawal of Vioxx® (rofecoxib) by the manufacturer after DSMB for the Adenomatous Polyp Prevention on Vioxx® (APPROVe) trial recommended that the study be halted because of an increased risk of serious cardiovascular events.[12]

The role of the IRB is not limited to initial review of studies. At minimum, the IRB must review each active study annually. The review period could be a shorter time and this is set at the time the IRB initially approves the research application. The IRB may determine that studies of higher risk may require review more frequently than annually.

Emerging Issues

Among the important emerging issues that impact the protection of human subjects in clinical research are certification of researchers and of IRB members and the development of networks for research in private practices. In 2000, the National Institutes of Health (NIH) mandated required education for all key members of research teams submitting NIH grant applications or those already receiving NIH grant funding.[13] The NIH provides an online tutorial through which researchers may receive their certification.[13] More recently, it has been proposed that a program for accrediting IRBs be developed[14] (Committee on Assessing the System for Protecting Human Research Subjects, 2001, No. 15). This would be a further step in creating quality IRBs and, hopefully, ensure quality IRB reviews.

A recent trend that has great promise for increasing the involvement of PAs in research are practice-based research networks.[15] Medical research traditionally has occurred in academic health centers, although most clinical care is delivered in office and community-based practice settings. One example is the Virginia Ambulatory Care Outcomes Research Network (ACORN) of primary care practices in Virginia in which data are collected on the health status of primary care patients and on the effectiveness and quality of the care they receive.[16] There is no doubt that this opens a research door to PAs, but with that opportunity comes the responsibility of understanding and applying rules that govern research.

How shall practice-based research be regulated to protect the subjects? Several options exist. If the research is directed from an academic health center, that center's IRB will review it. For studies not based in an academic center, independent IRBs can be used on a contract basis. Sponsoring or funding agencies may also use a central IRB to review practice-based research.[17]

Conclusions

Protection of human subjects in medical and behavioral research is the responsibility of all members of the research team, not just the principal investigator or study director. The inclusion of research in PA educational programs at the master's level has increased the research expertise of PAs in clinical practice. PAs can become a significant force in the conduct of ethical, practice-based clinical research. PAs must learn and be involved with the processes that govern research involving human subjects.

Case 1: The randomized, double-blind clinical trial is considered the "gold standard" of clinical research design, providing the best evidence for assessing the efficacy of treatment. If subjects are aware of their specific treatment, particularly for psychiatric conditions, such as the example of obsessive–compulsive disorder, the possibility of a placebo effect is high. If a placebo effect cannot be ruled out in a study then the potential benefit of that study has been reduced. Thus, the ethical principle of *beneficence* comes into play. The generally accepted view is that the principles of respect for persons and beneficence can both be satisfied if the subjects are clearly informed that they may or may not receive a particular treatment. Inform the subjects they have a 50 percent chance of receiving the interventional drug and a 50 percent chance of receiving the standard treatment. The information needs to be presented using language appropriate for the subjects. For example, tell the subject that assignment to treatment conditions would be akin to flipping a coin.

Case 2: Would this study fall into a category of research exempted from federal regulation? One could argue the study is an example of research conducted in established or commonly accepted educational settings, involving normal educational practices. On the other hand, students are a potentially vulnerable population susceptible to the influence of the faculty member. Can the students truly function as autonomous agents in giving their consent? The recruitment procedures could be modified to remove any undue influence by the faculty member. The change could be as simple as not recruiting subjects in the classroom and having the questionnaires returned in an anonymous manner. This case is a good example of why many universities do not exempt educational research from IRB review in order to ensure that students are not subjected to undue influence or coercion.

Case 3: Consent to treatment and consent to participate in research are separate issues and should not be confused. Protection of the rights of human subjects is not just a responsibility of institutions, but of the investigators. As a matter of maintaining a relationship of trust, the surgeons would be advised to obtain informed consent of their patients to participate in the study. The PA could suggest an outside review by an outside ethical consultant or a review by an independent IRB. Either approach would be very helpful for clinicians less familiar with research ethics than clinical ethics.

References

1. American Academy of Physician Assistants. Guidelines for Ethical Conduct for the Physician Assistant Profession. Available at: *http://www.aapa.org/policy/ethical-conduct.html*. Accessed October 13, 2004.

2. Penslar RL, Porter JP. *Protecting Human Research Subjects: Institutional Review Board Guidebook*. Pittsburgh, PA: United States Government Superintendent of Documents; 1993. Available at: *http://www.hhs.gov/ohrp/irb/irb_guidebook.htm*. Accessed October 13, 2004.

3. United States Government Printing Office. Trials of War Criminals before the Nuremberg Military Tribunals under Control Council Law No. 10. Vol. 10. Washington, DC; 1949:181–182.

4. Jones JH. Bad Blood: The Tuskegee Syphilis Experiment. New York: Free Press; 1993.

5. Department of Health and Human Services. Health and Human Services Policy for Protection of Human Subjects; Final Rule, 59 Federal Register 13273 (1994) (codified at 45 CFR §45).

6. National Research Act; 45 CFR §46 (1974).

7. National Commission for the Protection of Human Subjects of Biomedical and Behavioral Research. Ethical Principles and Guidelines for the Protection of Human: Subjects of Research 1979. Available at: *http://www.hhs.gov/ohrp/humansubjects/guidance/belmont.htm*. Accessed October 13, 2004.

8. Health Insurance Portability and Accountability Act, 42 USC §201 (1996).

9. National Institutes of Health. Guidelines on the Inclusion of Women and Minorities in Clinical Research. Available at: *http://grants2.nih.gov/grants/funding/women_min/guidelines_amended_10_2001.htm*. Accessed October 13, 2004.

10. AS Food and Drug Administration. Protection of Human Subjects, 45 Federal Register 36390 (1980) (codified at 21 CFR 50); 1980.

11. National Institutes of Health. Required Education in the Protection of Human Research Participants. Available at: *http://grants.nih.gov/grants/guide/notice-files/NOT-OD-00–039.html*. Accessed October 13, 2004.

12. US Food and Drug Administration CfDEaR. FDA Public Health Advisory: Safety of Vioxx; 2004. Available at: *http://www.fda.gov/cder/drug/infopage/vioxx/default.htm*. Accessed October 13, 2004.

13. National Institutes of Health. Human Participant Protections Education for Research Teams. Available at: *http://cme.cancer.gov/clinicaltrials/learning/humanparticipant-protections.asp*. Accessed October 13, 2004.

14. Koski G. Changing the paradigm: new directions in federal oversight of human research. Journal of Pediatric Gastroenterology & Nutrition 2003;37:S2–6.

15. Lindbloom EJ, Ewigman BG, Hickner JM. Practice-based research networks: the laboratories of primary care research. Medical Care 2004(Apr):III45–49.

16. The Virginia Ambulatory Care Outcomes Research Network (ACORN). 2004. Available at: *http://www.acorn.fap.vcu.edu/*. Accessed October 13, 2004.

17. National Cancer Institute. The Central Institutional Board Review (CIRB) Initiative. 2004. Available at: *http://www.ncicirb.org/*. Accessed October 13, 2004.

chapter 16

Writing Clear, Compelling, and Convincing Grant Applications

William D. Hendricson, MA, MS

Chapter Overview

Writing a grant is an intellectually challenging, time-consuming, and emotionally intensive task. It is a high-risk endeavor. There are no guarantees of success; in fact, failure is common, although the percentage of grants that ultimately receive funding is higher than grantsmanship mythology would lead one to believe, especially for investigators who are persistent. However, grant writing also yields high rewards. It is estimated that in 2003, **35 billion dollars** of funding from various sources was provided to grant seekers. It is estimated that more than a million grants are submitted to various types of funding agencies every year in the United States ranging from small family-based foundations (e.g., the Joe and Sally Smith Charitable Trust) to the National Institutes of Health (NIH) and other federal organizations. Numerous sources of funding lie in between small private foundations and the NIH including church-based foundations; professional associations; the military; the business sector; nonprofit organizations; and government agencies at city, county, and state levels. In addition, many colleges and universities and state higher education coordinating boards operate grant programs to stimulate research or educational innovation.

The information presented in this chapter is drawn from four sources: (1) my own experiences as a grant writer over the past 30 years; (2) my personal favorites among the literature on grant writing which is massive; for example, a Google search in June 2004 yielded 2.3 million citations for "books—grant writing"; (3) a 2-day grant writing workshop that I have conducted for the past 13 years at my home institution, the University of Texas Health Science Center at San Antonio (UTH-SCSA), and at approximately 50 other universities; and (4) a fellowship program on writing grants that I have conducted for the past 9 years for the American Academy of Family Physicians.

Although the major concentration of this chapter is on the NIH format, the information can be used for any type of grant application.

Introduction

There are many categories of grants in the biomedical sciences and health professions education including *training grants* designed to support educational programs for health-care providers; *program development grants* designed to help institutions establish centers of excellence that promote research, education, and community service in focused areas, often centered on a public health problem (diabetes, alcoholism, health problems of the elderly, rural access to care); *infrastructure grants* designed to help schools create core support services and facilities that will enhance research or education for the entire campus; *career development grants* of many types that are designed to enhance the professional growth of faculty and help establish research careers; and a multitude of *research grants* designed to support investigations of scientific unknowns in the basic, clinical, and behavioral sciences as well as to explore research questions pertinent to health services delivery, public health issues, organizational dynamics within health-care service institutions, and best practices for educating health-care providers and patients.

This chapter focuses on the development of research grants because many of the writing strategies that are critical for creation of a competitive research application are also essential for other types of grant proposals. We will address several grantsmanship issues, but the primary focus of the chapter is on writing strategies that can make your grant application Clear, Compelling, and Convincing: the 3Cs of grant writing. The 3Cs are universal principles that apply to telling your story in any type of grant application. Your primary job as a grant writer is to communicate the scientific plan in an easy to understand and persuasive manner so your grant application stands out from the many other proposals that a reviewer is likely to be critiquing in the same period of time.

The grant writer's goal: communicate your scientific plan with the 3Cs

Clear
: Your grant application is reviewer friendly. It is succinct, easy to comprehend, well organized, and easy to follow.

Compelling
: Your application presents a persuasive case for the importance and value of the project.

Convincing
: Your description of the project makes it seem exciting and unique. The proposal grabs the attention of reviewers and makes them want to be an advocate for your research question—"Why hasn't this been studied before?"

Figure 16–1 communicates the three components of a successful grant application. First and foremost, a *clear need* must exist for the project proposed in your application. In the biomedical world, needs often involve deficits in our understanding of "how things work" ranging from gaps in our knowledge of how breakdowns in cellular mechanisms or genetic structure can trigger disease to lack of understanding about how to effectively implement health-care services for the public. Your success as a grant writer hinges on your ability to clearly articulate a knowledge gap and convince reviewers that this gap needs to be addressed now. A second ingredient in the formula for a successful grant application is *good science*; using up-to-date and appropriate scientific principles and methodology to investigate the knowledge gap. The third ingredient is *persuasive communication*; your use of language to communicate the need for the project (e.g., the knowledge gap) and the scientific plan in a clear, convincing, and compelling manner that distinguishes your proposal from all other applications that are being considered.

The first section of this chapter reviews three important "getting into the grant writing game" considerations, often known as grantsmanship, including looking at grant writing from the reviewer's perspective. The second section presents writing strategies for the six major sections of a research grant application: the abstract, specific aims (e.g., project objectives), background and significance, preliminary studies, research methods, and the budget justification. The format and level of detail for the budget section of grant applications varies considerably depending on the nature of the funding agency. Therefore, the material on budget in

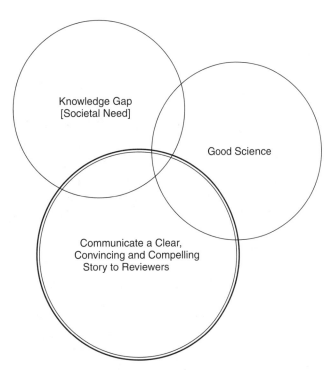

FIG. 16–1. Components of a successful grant application.

this chapter focuses primarily on how to write compelling justifications for project personnel using a template I have found to be effective. Format requirements (i.e., page length, word count, or sequencing) for the other components of a research grant proposal also vary depending on the funding agency, but the core information that needs to be provided in each section is basically the same whether you are applying for a $5,000 start-up grant from a county public health department or requesting a million dollars from NIH or the National Science Foundation. We will examine the grant writer's goals, writing strategies (i.e., presentation and sequencing of ideas), and critical red flags to avoid for each of the "narrative" components of a research grant application. I use the term narrative because your primary task is to employ the written word to explain your conceptualization and rationale for the project proposed in the grant application. Successful grant writers tell a story with words that builds a compelling case for the project.

Getting into the Grant Writing Game

In this section, we address three questions: What is a grant? What do I need to know about funding agencies? And, what do I need to know about reviewers? Let's start with the basics. *What is a grant?* A grant is basically a financial award given to you by an organization to help you implement a project that is consistent with the mission and priorities of the grantor (i.e., the organization that is awarding money to sponsor projects). Essentially, the agency that provides grant monies is making an investment in you. In return for the monies provided to support your research, the funding agency is anticipating a pay-off on its investment in terms of answers to scientific unknowns or better ways to provide health-care services for the public. Grantors may also expect to garner notoriety and enhanced public image from their support of a project. A grantor in the business sector, such as a company that makes medical instruments, may expect to gain a marketplace advantage over competitors as a result of products that evolve from research that they support. Thus, grants provide recipients with the financial support to conduct a project under conditions that meet the expectations and desired outcomes of the grantor. There are many award mechanisms that are globally called "grants." The three most common award mechanisms are (1) grants, which can be either unsolicited or submitted in response to a solicitation (request) for applications; (2) contracts; and (3) cooperative agreements. The key characteristics of each mechanism are described in Table 16–1.

For Requests for Applications (RFAs) and Requests for Proposals (RFPs), it is important to carefully analyze what the funding agency wants and absolutely critical to construct your grant application so that it "gives them what they want." Many applications submitted in response to an RFA are rejected because the grant writers apparently paid scant attention to the information in the solicitation announcement. RFAs can be quite detailed—often 10 to 15 pages in length—and many are prescriptive in describing what types of projects they want and the conditions under which the research should be conducted. Failing to respond to the "wish list" communicated in the announcement of the RFA is usually fatal. If you have not seen a RFA announcement, go to the NIH Web site for the Office of Extramural Research at *http://grants.nih.gov/grants/guide/index.html*. This link takes you to the Funding Opportunities and Notices page. Click on Requests for Applications (RFAs) under "Browse Funding Opportunities." Dozens of currently active RFAs are listed at this site and can be reviewed online. Box 16–1 illustrates the type of information typically available in an RFA including the goal of the solicitation (which should be read carefully and addressed directly in your proposal), level and duration of support, key project design considerations, guidelines for creating the research plan (ignoring these is fatal), and examples of research questions that the funding agency would like to see answered by funding projects. The research questions presented in your proposal should closely paraphrase (not verbatim) one or more of the questions that appear in the RFA.

What Do I Need to Know About the Funding Agency?

In a word—*everything*. One of the most common reasons for rejection of grants at all levels below NIH is that the topic (i.e., area of emphasis) and goals of the proposal do not match the mission and priorities of the funding agency. I coordinated the peer review process for a philanthropic foundation with a substantial grant program for more than 10 years. In that period of time, nearly 33 percent of submitted proposals were not even distributed for peer review because they were completely off-target in relation to the core mission of the organization and our funding categories and priorities. Unfortunately, mismatches between proposal goals and agency mission are more common than you would think even at the federal level. A former university colleague who now serves as a peer review coordinator for one of the NIH institutes, and who works closely with the institutes' study sections (i.e., peer review panels), indicates that proposal–mission mismatches account for 20 percent of the applications that are judged to be not worthy of peer review in the prescreening (triage) system employed by

Table 16–1
Characteristics of Funding Mechanisms

Grant—unsolicited	• The grantor (funding agency) agrees to support a project that has been proposed by the applicant.
	• The research question, project conceptualization and methodology are originated by the applicant.
	• Recipients of unsolicited grants typically have considerable freedom to configure and conduct the project as they see fit.
	• The funding organization typically plays no active role in project implementation other than to receive progress reports.
Grants—solicited	• Solicited grants are often called RFAs which stands for Request For Applications.
	• The funding agency has already identified a problem or issue that needs to be studied.
	• The agency sends out a request for applications to solicit projects to study the problem or issue.
	• Generally RFAs come with certain stipulations to guide grant writers in creation of their proposals; for example, types of research protocols that are acceptable, specific aspects of the overall problem that are higher priority, study populations that need to be addressed, and health-care providers that need to be involved in the project.
	• Awards made in response to RFAs are typically monitored more closely that unsolicited grants, but investigators often have a fair degree of latitude in structuring the project.
Contracts	• The agency solicits proposals to perform specified tasks that are often tightly prescribed. Contract-based solicitations are often called RFPs – Request For Proposals.
	• Contracts are frequently issued for applied research; for example, implementation of projects that attempt to incorporate a biomedical science breakthrough into clinical practice or to evaluate the "real world" effectiveness of a technique that has had promising results in an experimental and well controlled environment.
	• The funding agency is often more involved in the day to day details of a contract-supported project than in a project supported by a grant.
	• The funding agency expects stricter financial accountability and project reporting than with grants.
Cooperative agreements	• Cooperative agreements are similar to RFAs (solicited grants) except that the funding agency works closely with investigators on project implementation details, basically functioning as co-investigators.
	• This funding mechanism is used by NIH and by many state agencies to pursue research in specific areas where pooling of resources is needed.
	• Conceptually, a project supported by a cooperative agreement is a shared research protocol between the grantor and grantee.
	• Most faculty are not likely to be involved in a cooperative agreement project unless they are well established investigators in their discipline.

the NIH. For example, a common misconception is that the scientific mission of the NIH is to support biomedical research when in fact the actual mission of the NIH is to "improve the health of the people of the United States."[1] NIH study section reviewers are not likely to endorse a project if they cannot see a connection between the research question and how the answer to that question can be implemented to enhance the public health.

In this electronic era, grant writers can obtain a wealth of information about almost any potential funding source in local, state, and federal government, among the thousands of private foundations that have grant award programs and among the numerous corporations in the business and industry sector that support biomedical research. Various military agencies also operate award programs (e.g., RFP contract mechanisms) to support biomedical research. An entire book could be written on the topic of search strategies to find sources

of funding to support research. Here are three strategies to get you started:

1. **Make voice contact**, either in-person or by phone, with the grant program managers at the funding sources you have identified as potential recipients of your grant application.

2. **Do your homework**—learn everything you can about the funding sources you are considering.

3. **Be proactive**—take advantage of online resources and searchable databases to stay up-to-date and informed about funding opportunities and stay in the loop about what your competitors for grant dollars are doing.

THE FIRST RULE OF GRANTSMANSHIP

The first rule of grantsmanship is to never submit a grant application to any organization, including NIH,

---

BOX 16-1

Summary of Information Available to Grant Writers in an RFA—EXAMPLE

Title: Interventions for Control of Asthma Among African American and Hispanic Children

Goal: Develop reproducible model programs that reduce asthma morbidity, decrease inappropriate use of health resources, and increase quality of life of asthmatic patients and families among target populations.

Support: $1.6 million annually for four grants. Awards for up to 5 years.

Key project design considerations:
• Seek multidisciplinary approaches involving medicine, public health, and behavioral sciences
• Applicants must demonstrate access to target populations.
• Projects should focus on children up to 18 years and parents and/or care providers.
• Interventions can include changing knowledge and behavior of health-care providers.

Research design should include:
• Well-defined population with asthma
• Reliable asthma assessment and long-term monitoring methods
• Appropriate theoretical basis for intervention
• Sufficient population for a control group
• Social and cultural characteristics of intervention population
• Health status and behavioral change measurements
• Follow-up data for two years post-intervention

Examples of questions that could be answered by programs developed through this solicitation include:
• How can patients at high risk be targeted for early intervention in order to avoid emergency room visits and hospitalizations for asthma?
• How can patient education be integrated into health-care systems used by these populations?
• How can education of health-care providers contribute to improved management of asthma among minority children?
• What strategies are needed to ensure that patients receive an appropriate treatment regimen?
• What are the relationships between interventions and medical outcomes?
• What is the effect of intervention on quality of life and family functioning?
• What interventions are most effective among Hispanic and Black populations?

Source: NIH-95-HL-11-L (RFA Number)
National Heart, Lung, and Blood Institute
Original application date: December 1, 1995

---

without talking to a grant program coordinator about your proposed project. It is essential to make sure that the funding agency has an interest in your research idea before you invest your time in proposal development. It's also important to determine if the agency has particular interests within the general topic area of your research that may help you focus your proposal on a specific aspect of the overall topic. With private foundations and with county and state government, it is critical to determine if they have recently funded projects that are similar to your proposal. Your research idea may have great merit and address a clear need, but if the agency has funded several projects in the past couple of years that are somewhat similar, they may be hesitant to provide financial support for yet another project in the same area. My approach strategy for foundations is to contact the grant program manager (who is usually listed on the Web site) by phone to discuss my project ideas. If the grant manager is encouraging, I follow up within 24 hours by sending a one-page synopsis by e-mail attachment. This e-mail is followed by a second phone call within 48 hours to determine if the project still seems to fit with the objectives of the foundation's award program now that the grant manager has a better appreciation of project details. Most grant program managers will be candid and tell you if your idea does not fit, but their responses may require reading between the lines. In general, my experience is that any degree of hesitancy about a project synopsis is not a positive sign.

THE SECOND RULE OF GRANTSMANSHIP

The second rule of grantsmanship is to do your homework. This means spending the time to identify and research potential funding sources. Here are suggestions for identifying potential sponsors among philanthropic foundations, the private sector (business and industry), and the federal government, including the military, and recommendations for communicating with foundations and private businesses. I did not include pharmaceutical companies, a major source of funding for biomedical research, because I have no personal grantseeking experience with this type of business enterprise.

Philanthropic Foundations

There are a wide variety of print and electronic resources to help you find "best fit" targets for your grant applications among foundations. Box 16–2 describes several print resources that I have found to be helpful; most of these have companion electronic versions that can be accessed online. The bible of information about private foundations is *The Foundation Directory*, which is updated annually and now includes information on more than 20,000 foundations with award programs. This is a searchable database that you can use to pinpoint potential targets for your proposal. Access to this database requires a subscription. The Foundation Center, which publishes the Foundation Directory, has an elaborate Web site with links to other directories, literature on grant writing, support services, and training opportuni-

ties available through the center. The Foundation Center link is *http://fdncenter.org/*. The Foundation Center's link to "Medical Research" at its RFP Bulletin page is *http://fdncenter.org/pnd/rfp/cat_medical_research.jhtml*. This is a valuable inventory of information about recently announced solicitations from a wide variety of foundations and other nonprofit organizations and it can be accessed without a subscription fee.

There are organizations within virtually all states that print directories of state-based foundations, and many of these are available online as well as in print. Directories of state and national foundations are usually available in university libraries. An example is the 2003 Directory of Texas Foundations which is listed in Box 16–2. This directory is produced by the Nonprofit Resource Center of Texas *http://www.nprc.org/* located in San Antonio, Texas, which also offers personal consultation on search strategies to help grant writers find funding sources. Most major metropolitan areas have similar organizations that function as grant information clear-

---

BOX 16–2

Funding Resource Directories in Print

The Foundation Directory New York: Sage

This annual publication provides information on the finances, governance, and giving interests of the nations' 10,000 largest grantmaking foundations. Information is arranged by the state where the foundation is located. Entries explain each foundation's purpose and activities, fields of interest, type of support, and limitations. Many entries list examples of grants funded in the last reported year.

Annual Register of Grant Support Medford, NJ: Information Today, Inc.

The Annual Register describes nearly 4,000 grant support programs including government agencies, public and private foundations, corporations, community trusts unions, educational and professional associations, and special interest organizations. Eleven broad categories, including "Life Sciences," are subdivided into more specific fields, including *Medicine (multiple disciplines); Dentistry; Nursing; Pharmacology;* as well as *allergy, immunology, infectious diseases* and several other specialties.

Directory of Texas Foundations San Antonio: Nonprofit Resource Center of Texas

Information about nearly 2,500 foundations located in Texas is listed alphabetically in the Directory of Texas Foundations. Indexes include areas of interest and type of support, headquarters city, trustees, and officers. This directory also includes information about foundation support in geographical areas of the state and a breakdown of types of grants given in each city (e.g., Medical Research received 7.7 percent of grants given in San Antonio in 2003). It also includes analyses of the top 100 Texas foundations, breaking down the types of grants given by each foundation.

Guide to U.S. Foundations, Their Trustees, Officers, and Donors New York: The Foundation Center

This publication includes entries for nearly 60,000 large and small foundations. Foundation listings are arranged alphabetically by state. Within each state, foundations are listed in descending order by total grants awarded. Indexes include lists of trustees, officers, and donors; a foundation name index; and a locator for independent, company-sponsored, and operating foundations and a community foundation name index and locator for community foundations.

Directory of Biomedical and Health Care Grants Phoenix: Oryx Press

More focused in scope than other directories, the Directory of Biomedical and Health Care Grants includes brief information on 2,500 funding programs. Arranged alphabetically, each entry explains the foundation's purpose, requirements, restrictions, grant amounts, and contact and sponsor information. Indexes include subject listings, program type, and sponsoring organization, in addition to a geographic (by state) index.

inghouses and sources of consultation or training. Foundations typically provide detailed information about their grant programs at their Web sites. Usually, the banner running vertically along the left margin of the Web site or horizontally across the top of the page includes a link labeled as one of the following: Grant Program, Grants, Award Program, or Funding Opportunities. Following this link will lead to you to information about the foundation's grant mechanisms. Whether you use one of the foundation directories, either print or online, or go directly to a foundations Web site, you should be able to find answers to most of the following questions. If you cannot answer these questions, contact the foundation directly to seek answers prior to spending much time writing your proposal.

- What is the overall purpose or mission of the grant program? Does the foundation have a priority list of problems, issues, and topics?

- Does the foundation have geographic limits on funding? For example, awards may be limited to specific counties within the state. Will the foundation fund out-of-state projects?

- Does the foundation provide grants to support higher education and specifically, health professions education?

- Does the foundation target certain population groups?

- Does the foundation have specific areas of interest? For foundations that support health professions education or research in the biomedical sciences, certain public health issues, such as alcoholism, or diseases such as diabetes, are often identified as high priorities.

- What types of projects does the foundation support? Foundations may support many of the following categories of grants or may focus on just one or two types: education and training, research, community service, scholarship programs, capital improvement projects, physical plant renovations, endowment funds, start-up funding (seed money), land acquisition, equipment purchase, endowed chairs in academic institutions, continuing education for professionals, and public education campaigns.

- Are there any specific restrictions on who can receive grants? For example, many foundations will not award grants to individuals who are not affiliated with an institution and may not make awards to religious organizations.

- How many grants are awarded annually and what is the range in funding provided to applicants?

- What were the titles of grants awarded in the past 2 to 3 years and what organizations received these funds?

- What is the application process including deadlines?

- Most importantly, who is the person identified as the grant program director for the foundation?

The answers to these questions will help you determine if a particular foundation is a best fit for your proposal. You should not submit a grant application to an organization unless you know the answers to these questions.

Business and Industry

Strategies for securing funding support from the private sector are generally similar to those employed with foundations. However, finding information on corporate award programs will be more difficult. There are fewer directories of corporate grant programs; and priorities and availability of funds shift in concert with marketplace factors. Generally, you will need to go directly to the Web site of the corporation to look for information about award mechanisms. A starting point to get to these Web sites is the corporate funding Web site of the Foundation Center. The URL is *http://fdncenter.org/funders/grantmaker/gws_corp/corp1.html*. As with foundations, personal contact with the grants program manager is extremely important. Before approaching a private company, ask yourself this question: How can my project benefit this company? In other words, why would they want to invest in me? In general, corporate entities are not likely to sponsor biomedical research unless it opens the door to a new and potentially profitable product line, provides them with resources (e.g., you and your expertise) that give them a competitive edge over marketplace challengers, or enhances their image within the business community or among the public.[2] Therefore, you need to do your own market analysis before approaching a company that you have targeted as a potential sponsor of your research. The business sector is not likely to fund a project that is "starting from scratch." They will expect to see that the project is already underway and has produced tangible products or outcomes. The decision-making process about your proposal in the private sector can range from a single empowered corporate officer making the "call" to a deliberate and well-researched process that parallels NIH peer review. In contrast to communications with private foundations, the first approach should be a brief personalized letter sent to an individual responsible for the company's grant program. The letter should include four components: define your product or concept, identify commercial potential for the company, discuss progress that you have already made on your own, and outline the next steps in development and thus your need for collaboration. An example of a hypothetical "first approach" letter to a private company appears in Figure 16–2. A writing template for composing this approach letter appears below.

October 22, 1998

Douglas Morgan, PhD
Vice-President for Research & Development
Silver Star Biotechnologies
2344 S. 31st Street
Carson City, Nevada 77011

Dear Dr. Morgan:

This letter is a follow-up to our meeting at the Western States Conference in Portland. We appreciated your willingness to meet with us. As you may recall, we are attempting to produce a safe, effective and commercially viable vaccine against respiratory syntial virus (RSV), the primary cause of lower respiratory tract infection among children under six years of age. RSV disease is now the leading cause of morbidity and mortality worldwide among children in this age group. In the past decade, there also has been a marked increase in deaths from RSV disease in the United States, Germany, Spain and Great Britain. There have been many attempts to produce a vaccine against RSV but all efforts to manufacture such a vaccine have been unsuccessful including attempts to use a formalin inactivated virus vaccine in the 1970's and efforts in the 1980's to use attenuated temperature sensitive mutants. Advances in biotechnology now provide legitimate opportunities for the production of a RSV vaccine that will embrace an international market due to the incidence of RSV disease throughout the world.

Because of Silver Star's commitment to vaccine development, and your collaboration with the World Health Organization's vaccine research team, we thought you would appreciate an update on our progress since we met in Portland. The goals of our project are to produce a RSV vaccine that: (1) can be administered to infants as young as 6 months, (2) has minimal immune response side effects, and (3) is economically viable as a mass vaccination in both developing and industrialized nations.

Viral proteins with well-defined sequences can be produced using recombinant DNA technology. During phase I of this project, we produced noninfectious RSV-like particles (virus like particles; VLPs) without the RSV genome. As you are aware, creation of such particles is a goal of the WHO's vaccine development team. This task was accomplished by coexpressing the envelope glycoproteins (F and G), and the envelope matrix proteins (M1 and M2) in cells using vaccinia virus (VV) recombinants. We then used Western blot analysis and immunoelectron microscopy to characterize the VLPs for the presence of four RSV proteins, and the presence of vaccinia virus and cell proteins. We are now determining the immunogenicity of the VLPs by immunizing rabbits.

Phase I has been supported by institutional seed money, departmental resources and two foundations that underwrite biomedical research but at modest funding levels. To continue with this project, we are seeking a collaborator in the private sector with similar research priorities. Phase II of this project will involve three tasks:

- Evaluate the humoral (mucosal and systemic) and cell-mediated immune responses induced by RSV-like particles with novel adjuvant/delivery systems such as dehydroepiandrosterone (DHEA) and vitamin D3.
- Evaluate the degree to which this immune response protects the respiratory tract after virus challenge.
- Determine whether this immune response will exacerbate the disease or induce significant side effects.

A prospectus is attached that reviews our phase I accomplishments and describes the objectives, methodology, needed resources and timetable for phase II. Two abstracts describing our progress to date are also enclosed. They will be presented at next month's North American Virology Conference. We look forward to continued discussion of our mutual interests in production of a RSV vaccine.

Sincerely,

James Bosworth, PhD   Janet Gunderson, MD
Associate Professor   Associate Professor
Division of Virology   Division of Pulmonary Medicine

FIG. 16–2. Example of an approach letter to a private company.

- Letter is addressed to a specific individual in a "decision position" within the company

- Mention any previous contact in first paragraph (indicate where and when you met)

- Style—brief (two pages maximum), clearly written, informative without making grandiose claims or boasting, and avoid overly technical language

- Discuss why the company should be involved in product development (market expansion, "edge" over competition, potential "breakthrough" product)

- Describe the status of work in progress (show that project is ready for expansion)

- Outline future plans (illustrate why support is needed)

- Request opportunity to meet in person without sounding "pushy"

Within 7 days, follow up with a phone call to the company's grant program manager to make sure the letter was received, elaborate on the letter, answer questions that hopefully will arise (questions are a good sign), and offer to send additional information. If the grant manager is receptive to receiving additional information, be sure to send these materials within 24 hours. Follow-up materials can include reports detailing work accomplished to date, reprints of publications, newspaper articles, pictures of your product, and links to Web sites. Reports should be professionally packaged because corporate mangers are accustomed to receiving polished and attractive documents. After another 7 days, follow up with a second phone call to make sure the materials were received and answer any questions. Hopefully, you will be invited for a meeting at this point in the process. If you are not, you should turn your attention to another potential source of funding. If a meeting is scheduled, bring two items:

1. A development budget that specifically identifies the financial support needed for clearly defined future tasks and

2. Any new products, outcomes, or reports that have evolved since the start of communication with the company. During the meeting, request a timeframe for making a decision about your funding request.

Federal Government

Box 16–3 describes online resources that can be used to stay abreast of funding opportunities at the federal level. I have found Grants.gov and GrantsNet to be particularly helpful. You can also arrange to have the NIH Guide for Grants and Contracts sent to you weekly by e-mail. The Guide announces the availability of NIH RFAs for biomedical and behavioral research and for

research training and also disseminates policy and administrative information. The link to the Web site for the NIH Guide to Grants and Contracts is *http://grants.nih. gov/grants/guide/description.htm*. Directions for subscribing to the Guide are available at this Web site. There are a number of online sources of information about military-sponsored research, which is more substantial than most people realize. For example, the link to Department of Defense Medical Research programs is *http://cdmrp.army.mil/* The US Army Medical Research and Material Command can be accessed at *http://www. usamraa.army.mil/pages/index.cfm*.

THE THIRD RULE OF GRANTSMANSHIP IS TO BE PROACTIVE.

This can be accomplished by having information about funding opportunities sent to you automatically online so you stay in the loop. An excellent way to stay up-to-date is to subscribe to SPIN.PLUS,™ which stands for Sponsored Projects Information Network, and its associated funding alert system known as SMARTS™. SPIN was developed by InfoEd International and is a searchable database that provides information on more than 1,000 sponsoring agencies and more than 10,000 separate funding opportunities. All of the information on SPIN is obtained directly from the funding agency and is updated frequently. Investigators can enter a detailed profile of their research interests and priorities, with both linked to keywords, in a companion system known as GENIUS Investigator Profiles. SPIN conducts automatic daily searches of its database using the research interest information supplied to GENIUS and sends daily e-mails to SPIN registrants that contain announcements of RFAs, RFPs, and other research support opportunities. SPIN is typically available free of charge through the grants management office of universities or sometimes through the library. A vast array of other funding alert systems are available online. Most are proprietary and they vary greatly in quality and accuracy so the admonishment "buyer, beware!" applies.

You can also practice proactive grantsmanship by taking advantage of a powerful database known as CRISP, which stands for Computer Retrieval of Information on Scientific Projects. CRISP is a searchable database of federally funded biomedical research projects conducted at universities, hospitals, and other research institutions. At the present time, you can search back to 1972, using key words to define research topics, to locate the titles, federal grant numbers, and names of the principal investigators for current or previously funded research projects. The database, maintained by the Office of Extramural Research at the National Institutes of Health, includes projects funded by the National Institutes of Health (NIH), Substance Abuse and Mental

BOX 16–3

Online Sources of Information About Federal Grants

The Catalog of Federal Domestic Assistance (CFDA) *http://12.46.245.173/cfda/cfda.html*
The Catalog of Federal Domestic Assistance (CFDA) is a government-wide compendium of federal programs, projects, services, and activities that provide assistance or benefits to the American public. It contains financial and nonfinancial assistance programs administered by departments and establishments of the Federal government.

Federal Register; National Archives and Records Administration
http://www.archives.gov/federal_register/index.html

The Federal Register is the official publication for Presidential Documents and Executive Orders as well as Notices, Rules, and Proposed Rules from Federal Agencies and Organizations. Many federal programs and deadlines are announced in the Federal register.

Grants.gov *http://www.grants.gov/*

Grants.gov is the electronic storefront for federal grants. The Department of Health and Human Services is the managing partner for the federal E-Grants initiative, designed to improve access to government services by the Internet. Grants.gov is a single access point for more than 900 grant programs offered by the 26 federal grant-making agencies. Grants.gov allows organizations to electronically find and apply for competitive grant opportunities from all Federal grant-making agencies.

GrantsNet *http://www.grantsnet.org/*

GrantsNet is a searchable database of Funding Opportunities for Training in the Biological and Medical Sciences. The American Association for the Advancement of Science—AAAS and Howard Hughes Medical Institute—HHMI created this searchable database of biomedical funding options aimed at scientists in training—graduate students, postdoctoral fellows, and junior faculty members

Guide to US Department of Education Programs and Resources
http://web99.ed.gov/GTEP/Program2.nsf

The Guide to US Department of Education Programs and Resources provides information about programs and resources administered by the US Department of Education. You will also find information on financial assistance offered to state and local education agencies, institutions of higher education, postsecondary vocational institutions, public and private nonprofit organizations, and individuals to help serve a variety of education needs including those of students, teachers, administrators, and researchers. It also includes information about laboratories, centers, and other research-oriented entities that produce resources important to education.

NIH Guide to Grants & Contracts
http://grants.nih.gov/grants/guide/index.html

The official publication of NIH policies, procedures, and availability of funds. At this site, one can search NIH Guide issues beginning with 1992.

NSF Guide to Programs; Funding Opportunities *http://www.nsf.gov/home/programs/recent.cfm*

The Guide to Programs lists funding opportunities offered by the National Science Foundation (NSF) for research and education in science, mathematics, engineering, and technology. The Guide includes broad, general descriptions of programs and activities for each NSF Directorate, as well as sources for more information. It also offers links to various NSF websites, program announcements, and solicitations that contain additional proposal or eligibility information and the NSF E-Bulletin for proposal deadline.

Health Services (SAMHSA), Health Resources and Services Administration (HRSA), Food and Drug Administration (FDA), Centers for Disease Control and Prevention (CDCP), Agency for Health Care Research and Quality (AHRQ), and Office of Assistant Secretary of Health (OASH). CRISP can be used to search for scientific concepts, emerging trends, or identify specific projects and/or investigators. The CRISP website is *http://www.crisp.cit.nih.gov/* For example, a CRISP search run in July, 2004 with the key words "screening" and "diabetes" identified 247 current or previously funded grants. You can select specific titles from the CRISP hit

list; in this case I selected one of the projects that the CRISP system rated as a close match to my keywords and printed the abstract that appears in Figure 16–3. Although not displayed in this figure, the CRISP search indicates the names of the investigators for each project that appears on the hit list. The thesaurus terms listed with the project abstract can serve as a guide to help you further refine and focus the search.

Up to this point we have addressed the questions, What is a grant and what do I need to know about the funding agency? Next, we'll consider the reviewer's perspectives about the world of grants.

Title: Screening for IGT: Glucose Challenge vs. Predictive Model
Source of Funding: National Institute of Diabetes and Digestive and Kidney Diseases (NIDDK)

NIDDK and the American Diabetes Association recommend routine screening for "pre-diabetes"—a major public health problem—but we do not know how best to detect it. The U.S. is experiencing a dramatic rise in both type 2 diabetes and its antecedent, "pre-diabetes" (mostly impaired glucose tolerance, IGT). Diabetes Prevention Program results show that progression from IGT to diabetes can be decreased, but patients can only be directed to risk reduction programs if they are recognized; detecting IGT will be especially important for minority populations such as African-Americans, who suffer disproportionately from diabetes. However, since we don't screen for IGT, many IGT patients progress to diabetes, and already have complications and increased cardiovascular risk when they are finally diagnosed. Risk factor-based "predictive models" might identify individuals who should have an OGTT to detect IGT, but such approaches may have limited applicability, and are generally not used to screen for gestational diabetes, where the metabolic defect is similar to IGT. Hypotheses: Two-step screening by a one hour oral glucose challenge test (GCT) followed, if abnormal, by an OGTT will have good predictive ability to identify IGT, and will be superior to "predictive models" in both diagnostic efficiency and cost-effectiveness. **Specific Aims:** (1) To validate the GCT as a reliable predictor of IGT, we will perform both the GCT and an OGTT in a large number of African-Americans and Caucasians, with two objectives: (a) to identify cutoff levels which provide optimal test characteristics in both groups despite variation in prandial status or time of day; (b) to determine how predictive ability is modified by the presence of potential risk factors (age, ethnicity, family history, BMI, waist-hip ratio, dyslipidemia, hypertension, etc.); (2) To compare GCT screening to "predictive model" screening, we will evaluate both predictive ability and cost-effectiveness. Fulfilling the potential of the DPP demands a highly generalizable, low-cost screening strategy; our multidisciplinary team will translate approaches proven beneficial for gestational diabetes into a cost-effective method to identify individuals who could benefit from programs to decrease progression from IGT to diabetes, and reduce cardiovascular risk. Starting management soon enough is a major problem in diabetes care-particularly for minorities which suffer disparities in health. By applying existing knowledge to disease control and prevention, our **Specific Aims** are the critical first steps to solve this problem.

Thesaurus Terms:

Diagnosis design/evaluation, diagnosis quality/standard, glucose tolerance test, noninsulin dependent diabetes mellitus, oral administration, pathologic process, prediabetic state, prognosis, rapid diagnosis, African American, caucasian American, cost effectiveness, diabetes mellitus genetics, disease/disorder prevention/control, disease/disorder proneness/risk, early diagnosis, gender difference, glucose metabolism, health disparity, obesity, clinical research, data collection methodology/evaluation, human subject.

FIG. 16–3. Example of abstract obtained by CRISP search of funded projects.

What Do I Need to Know About Reviewers?

Put yourself in this situation. You review grants for a state agency. You were assigned 15 grants to critique. They are each at least 30 pages long. You received the box of proposals last week but you are extremely busy with many other patient care and administrative responsibilities. It is now 10:30 P.M. on Wednesday evening and all 15 reviews are due Friday. You are still at your office after a long day in the clinic. You are tired and your back hurts. Your spouse called an hour ago and said that the air conditioner is blowing only hot air and the compressor unit is making a lot of weird noises. You have finished seven of the reviews and pick up the eighth grant in the box. Welcome to the reviewer's world. I review approximately 50 grants a year for various organizations. I am perpetually behind schedule and constantly pushing to finish my critiques in the 24 hours before the deadline. I complete most of my grant reviews in the

following situations: between 5:00 and 7:00 A.M. sitting at my kitchen table before showering and getting dressed for work, late at night after the evening news, on Saturday mornings before the rest of the family gets up, on airplanes while flying to and from meetings, and propped up in my hotel room bed in evenings after attending conferences during the day. Again, welcome to the real world of grant reviewers. Grant reviewers are just like everyone else—overworked, often fatigued, distracted with job and family responsibilities, struggling to maintain a hobby, trying to have a social life, and scrambling to make it all fit together as best as possible. Reviewing grants is extra work for the already overworked. Given these circumstances, reviewers tend to focus on what they don't like about a proposal (i.e., red flags) as much as what they like about the proposal. Red flags are warning signals that raise the reviewer's level of alertness for other deficiencies in the proposal. Tired and distracted reviewers have a low tolerance for applications that require hard work (i.e., reading and re-reading) to understand what the grant writer is trying to say. One of the grant writer's top priorities is to write a "reviewer-friendly" proposal. Your job is to communicate your scientific plan and underlying rationale for the project in a clear, compelling, and convincing manner, with a major emphasis on clarity, and the reviewers' job is to provide an objective, scientifically sound, and thoughtful critique of your proposal. If you make it difficult for reviewers to do their job, you will decrease your chances for a favorable review. So, another critical goal of effective grantsmanship is to make it easy and painless for reviewers to critique your grant—help yourself by helping reviewers do their job. To accomplish this critical goal, it's important to understand what annoys reviewers and puts them in a negative frame of mind as they struggle through a proposal that is not reviewer friendly. An annoyed reviewer is much more likely to be a picky reviewer who is looking for excuses to "go south" (i.e., reject) a grant application. The initial impression, or curb appeal, of the application package can be critical. When I pick up a proposal, the first thing I do is flip through the pages to inspect the overall layout and to estimate how much effort will be required to complete the review. Does the proposal look like it's going to be a hard read—for example, page after page of dense single-spaced text, typed in 10 point font, without any paragraph breaks, white space, bold-fonted section titles, or tables and figures? During my flip-through, I often randomly pick out a page in the Methods section and read it to get a sense of the writing style. Within a few lines of text, I'll know if reading the grant will be a painful experience. A tired reviewer trying to slog through a poorly written proposal at 10:30 at night is not an ideal formula for a positive critique.

What annoys reviewers? Here are six annoyances that are prominent on my list. First, reviewers are highly sensitive to a red flag known as *detail drift*, which is sometimes called sliding precision or moving targets. For example, in the abstract, the grant writer states that a study will be conducted at six community-based clinics in three cities, involving a total of 200 patients. However, in two subsequent sections of the proposal the number of clinics and patients is reported differently each time. Detail drift is disconcerting for reviewers and can lead them to question whether the investigators have their act together. In addition, sloppiness with key details in the proposal may lead reviewers to conclude that the project may be managed in a similar sloppy manner. Second, *lack of precision* in explaining project implementation (i.e., the "who, what, where, when, and how" details) is annoying and prevents reviewers from doing their job. Third, a *convoluted and obtuse writing style*, especially in the explanation of concepts or project rationale, is potentially fatal. When I

am reviewing grants, the most frequent editing comment I write in the margins of proposals is the acronym S-A-T, which stands for **S**top **A**nd **T**hink. SATs mark sentences or entire paragraphs of text that are simply not clear; the reviewer has to stop, re-read the offending text, and then decipher what the grant writer is trying to communicate. Grant proposals laden with SATs that force reviewers to guess about the writers' intended meaning rarely result in a positive review. Liane Reif-Lehrer's famous statement about grant writing is well worth remembering: "The best writing cannot turn a bad idea into a good grant proposal. However, bad writing can turn a good idea into a poor grant proposal."[3] A fourth catalyst for reviewer annoyance are *unsupported assertions* that are authoritatively stated as fact but not backed up with evidence or citations to the research literature. The reviewer is left to guess: Is this contention the opinion of the investigators or is there unstated research support that the writer assumes the reviewers will know? The acronym A-S-K, which represents **A**ssumed **S**hared **K**nowledge, is one of the most frequent editorial "red flags" I write in the margins of grants, usually in response to unsupported assertions or in reaction to unexplained models, theories, techniques, or equipment. Fifth, reviewers react poorly to *surprises* that suddenly pop up in the later stages of a proposal. Consider this scenario: A reviewer has devoted 3 hours while sitting in a cramped coach class airplane seat diligently reading through a grant application and believes that he or she has a firm grasp on the details of the protocol. Near the conclusion of the Methods section, new and previously unmentioned ideas and techniques start to appear in an "oh, by the way, we're also going to conduct a test to …" which may strike the reviewer as a sign that the investigators do not know what they want to do or may manage the project in a similar ad hoc manner. The sixth writing red flag is a *"hide and seek" organizational structure* that makes the grant painful to read. Sometimes the flow (e.g., sequencing) of ideas in grant applications is so obtuse and disorganized that it almost seems intentional as if the writer is challenging the reviewer—"let's see if you can figure out the details of this project on your own."

When writing a grant application, I assume that the following statements are true to remind myself to write as clearly as possible:

- Most reviewers will not read my application completely, and many will only skim it.

- Some reviewers will only read my abstract and specific aims (project objectives) and make a decision about the merits of the grant based on these two sections (more about this phenomenon later).

- Some reviewers will be only remotely familiar with the area of research proposed in the grant.

- No reviewer will understand the project as well as I do.
- Some reviewers will misinterpret or simply forget key elements of my proposal.
- **But,** I will not be sitting beside the reviewers when they read my grant to answer questions and will not be in the room when the entire review committee meets to provide missing details or clarify misconceptions. The fate of my grant rests on the clarity of the story told in the grant application and the strength of the case that I build for the project. This leads to the final take-home message in relation to reviewers: you are competing for the reviewer's attention. Do not assume that you automatically have captured the reviewer's attention. You have to earn it with clear, compelling, and convincing writing.

Before leaving the reviewer's world, here are four closing recommendations for enhancing your grantsmanship skills:

1. Become a reviewer yourself. My grant writing skills, and success, increased dramatically after I started serving as a reviewer. As we have discussed, grant reviewing can be "more work for the already overworked" but it can also be a powerful learning tool. There is no better way to see what works and what doesn't work than to critique grant applications of various formats and quality, noting the characteristics of grants that are funded and those that "go south."

2. Be aware of the so-called "fatal seven" red flags that are listed below. The NIH periodically analyzes reasons for grant rejection and publishes these findings; the fatal red flags below have not substantially changed for many years.[4] Several of these red flags evolve from problems in the conceptualization of the overall research design, use of inappropriate statistical techniques, or scientific principles and methodology that are out of date or discredited. These big picture issues are beyond the scope of this chapter, but few research grants will be approved for funding if the underlying scientific foundation is weak even if the proposal is communicated with persuasive use of the 3Cs.

Seven Fatal Red Flags

1. The proposed research is not unique, novel, or innovative. For example, the research plan addresses questions that have already been answered or are no longer of scientific interest.
2. The proposed project is not conceptually significant. Even if the protocol is successfully implemented, the results of the project will not produce a substantial finding that will enhance understanding of disease mechanisms or improve the public health.
3. The proposed methodology is not feasible; the study cannot be implemented given the resources of the institution.
4. The principal investigator lacks expertise or experience in the topic area.
5. Methods, equipment, and procedures are not state of the art.
6. The research design or statistical methods are not appropriate.
7. The proposal is not communicated clearly; for example, reviewers cannot understand the purpose of the project and the methodology after reading the synopsis (abstract) and specific aims (objectives).

3. Red flag number 4—investigator lacks expertise or experience—becomes more and more fatal as you move upward in the hierarchy of funding sources toward the NIH level. At the federal level and among the major foundations (e.g., Robert Wood Johnson, Pew, Macy, Kellogg), my experience is that review panels will almost always fund the grant application with the most experienced PI when choosing among several well written applications that have equal scientific merit. Young investigators and other individuals who have considerable professional experience but a limited research track record need to think "TEAM" when preparing grant applications. Reviewers will expect that you will partner with individuals who have established records of publication and funding in critical areas of your protocol. In particular, it is essential to have partners (e.g., co-investigators) who will be perceived by reviewers as bonafide subject matter experts in the biomedical problem that is addressed in your grant. For example, if your proposal addresses juvenile arthritis, at least one of your co-investigators needs to be an established investigator with 5 to 10 publications, and hopefully, previous funding, related to this disorder.

4. Purchase and read *Grant Application Writer's Handbook* (4th ed)[7] by Liane Reif-Lehrer (National Book Network, 2004). This book is an outstanding resource, focuses exclusively on writing grants in the biomedical sciences, and contains many useful examples of effective writing strategies for the various components of a grant application. Although the examples are geared toward NIH, most of the principles and recommendations described by Reif-Lehrer apply to other types of funding sources. Three other valuable resources that I recommend are given in references 8–10.

Writing Strategies for the Six Major Narrative Sections of Research Grant Applications

Figure 16–4 displays the six sections of a research grant application where you have an opportunity to tell the story of your proposed project. Reviewers will read each of these sections seeking answers to specific questions that are indicated on the right side of Figure 16–4. Our job as grant writers is to help reviewers do their job by making the answers to these questions as obvious and convincing as possible. For applications submitted to NIH, and for most other funding agencies, the first and most critical section, the abstract, is a stand-alone item that appears on the second or third page of the application package. Sometimes the abstract is called the project synopsis, and the official NIH term for the abstract is project description. In the middle of the application package, often following the budget, resumes of key personnel, and several pages of information about institutional resources, four sections are typically packaged together as the research plan: specific aims, background and significance, preliminary studies, and research design and methods. The research plan is the "guts" of your proposal and you typically are allowed from 10 to 25 pages to communicate your story, or stated another way, approximately 6,000 to 15,000

words in a proposal that is single spaced with one-inch margins and typed in 11-point Arial font. The sixth narrative component that we will discuss, the budget justification, appears in the financial section of the proposal following the budget request. The justification for personnel and other expenditures is often written haphazardly as an after-thought, which is a substantial mistake because this section provides an opportunity to convince reviewers of the expertise and credentials of your team. The following pages describe what grant writers need to do in each of these sections to sell your project and to help reviewers do their job. After reviewing writing goals and organizational strategies for each of these components, several "never do these" red flags are presented as a summary. As a final note before moving on, the terminology used to describe the narrative components of a grant application is linked to the Public Health Service Form 398 (PHS 398), which is the most commonly used application for federal grants. The PHS 398 application package and directions are available online at the NIH Forms and Applications Web site at this URL *http://grants1.nih.gov/grants/forms.htm*.

Abstract

Development of the abstract is the single most important piece of writing that you will do when preparing a

Component	Questions that reviewers want to answer
Abstract	What is the overall purpose and methodology of this project?
Research Plan	
A. Specific aims	What do you intend to do? (what are your objectives?)
B. Background and significance	* Why is the work important? * What knowledge gap does this project address? * What is innovative and unique about this project?
C. Preliminary studies	What has already been done by your team?
D. Research design and methods	* What is the underlying model/concept? * How are you going to do the work? Who? What? How? When? Where?
Budget justification	* What personnel are needed and why? * How much time will personnel devote? * What supplies/equipment are needed and why?

FIG. 16–4. Principal narrative components of a research grant application.

research grant application. It is the 200 to 400 words, depending on the application package format, in the entire proposal that you should spend the most time massaging to make sure every word counts and every sentence clearly communicates information that reviewers want to read. The abstract should also be critiqued by numerous other people who should be vigorously quizzed to obtain their feedback and wordsmithing (editing) recommendations. A critical question when debriefing individuals who have read your abstract is: *Describe my project to me.* If these individuals cannot coherently explain the details of your project, your abstract needs more work. The abstract provides the critical first impression that will linger with reviewers while they read the rest of the proposal. My experience is that abstracts stimulate two reactions that flavor my overall approach to the critique of the proposal. After reading the abstract, I am either excited, or at least intrigued, about the central concept of the grant and eager to read more, or conversely, I am almost immediately skeptical about the merits of the project and find myself reading the rest of the proposal with the somewhat jaundiced attitude of "you've got to prove to me" that this proposal has value. The damage that can be caused by a sloppily written and unclear abstract cannot be overestimated. Thus, the abstract needs to contain your best writing in the entire proposal. Unfortunately, many abstracts are thrown together at the last minute, literally in the final moments before the grant applica-

tion is submitted electronically or sealed into the FedEx package.

The overall purpose of the abstract is to provide an executive summary of the entire research study. The abstract is often referred to as the "box" because the text appears within a prescribed space that literally limits the number of words that can be typed. What questions do reviewers want answered by the words in the box? An informative abstract that helps reviewers do their job should provide answers to the six questions below. These questions should form the template for constructing your abstract and for allocating the 200 to 400 words that you have to tell your story.

1. What problem will be addressed, and in what population? The problem statement should identify an unknown—a phenomenon we do not understand or something that we do not know how to accomplish.
2. What is the purpose of the project? What, specifically, do you propose to do?
3. What research question(s) will the project answer? OR What hypothesis will be tested?
4. What methods will be used to answer these questions or test the hypothesis?
5. What outcomes will be measured? (i.e., what data will be collected?)
6. What will we learn if we conduct this project? (i.e., what is the benefit?)

Problem: Hispanic children experience asthma with equal frequency as the general population but have greater morbidity. Education is proposed as the key to asthma management, but no studies have evaluated the effectiveness of educational interventions for Hispanic children in outpatient settings. **Purpose:** This study will evaluate an outpatient intervention for Hispanic children with asthma that includes physician and patient/family education. **Research questions:** 1) Will physician education improve medical management of Hispanic children with asthma in an outpatient clinic? 2) Will an educational intervention for Hispanic children with asthma and families decrease morbidity and improve quality of life? **Methods-physicians:** Prior to patient enrollment, pediatric residents will participate in an educational intervention including case conferences, workshops, role modeling by attending physicians, pocket cards depicting asthma management algorithms, convenient access to peak flow meters and spirometry, computer-based asthma management simulations and asthma knowledge self-tests. **Methods-patients:** 160 Hispanic children with asthma, ages 6-15 years, receiving care in a continuity clinic, will be enrolled. A research associate will interview parents and children separately using standardized questionnaires to obtain data about health beliefs/behaviors, asthma knowledge/attitudes, functional morbidity, acculturation, and sociodemographic factors. A research nurse will perform spirometry on subjects. Medical records and school attendance logs will provide additional information. Patients will then be randomized into treatment and control groups. The treatment group will participate in the intervention to learn asthma self-management, use of inhalers and peak flow meters and peak flow charting. Patients/parents will participate in four educational modules conducted by a bilingual nurse educator. Patients/parents will view videotapes that provide peer role modeling by showing Hispanic children performing asthma self-management tasks. Patients will review asthma management skills with a research nurse at appointments 6, 12, and 24 months following enrollment. **Physician outcomes:** The physician education outcomes will be measured by asthma knowledge tests, chart audit and computer-based patient simulations administered pre and post intervention. **Patient outcomes:** Longitudinal data will be obtained by interview, medical record review and spirometry at the 6, 12 and 24 month visits. Intervention and control groups will be compared for morbidity (ER visits, hospitalizations, school days missed), quality of life (Stein's Impact on Family Scale and Functional Status Measure), asthma knowledge/beliefs and pulmonary function (FEV_1). **Benefit:** This project will enhance knowledge of outpatient asthma education strategies for physicians and for patients and their families.

FIG. 16–5. Example of abstract for an application written in response to an RFA.

The abstract displayed in Figure 16–5 is organized around these six questions and provides answers to each question. This abstract also demonstrates two other desirable techniques. I encourage grant writers to use "gap" language in the sentences describing the problem. Gap language includes phrases such as "is not known," "has not been investigated," "do not understand," and "no studies have evaluated" which are designed to focus reviewer attention on the knowledge gap. The second sentence of the abstract contains a good example of an attention-grabbing gap statement: "Education is proposed as the key to asthma management, **but no studies have evaluated** the effectiveness of educational interventions for Hispanic children in outpatient settings." This abstract also includes eye-catching "headers" (bold-fonted bullets) linked to the six questions. I strongly encourage grant writers to insert bolded headers into the abstract to help guide reviewers through the text and focus their attention. Headers can be placed where they naturally fall in the text as demonstrated in Figure 16–5 or they can all be placed at the left margin which I prefer, but which reduces, by about 20 words, the amount of text that can be typed into the box.

I try to follow these assumptions and guidelines when writing abstracts.

Assumptions:

- Assume that reviewers will read *only* this page.
- Assume that the proposal will be judged *only* on the information communicated in the abstract.
- Assume that reviewers will make an initial "snap" judgment about the merits of the proposal based only on the abstract and will read the rest of the proposal either with enthusiasm or with a skeptical "show me" attitude.

Writing guidelines:

- Do not waste words telling reviewers about things they already know, especially for RFAs and RFPs. Abstracts often contain articulate and thoughtful descriptions of problems that need to be explored or resolved, but these problem statements consume much of the text in the abstract box, leaving only a few sentences to sketchily describe how the project will be conducted. Reviewers who are critiquing applications submitted in response to a solicitation already are well informed about the scope and severity of the problem; they want to read the details of how you propose to study the problem. Even with unsolicited proposals (i.e., investigator initiated), grant writers tend to devote too many words to explaining the problem and too few words to describing the "plan of attack."
- Related to the previous guideline, use at least 50 percent of your words to describe the methods and outcomes with as much specificity as you can squeeze into the abstract box. As in almost all areas of science and research, "the devil is in the details" and reviewers will want to be convinced that you know what you are doing. Starting with the abstract and continuing throughout the research plan, one of your primary goals is to convince reviewers that you have a well conceived plan for implementing the project.

- Clearly state the outcomes to be measured and name the measurement instruments that will be used to obtain the outcomes data. In other words, be precise by naming names. For example, in the abstract in Figure 16–5, instead of using a global term such as "spirometry" to measure pulmonary function, the grant writer named a specific test, FEV_1. In the same abstract, the writer named a specific instrument to measure impact on family, Stein's Impact on Family Scale, rather than using global language such as "functional status and family impact will be examined."

- Do not leave unanswered questions in the minds of reviewers. Avoid S-A-Ts at all costs. If a reviewer is confused after reading the abstract and annoyed by having to ponder numerous SATs, you will have lost your opportunity for a positive first impression. Intense critique of your abstract prior to submission by many "extra sets of eye-balls" will help identify areas that need better clarity and more detail.

- Be careful to avoid detail drift between the abstract and the Methods section. The description of the "who, what, when, where, and how" details should be precisely the same in the abstract as they are in the Methods section. It's not uncommon for grant writers to make a flurry of tweaks to the methodology, often at the last minute before submission, and forget to modify the description of these details in the abstract. In addition, make sure that the exact text used to state the research questions or hypotheses in the abstract is repeated verbatim throughout the remainder of the proposal. Again, it is not uncommon for grant writers to tweak the research questions each time they are written in the proposal with the result that reviewers may literally read several versions of research questions, or other key statements, as they proceed through the grant. Lack of precision rarely strikes reviewers as a positive attribute.

- Allocate your words wisely. Using 11-point Arial font, roughly 380 words will fit in the current NIH abstract box. Table 16–2 provides a guideline for allocating these words in abstracts written in response to an RFA and in abstracts for unsolicited proposals. For an RFA, I recommend using no more than 20 percent of the total text, 70 words conveyed in two or three sentences, to describe the problem and state the overall purpose of the project. In an unsolicited proposal, the writer needs to do more case building when de-

Table 16–2
Template for Allocating Words in Abstracts for NIH Grant Applications

	Response to RFA		Unsolicited	
	%	Words	%	Words
Problem & purpose	20%	72	40%	144
Research questions	10%	36	10%	36
Methods & outcomes	60%	216	40%	144
Benefit	10%	36	10%	36
Total	100%	360	100	360

scribing the problem and purpose, but I recommend allocating no more than five sentences to this part of the abstract, which equates to roughly 140 words or 40 percent of the text. A research question or hypothesis (depending on the nature of the research) should be stated next using approximately 10 percent of the abstract text for either type of grant. In an abstract written for a RFA response, 60 percent of the text should be devoted to detailing the methodology and outcomes. In an unsolicited proposal, the writer should allocate at least 40 percent of words to methodology and outcomes. The abstract displayed in Figure 16–5, which was written in response to an RFA, has the following word allocation: problem and purpose—60 words (15 percent), research questions—37 words (10 percent), methods and outcomes—268 words (70 percent), benefit sentence—19 words (5 percent).

- Say something meaningful in the last sentence of the abstract that is designed to address the question: What will we learn if we conduct this project; that is, what is the benefit? Even a brief 20-word sentence consumes 5 percent of your abstract text so it needs to contribute to the overall, and hopefully positive, impact of the abstract. Benefit sentences often start with the phrase, "if successful," which should be avoided; why remind reviewers that the project may not work? Instead, remind reviewers what can be learned if we explore the research question. I recommend starting the benefit sentence with the words, "This project will enhance our knowledge of …". Conclude the sentence by describing what we don't understand or don't know how to do (i.e., the knowledge gap that was articulated early in the abstract). For example: This project will enhance our knowledge of strategies to provide prompt emergency care services in rural communities (17 words). The concluding benefit sentence in the abstract displayed in Figure 16–5 follows this format.

RED FLAGS—ABSTRACT

In summary, here are several red flags that should be avoided at all costs in your abstract.

- Abstract fails to answer the six questions that reviewers want addressed.

- If responding to an RFA, the abstract "belabors the obvious" with too much background information about the problem that reviewers probably already know.

- Inadequate narrative is devoted to methodology so reviewers must guess about key "who, what, where, when, and how" details.

- Lack of eye-directing "headers" within the text.

- Detail drift: The description of "who, what, where, when, and how" details and other key information in the abstract does not match the description of these details in the Methods section of the proposal.

Specific Aims

In NIH grant applications, the statement of the project objectives is known as the *specific aims,* as in *"This is what we aim to do during this project."* The statement of the specific aims for the project is section A of an NIH research grant application—the first section of the research plan. The expectation in an application submitted to NIH is that you will use only one page to communicate the specific aims, which leads to the common use of the term "the aims page." Other non-NIH funding sources may use different terminology for this page, such as project goals and objectives, project purpose, or project outcomes, and allow you more or less space to communicate this information. No matter what terminology is used, your goal as a grant writer is to clearly answer this question: *What will we do to answer the research questions or test the hypothesis that we propose to study?* Another way to say this is, What are we going to do to produce the data needed to answer the research question or test the hypothesis? One of your primary goals when writing the aims page is to establish a direct link between the aims and the research question in the reviewer's mind. I conceptualize the specific aims page as my contractual agreement with the funding agency; that is, in return for your sponsorship, I will undertake the following tasks to investigate this research question. Ultimately, the evaluation of the success or failure of the grant will hinge on the degree to which each aim (task) is accomplished. There are two strategies for writing specific aims. Which one you use may in large part depend on your personal style, but may also depend on the nature of the research you propose to conduct. One strategy for writing aim statements is specific and contains "what, how, and who" details within the text of the sentence. The other strategy is more general and basically resembles a goal statement you would write for a course syllabus. An aim written in the "what, how, and who" format includes information to help reviewers answer three questions: What task will be performed to collect needed data? How will this task be accomplished? Who are the subjects (e.g., in what populations will this task be performed)?

Here is an example of a specific aim from a funded NIH grant written in the "what, how, and who" format followed by a breakdown of the text into the three components.

Assess the impact of an evening home visit (EHV) program conducted by internal medicine resident—RN teams by comparing ED visits and hospitalizations 12 months prior to the intervention to the 12-month intervention period among elderly patients enrolled and not enrolled in EHV.

Breakdown

What? … Assess the impact of an evening home visit (EHV) program conducted by internal medicine resident—RN teams …

How? … by comparing ED visits and hospitalizations 12 months prior to the intervention to the 12-month intervention period …

Who? … among elderly patients enrolled and not enrolled in EHV.

An aim written in a more broadly stated "goal" format includes information to help reviewers answer two basic questions: (1) What are you evaluating? and (2) In what population? Here is an example of the same aim about the evening home visit (EHV) program written in the goal format followed by a breakdown into the two components:

Determine if an evening home visit program by internal medicine resident—RN teams decreases ED visits and hospitalizations among home-bound elderly individuals.

Breakdown:

What are you evaluating? … Determine if an evening home visit program by resident—RN teams decreases ED visits and hospitalizations …

In what population? … among home-bound elderly individuals.

One way to make your specific aims (or objectives) reviewer friendly is to use the active voice, which means that the first word of the aim statement should be a verb that clearly communicates the task: calculate, develop, analyze, measure, perform, evaluate, compare, and so forth. Avoid vague language in aims statements such as, "This projects seeks to understand mechanisms that influence …" " learn about the interaction of …" or "continue exploration of factors that predict …".

How should you organize the specific aims section? I recommend the following format which is displayed in the example in Figure 16–6. Start this section with an overview paragraph, labeled as "project overview" by a bold-font header, which consists of approximately 80 to 100 words (four or five sentences) and that serves as an "abstract of the abstract." The purpose of this mini-abstract is to remind the reviewer of the knowledge gap addressed by this project, and the overall purpose of the study. Next, state the research questions or hypotheses that you will investigate. State the research questions/hypotheses with exactly the same words you used in the abstract. Insert a bold-font header that directs the reviewer's eye to the research questions/hypotheses statements and provide "white-space" before and after these statements to further focus attention. Write a bridging, or transitional, sentence that links the research questions to the specific aims. The bridging sentence that I often use is: *To investigate these research questions, we will complete the following tasks, which are described in the specific aims.* Using one of the formats previously described, state each of the specific aims as demonstrated in Figure 16–6 and below by numbering each aim along the left margin with a distinct bold-font header and begin each aim statement with an action verb.

- **Aim 1:** Identify …
- **Aim 2:** Categorize …
- **Aim 3:** Evaluate …

Most reviewers will expect to read three or four aims statements. More than four aims will wave a red flag that the investigators may be biting off more than they can handle or the application is a grab-bag of projects. The tasks communicated in the aims statements should flow logically from one to the other in a progressive stair-step fashion, with the first aim being the most foundational and subsequent aims building on the outcomes derived from accomplishment of that aim.

A. Specific Aims

A.1 Project overview

Acute otitis media (AOM) is one of the most common indications for antibiotic prescriptions in the outpatient setting, but it is not known if antibiotic therapy provides any advantage over non-pharmaceutical approaches. In Europe, an approach called watchful waiting is utilized instead of routine antibiotic therapy. Under watchful waiting, antibiotics are withheld unless symptoms persist for several days. It is unclear which approach is the most cost-effective. To explore this issue, we will perform a cost-effective analysis of watchful waiting versus antibiotic therapy.

[Four sentences; 83 words including a "gap" statement: "but it is not known"]

A.2. Research questions

1. In children with acute otitis media, does watchful waiting in comparison to antibiotics produce equivalent clinical outcomes at less cost?

2. What is the cost of antibiotic-resistant *Streptococcus pneumoniae* when AOM is routinely treated with antibiotics?

To investigate these research questions, we will complete the following tasks described in the specific aims below. **[Bridge sentence]**

A.3. Specific aims

AIM 1:   Develop a decision analysis model using efficacy-of-treatment probabilities from the AHRQ Evidence Report that outlines the management options and their range of outcomes for AOM if: 1.) managed by watchful waiting or 2.) treated with antibiotics.

AIM 2:   Calculate utilities from the Quality of Well-Being Index (QWB) and compute quality adjusted life years (QALYs) to produce outcomes for the decision analysis in AIM 1.

AIM 3:   Perform a cost-utility analysis of watchful waiting compared with antibiotic treatment using the outcomes from the decision analysis model developed in AIM 1 and AIM 2 and cost-of-therapy estimates obtained from the literature.

AIM 4:   Estimate costs of antibiotic-resistance *Streptococcus pneumoniae* attributable to antibiotic treatment for AOM. Repeat the AIM 3 cost-utility analysis with this estimate to determine effect of antibiotic-resistant *S. pneumo* on cost-to-utility ratio.

FIG. 16–6. Example of layout for the specific aims page.

One of your most important writing goals for the aims page is to help reviewers "lock-down" three critical pieces of information that they will need to remember for the next several hours of reading: the knowledge gap (e.g., the unknown), the research questions, and how you are going to produce the data needed to answer the research question or test the hypothesis (i.e., your specific aims). Taking the time to carefully lay out the aims page in the manner displayed in Figure 16–6 will help you accomplish this goal and also convey an important subliminal message to reviewers that you are organized and have a well-thought-out research plan.

This chapter focuses on strategies to communicate your scientific plan with the 3Cs and is not intended to review research design, but one critical element in the clarity component of the 3Cs overlaps with design considerations: your research questions, which drive the overall study, must be stated with precision. Research questions that are vague and S-A-T–inducing rarely lead to positive critiques. One strategy for writing clear and precise research questions, especially for studies that compare different approaches (e.g., controlled trials) is called the P-I-C-O format.[11] P-I-C-O (pronounced "Pie .. Co") stands for **P**roblem in a particular **P**opulation, **I**ntervention, **C**omparison, and **O**utcome. The first research question in Figure 16–6 is stated in the P-I-C-O format: *In children with acute otitis media, does watchful waiting in comparison to antibiotics produce equivalent clinical outcomes at less cost?* The breakdown of this question into the P-I-C-O components appears in Table 16–3.

RED FLAGS—SPECIFIC AIMS

In summary, here are several red flags that should be avoided on your specific aims page.

Table 16–3
Breakdown of Question in Figure 16–6 into P-I-C-O Components

Population/ Problem	Intervention	Comparison	Outcome
In children with acute otitis media	Does watchful waiting	In comparison to antibiotics	Produce equivalent clinical outcomes at less cost

- Aims are not clearly linked to the hypothesis or research question. Reviewers fail to see that the aims describe how data will be collected to answer the research question or test the hypothesis.
- Too many aims; project looks overly ambitious or poorly planned.
- Aims statements lack precision and are difficult to understand.
- Aims do not start with action verbs that give the reviewer a clear sense of the task to be performed.
- Aims are not integrated with each other (e.g., the aims give the impression of a "grab-bag" of unrelated projects).
- Aims page does not start with a brief 100-word project overview to help reviewers remember the knowledge gap and overall purpose of the project.

Background and Significance

Your primary goal in the background and significance (B & S) section is to "sell" reviewers on the merits of your project. In other words, turn them into advocates for your project so they read the remainder of the proposal looking for reasons to give it a good score versus looking for reasons to throw it into the reject pile. When I'm reviewing a grant and "buy" the underlying premise or rationale for a project, I am more likely to overlook flaws and leaps of logic in the proposal and consequently less likely to look for excuses to go south on the proposal. Unfortunately, many grant writers see this section as merely the "literature review" which is a mistake. True—one of the purposes of the background component of this section is to trace the evolution of the problem and the corresponding research (which hopefully is both skimpy and inconclusive) that lays the groundwork for the current proposal. However, a second and more critical task is to provide your strongest case-building arguments in the B & S section; this is the section where the compelling and convincing components of the 3Cs come into play.

The directions for the PHS 398 package suggest that the B & S section should be three pages. What questions do reviewers want answered in these three pages? When I review grant proposals I want to learn answers to these four questions in this section:

1. What knowledge **GAP** will this project address? What is the unknown?
2. Why is this work important? Convince me that this GAP needs to be investigated NOW.
3. What is unique about the investigators' approach? What makes this project stand out from all the others that I have read? Does the project **GRAB** my attention and make me eager to read more?
4. What is the deliverable? (i.e., what is the product or outcome?) What will the grantor and the scientific community **GET** as a consequence of this project?

I highlighted three words in the preceding list of reviewers' questions: GAP, GRAB, and GET.

My strategy for writing the background and significance, especially the introductory paragraph, is to structure the narrative around the *triple G formula*: focus reviewer attention on an unknown (*gap*) and convince them that it is important and under-studied; *grab* their interest with compelling data that provides a solid and convincing rationale for the importance of this research, and describe tangible outcomes that will evolve from the project so the reviewer will know what the sponsor will *get* in exchange for financial support.

Conceptually, the writing strategy for this section is illustrated in Figure 16–7. To use a marketing term, this is your "pitch" to the reviewers. For example, for a project designed to develop strategies that minimize barriers to primary care services among a specific underserved population, start by describing current health-care practice, and then identify documented deficiencies in current practice and provide evidence of substandard health outcomes. Next, "attack the gap" by clearly identifying an unknown (i.e., a causal factor) related to these barriers that needs to be investigated, or describe a proposed mechanism for alleviating barriers that has not been evaluated. Conclude by painting a picture with words of a potentially brighter future if we can enhance our understanding of underlying causal factors that inhibit access to health-care services.

The first paragraph in the B & S section is one of the most critical pieces of writing you will do in a grant proposal. It is an excellent opportunity to build a strong case for your proposal and hopefully convince reviewers to read this section carefully rather just skimming it, as many reviewers tend to do. The Triple G formula can be used to construct what I call an "Attack the Gap" paragraph. Figure 16–8 demonstrates how to structure this paragraph. Each sentence of this paragraph is written to address one of the questions that reviewers want answered in the B & S section. In the first sentence, the GAP sentence, your goal is to answer the question: What is the unknown? Several examples of lead-off gap sentences are presented in Figure 16–8 to demonstrate writing style. This first sentence should have a definite gap statement (see italicized text in Figure 16–8) and should be written in a succinct, to-the-point, style. For example, *Seventy percent of postmenopausal women at risk for osteoporotic fractures are not diagnosed despite availability of accurate screening tests.* Or, *The influence of cultural context upon the decision-making of urban low-income African-American women about infant feeding has not been studied.*

The second through the fourth sentences are the GRAB sentences designed to answer the reviewers' question: Why is it important to study this problem? These are the evidence sentences in which you present your most compelling and convincing data to document the societal and/or scientific consequence of allowing this problem to continue. The fifth and concluding sentence is your GET sentence to answer the reviewers' question: What will the grantor "get" from this application if it is funded? For illustration, the get sentence that appears in Figure 16–8 is linked to one of the gap sentences by the arrows. Ideally, the relationship between the gap and get sentences should be clearly established in the reviewers' minds as they read the remainder of the proposal.

The second paragraph in the B & S section should start a discussion of the pertinent literature related to the unknown addressed in this proposal. This is the

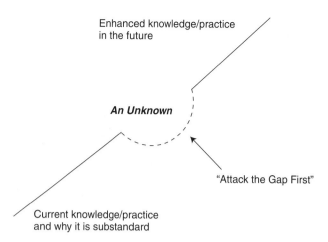

FIG. 16–7. Writing strategy for the background and significance section; your case-building "pitch" to reviewers.

classic literature review component of the grant application. Insert a signpost, or roadmap sentence, to signal the transition from your opening attack the gap paragraph to your synopsis of the work of other investigators. Here is an example of a signpost sentence that sets the stage for the upcoming literature review, and reinforces that little is known about this particular topic:

Our understanding of the factors that influence infant feeding decisions among low-income African-American mothers is based on only three cross-sectional studies conducted in the 1980s with small samples of subjects. These studies will be reviewed in the next section, followed by a discussion of questions that were not answered by these studies.

1st Sentence: Gap Sentence What is the unknown?

Several Examples

The etiology of Meniere's disease *is not known.*

Despite being one of the most detectable of cancers, the mortality rate for oral cancer is 53%. Strategies to increase early detection *have not been successful.*

Seventy percent of postmenopausal women at risk for osteoporotic fractures are *not diagnosed* despite availability of accurate screening tests.

The influence of cultural context upon the decision-making of urban low-income African-American women about infant feeding *has not been studied.*

2nd – 4th Sentences: Grab sentences Why is it important to study this problem?

Describe societal consequence: % households affected, morbidity and mortality, financial costs, resource consumption, missed school and work days, etc.

5th Sentence: GET sentence What will reviewers "get" from this application?

This project will develop a testable, conceptual model of how low-income African-American mothers in District of Columbia make infant feeding decisions. We will use qualitative methods and a collaborative partnership with the women in the community to develop this model.

FIG. 16–8. Writing strategy for an "attack the gap first" paragraph in the background and significance section.

Strategic use of signpost sentences guides reviewers through your proposal and gives them a sense of what is coming next. Another strategy to focus and guide reviewers through your discussion of the background literature is to insert full-sentence signpost headers that communicate the key concept (take-away message) of each paragraph. Box 16–4 displays the first page of a background and significance section and demonstrates the use of reviewer focusing headers. If reviewers remember only the signpost headers, they will retain the important messages about previous research pertinent to the problem. Box 16–4 also demonstrates another useful technique that can help reviewers do their job—use of a table to summarize several key studies. The table in Box 16–4 provides reviewers with a convenient capsule summary of previous studies indicating investigator name, date, research design, number and type of sub-

jects, type of intervention, and outcomes. Strategically placed tables such as this are welcomed by reviewers and also send the message that the proposal is well organized.

Close the B & S section with a strong "significance" paragraph that is labeled with a header typed in bold font to alert reviewers that this is the wrap-up paragraph. In many grant applications that I review, the B & S section simply ends, often with an inconclusive thud, when the grant writer runs out of literature to discuss. Instead, end this section on a positive note by reminding reviewers of the gap—what knowledge is missing—and by helping them answer the critical question: What is unique about this project? Figure 16–9 demonstrates how to structure the concluding significance paragraph for the B & S section of a grant application. Note how the grant writer reminds reviewers how little we know

---

BOX 16–4

Strategies for Reviewer Focusing Including Use of Signpost Headers and Summary Tables

B. Background and Significance
It is not known if depression treatment leads to improved metabolic control in patients with diabetes. Major depressive disorder is present in at least 20 percent of diabetic patients, and is associated with poor treatment adherence and with an increased risk of diabetes complications. Cross-sectional studies have linked depression with poor glycemic control. There are no prospective studies testing the effect of improved depressive symptoms on metabolic control. We will conduct a randomized, controlled trial to evaluate the metabolic results of treatment-related improvement of depression among adult patients with diabetes in primary care.

B.1. Depression is associated with poor diabetes outcomes
One in three people with diabetes has depression at a level that impairs functioning and quality of life, adherence to medical treatment, and glycemic control.[1] Depressive symptom severity is associated with poorer diet and medication regimen adherence, functional impairment, and higher health-care costs in diabetic patients[2] and it increases the morbidity and mortality of cardiovascular disease,[3] the leading killer of patients with diabetes.

B.1.1. It is not known if improvement in depressive symptoms results in better diabetes outcomes.
Only three published studies have examined the association of depression improvement with glycemic control. No studies have evaluated outcomes of equivalent importance to cardiovascular risk in diabetes (blood pressure and lipids). The methodology and outcomes of these three studies are presented in Table 2.

Table 2: Summary of interventions that have been implemented to improve glycemic control by treating depression

Study	Methods	Participants	Intervention	Outcomes
Lustman 1997	RCT	68 DM pts w/ new diagnosis of depression	Nortriptyline vs. placebo	At 8 weeks: Remission in 40 percent HbA1c unchanged despite hyperglycemic effect of nortriptyline
Lustman 2000	RCT	60 DM pts w/ new diagnosis of depression	Fluoxetine vs. placebo	At 8 weeks: Depression improvement 67 percent vs. 37 percent Remission 48 percent vs. 26 percent HbA1c better (trend)
Lustman 1998	RCT	51 referred DM-2 pts with depression	CBT (weekly × 10). vs control (both groups got DM education)	At 6 months ($n = 42$): Remission 70 percent vs. 33 percent HbA1c –0.7 percent vs. +0.9 percent Responders vs. persistent: HbA1c –1.0 percent vs. +1.7 percent

Project Significance

This study is unique in that no previous investigation has documented the rates of hospice utilization by minority groups compared to non-Hispanic Anglos in populations for which detailed social and demographic data are available. There have been only three studies, all involving small numbers of upper middle class African-Americans, that investigated hospice utilization among minority populations. No studies have described hospice utilization patterns among Hispanic/Latinos, Native Americans, or Asian Americans. There have been no studies comparing the factors associated with end-of-life hospice care between non-Hispanic Anglos and minorities. For example: What is the effect of racial concordance between provider and patient on hospice use? To address this lack of information about hospice decision-making among minority populations, we will analyze hospice use among an ethnically diverse urban population in three cities and evaluate the effect of racial concordance between provider and patient on hospice use.

Fig. 16–9. Example of a paragraph describing the significance of the project.

about the issue using phrases such as: "no previous investigation has documented," "there have been only three studies," and "no studies have described."

As a concluding note, your selection and discussion of literature should reveal your awareness of current, cutting edge research pertinent to your topic, and your knowledge of pivotal papers that are more than five years old. With the exception of classic and comprehensive review articles, the articles described in your review should represent the most recent work available. I become very uncomfortable when all of the citations are 10 or more years old, which makes me wonder if the investigators are up to date or just recycling an old grant that has been submitted previously. Include comprehensive reviews, where available, rather than discussing scores of individual studies. Assume that reviewers will be equally familiar with the literature as you are, if not more so, and will notice if you have omitted a key study or selected poorly designed studies to include in your review.

RED FLAGS—BACKGROUND
AND SIGNIFICANCE

Did the investigator: (NO = red flag!)

- Attack the gap? Did the grant writer provide a convincing argument that an important knowledge gap exists?   YES   NO
- Begin the B & S section with an "attack the gap" paragraph using the GAP—GRAB—GET format?   YES   NO

- Use reviewer-focusing section titles?   YES   NO
- Demonstrate real familiarity with the literature by selecting recent, pivotal, and well designed studies and cite comprehensive reviews rather than large numbers of individual articles?   YES   NO
- Write a concluding significance paragraph that reminds reviewers of the gap and why this project is unique?   YES   NO

Preliminary Studies

In this section of your application, reviewers want an answer to this question: What has been accomplished already by *your research team*? In the previous Background and Significance section, you summarized what is known and more importantly what is *not known* about the problem, focusing primarily on the work of other investigators. But in Preliminary Studies, the reviewers' attention turns to the work produced by **you and your research team**. My underlying concern when I read this section is: Are these investigators ready and able to conduct this project? Clear, convincing, and compelling descriptions of your preliminary studies can increase reviewer confidence that you have adequate experience with the techniques and equipment you propose to use, can design appropriate and well run experiments, and can present your results in an objective manner. Reviewers want to be convinced that you possess these attributes and it is your job to provide the evidence that will make them comfortable with your skills.

What are the grant writer's goals when creating this section of the proposal? To help reviewers do their job, I recommend that you concentrate on four writing goals:

- Convince reviewers that the proposed hypothesis is valid and testable by showing preliminary data that naturally "leads" to the next question which you will attempt to answer.
- Prove that you (PI) have appropriate training and experience to conduct the project.
- Demonstrate you have a *team* (including coinvestigators and support staff) capable of accomplishing project tasks.
- Answer feasibility questions by presenting pilot data that indicates that your project is "do-able."

The directions for the PHS 398 application package recommend six to eight pages for this section. However, my experience is that new investigators rarely have enough pilot studies to fill more than three or four pages, so do not resort to padding to "use up all the space." When presenting pilot data, communicate it in a professional manner using well designed tables and figures that are clearly labeled with a title that is cross referenced in the text. Write a one or two sentence legend that appears directly below the table and that explains in clear language what information is displayed in the table. Within the text, carefully describe the type of statistical analyses that were performed and summarize the key results. Do not rely on the motivation of reviewers to stare at tables and deduce the important results on their own without guidance from you. Present only pilot data that are directly relevant to the experiments proposed in this application. Above all, be objective and candid—*don't overstate outcomes* or make unsupported claims. Reviewers react poorly to blatant attempts to prematurely "declare victory." Reviewers also react very negatively to proposals in which the grant writer has simply placed copies of several reprints in an appendix rather than creating a fully developed preliminary studies section that educates the reviewer about the work that formed the pathway to the current proposal.

Here is one final suggestion that does not directly relate to writing the Preliminary Studies section, but may help you build an impressive inventory of preliminary projects and a tangible track record of scholarship. Make every effort to publish, even in abstract form, all aspects of your preliminary work. Over the years, I have observed countless faculty members and clinical practitioners conduct study after study and obtain notable results but never quite get around to "putting the words on paper" and getting their data into print. In academia and the world of research, publications are still the currency of the realm. The higher you go in the grant writing world, the harder it is to get funded without the expected quota of peer-reviewed publications. In many highly competitive disciplines, you are also expected to meet quotas in the "right" journals. For example, one of my sons does research in the intensely competitive world of brain chemistry, focusing on receptor sites and neural pathways that influence addictive craving. In this field of research, one publication in a certain highly respected and extremely selective journal is worth five publications in a so-called second-tier periodical. Participants in my grant writing courses often ask, How many publications do I need? My response: a rule of thumb is roughly one publication per $50,000. Thus, applicants for NIH start-up grants designed to support pilot work are typically expected to have two or three peer-reviewed publications when applying for the $100,000 start-up awards, known as R0-3s in NIH ter-

minology. When applying for a more substantial and multiyear award of $500,000, I would expect at least ten publications pertinent to the topic in solid, respected journals. But, to emphasize, these are just rough estimations of the scholarly productivity required to demonstrate readiness for funding.

I recommend that you use a book-end structure to organize the Preliminary Studies section; start with a "tone-setting" overview paragraph and conclude with a wrap-up paragraph that reminds reviewers how the various preliminary projects lead naturally to the current project. The first paragraph of approximately 100 words (four or five sentences) should summarize the pilot studies and other pertinent past work of your entire team. Frequently, new investigators focus exclusively on their own work but fail to mention research conducted by collaborators on the proposal. Remember—always think "team" when writing grants. In the overview paragraph, also identify past collaborations among members of your research team. As a reviewer, I am more confident about project feasibility when I know that the research team has a track record of previous collaborations and has had tangible success as demonstrated by previously funded grant applications and publications. The next to last sentence in this overview paragraph should state that the experience gained from these preliminary studies and past collaborations will enhance the quality of currently proposed project. The last sentence in the overview paragraph should be written very much like the final sentence in the overview paragraph displayed in Figure 16–10. The purpose of this final sentence is to provide a signpost sentence that alerts reviewers to the fact that they are now going to read summaries of a specified number of prior studies that demonstrate the capacity and readiness of the research team to undertake the project proposed in the application.

As demonstrated in the example of the first page of a preliminary studies section in Figure 16–10, each pilot project should be clearly labeled with a definitive title and described in one or two paragraphs as a distinct entity. Identify the principal investigator for each study and identify the source of funding as shown in the example. Below each description, provide a full citation to key publications that were generated by the project. I type these citations in 10-point font. Following the book-end format, conclude this section with a wrap-up summary paragraph of approximately 100 to 150 words that succinctly explains the key outcome of each preliminary study and "ends on a high note" by stating that the experience and knowledge gained in these pilot projects sets the stage for the proposed project. An example of a wrap-up paragraph for a Preliminary Studies section appears in Figure 16–11.

C. PRELIMINARY STUDIES

Overview: Several preliminary investigations demonstrate the expertise of this interdisciplinary research team and its ability to carry out the proposed scope of work. The team is led by an experienced health sciences researcher and includes co-investigators from informatics, oncology, family medicine, nursing, public health, health services, and journalism. The team has conducted research in five areas that are pertinent to the proposed study: (1) the role of the patient in healthcare decision-making, self-care and patient practice variation; (2) healthcare consumer guides and organizational performance reports in hospital care and managed care; (3) breast cancer and other chronic illness management; (4) clinical oncology; and (5) patient and employer use of healthcare information. These studies are described below.

C.1. Variations in Patient Practice. (A. Smith, XYZ Foundation, 1995-1997.)

This paper established the initial conceptual underpinnings of the theory that has guided our research on the role played by patients in their own healthcare, especially as it relates to chronic problems such as smoking and cancer, and other areas in which the patient plays the primary role, such as pre-natal care. The theory of patient practice variation is presented as the patient analogue to Wennberg's concept of "physician practice variation" and is applicable to how breast cancer patients make decisions about their healthcare options.

Smith A. Patient practice variation: a call for research. Medical Care 1993;31(5 Suppl):YS81-85.

C.2. Consumer Reports: Do they make a difference in patient care? (A. Smith, et al.)

This study, published in JAMA, is one of the few studies to evaluate the impact of consumer guides on the quality of patient care. It found that within one year of the Oregon obstetric report, of the hospitals that did not have a car seat program, formal transfer agreements, or nurse educators for breast feeding prior to the report, 50% instituted these services. Hospitals in competitive markets that did not offer one of these services at the time of the report were more likely to institute a service or were about twice as likely to consider improving service. Clinical outcome indicators, ultrasound rates, Caesarean delivery rates, and rates of vaginal delivery after Caesarean all improved in the expected directions.

Smith A, Green B, Black M, Blue D. Consumer reports in healthcare: do they make a difference in patient care? Journal of the American Medical Association 1997;278(19):1579-1584.

C.3. Nature, Process and Modes of Hospice Care Delivery. (A. Smith, PI; ABC Trust, 1992.)

This project evaluated the quality of care of hospices throughout the US to determine the extent to which hospices were able to meet national standards established by the JCAHO hospice accreditation program and HCFA reimbursement participation conditions. Among other factors, this national evaluation investigated issues of patient self-determination. The study methods included on-site data collection as well as the fielding of survey instruments by mail. The study resulted in revised JCAHO hospice standards and HCFA requirements for hospice care.

Blue D, Smith A, Green B. Do not resuscitate (DNR) policies in healthcare organizations with emphasis on hospice. Proceedings of the Annual Meeting of the American Society of Clinical Oncology, 1987;6:263.

FIG. 16–10. Example of organizational structure for the preliminary studies section.

RED FLAGS—PRELIMINARY STUDIES

Does the investigator: (NO = red flag!)

- Use a book-end writing structure?   YES   NO
- Present only preliminary studies that are pertinent to the research question?   YES   NO
- Describe preliminary results in an objective manner?   YES   NO
- Showcase the overall strength of the team?   YES   NO
- Provide a description of preliminary studies (vs. appending reprints without an explanation)?   YES   NO

Research Methods

At any level of grant writing, the Methods section will constitute the majority of your text. For an NIH grant application, as much as 60 percent of the 15,000 to 20,000 words in a fully developed 25-page research plan which comprises specific aims (1 page), background and significance (3 pages), preliminary studies (6 to 8 pages), and research methods (up to 15 pages) will appear in this section. What do reviewers want to learn when they read the methods section? When I read this section, I want answers to three questions: (1) At a conceptual level, how do you propose to organize this project? (2) Why did you decide to approach the project in this manner; that is, what is the underlying concept or

Summary—Preliminary Studies

In summary, the Flagstaff medication compliance study (Preliminary project 1), the UAHSC/IRGP study (preliminary 2) and TAHEC study (preliminary 3) will provide baseline information concerning patient morbidity and medical care problems prior to implementation of physician or patient interventions, and help identify barriers to optimal care and barriers to effective education. Preliminary study 4 (Pima-Kino Community Hospital focus groups) provided information from the patients' and parents'/care providers' perspectives about issues and skills to emphasize in asthma education. These preliminary studies will help us design relevant educational programs for physicians and patients. Preliminary study 5, supported by the Southwest Asthma Foundation and UAHSC Institutional Research Grant Program, will produce questionnaires pilot tested in Spanish and English with members of the target population. Each preliminary study is directly linked to a key component of the project proposed in this application and provided our research team will valuable experience that will be used to implement our new initiative.

FIG. 16–11. Example of a wrap-up paragraph for a Preliminary Studies section.

model that is driving the design of this project? and (3) How do you plan to do the work? In regard to the third question, I want answers to classic "who, what, when, where, and how" questions and I usually develop a grid with these words as column headers and try to find the answers as I read through the methodology. Empty columns or question marks in my grid are rarely associated with a proposal that gets a positive review.

What are your goals as a grant writer when developing the Methods section? From my perspective, there are five critical goals:

1. Demonstrate that your methodology is based on a recognized, sound, and appropriate model.
   In other words, what is the underlying framework for what you propose to do? Why did you decide to conduct the project this way?

2. Communicate your conceptualization of the project's experimental design. This is your chance to share your unique insight into the problem and show the sophistication of your approach.

3. Describe how you will design experiments to accomplish each specific aim.

4. Show your depth of planning by explaining:
   - the rationale for each experiment; that is, why it is an appropriate test for the specific aim?
   - the fine grain details of how you will conduct each experiment with the level of specificity that you would find in a manuscript published in a high caliber journal

   - how you will analyze the data
   - your plans for revising the study design, if needed, during the course of implementation

5. Help reviewers link tests and analyses to hypotheses or research questions and specific aims.

All of these goals are important, but I encourage writers to particularly focus on goal number 5. One of the most common reasons I go south on a proposal is that I simply cannot decipher the research plan. All too often, Methods sections require a massive amount of re-reading, note-writing, guessing and even drawing diagrams just to determine the relationships between the research questions, specific aims, data collection measures (tests), and statistical analyses. Thus, lack of coherent organization is a frequent and often fatal flaw in the Methods sections of grant proposals. Remember the scenario of our prototypical reviewer who starts to read a grant at 10:30 at night. By the time he or she reaches the Methods section, it will be past midnight. A tired, distracted, and increasingly annoyed reviewer who is struggling through a disorganized Methods section with countless S-A-Ts and no discernible organizational structure is a formula for failure. To avoid this scenario, how should the Methods section be organized to help reviewers do their job? Box 16–5 provides the organizational structure and sequence that I recommend for this component of your proposal. As with other sections, employ a bookends structure that begins the section with a strong "big picture" overview and concludes with a "pull it all together" wrap-up.

Devote the intitial two to three pages to an overview of the entire project so reviewers will understand how the whole project "hangs together" including the rationale for your decisions about research design. Start the overview with a one-paragraph synopsis of the entire project (i.e., another mini-abstract) that reminds our sleepy reviewer of the gap, research questions, and key methodology that will be used to attack the gap. Depending on the nature of the research, it might be appropriate to graphically display, in a figure, and also describe the underlying conceptual model for the design of the study. There's more discussion of the reasons for using conceptual models later in this chapter. Next state the research questions and/or hypotheses with exactly the same words as used previously in the proposal. At this point, I recommend presenting a table that graphically displays the overall study design. Table 16–4 is an example of a study design summary table. Tables like this are invaluable to reviewers and send the message that the research team is organized and has assembled a well orchestrated plan. I prefer a four column table as displayed in Table 16–4 with the columns labeled as aims, data to be collected, measurement methods/instruments, and statistical analyses. I recommend typing

BOX 16–5

Writing Outline for Research Design & Methods Section

- Overview of project design (two to three pages)
  - One paragraph synopsis of the entire project (100- to 150-word mini-abstract)
  - Conceptual model (if appropriate, depending on study objectives and design)
  - State research questions and/or hypotheses
  - Display the study design in a table and walk the reviewer through the table with one or two paragraphs of text (see example of a study design summary table in Table 16–4)
- Describe procedures/methods to accomplish each specific aim (10 pages)

Aim	Interventions	Data to be Collected	Data Collection Instruments	Statistical Analysis
Aim 1: Type full statement of the aim	Describe protocol	Describe types of data to be collected	Name instruments & methods used to collect data	Name statistical tests
Aim 2: full text	Protocol	Data	Instruments & methods	Name statistical tests
Aim 3: full text	Protocol	Data	Instruments & methods	Name statistical tests

- Describe how your team will interpret the results. What is your decision-making process? (1/2 page)
- Provide a "limitations" section. (1/2 page)
- Provide a "wrap-up" summary at the end of the section. (1/2 page)

the full aim statement in the left-hand column, rather than relying on the reviewer to remember the wording of the aims. If your study includes an intervention such as two different types of training for experimental and control groups, I recommend creating a five-column table with an intervention, or protocol, column inserted immediately to the right of the aims column.

After the overview, the bulk of the Methods section text is devoted to guiding reviewers through the fine-grain details of how you will accomplish each of the specific aims. Write a distinct section for each of your specific aims. The key take-home message for writing this part of the Methods section is: *organize around the aims*. Your writing task is to answer the who, what, when, where, and how questions that will be in the reviewer's mind for each aim. Tell the reviewers everything they need to know about aim one, then move on to aim two and describe the protocol in detail, and then describe your plan of attack for aim three. The description of the protocol for each aim should be similar in detail to what appears in the Methods section of a

Table 16–4
Example of a Study Design Summary Table

Table 2: Summary of Study Design

Aim No. and Text	Outcomes Data to Be Collected	Measurement Methods	Methods for Statistical Analysis
Aim 1: Type full text of the aim	Provider screening, identification & intervention	Chart abstraction Patient phone interviews	Fixed-effects logistic regression Chi-square test
Aim 2	Patient, community and expert viewpoints on patient outcome measures.	Mini-conference proceedings	Conference report
Aim 3	Effects of domestic violence over time.	Instruments that measure constructs of domestic violence severity, psychological sequelae, quality of life, and correlates of well being, and health-care utilization.	Logistic or linear regression
		Semi-structured qualitative interviews.	Thematic analysis
Aim 4	Cost categories for domestic violence.	Patient self-report and data obtained from community agencies.	Descriptive analysis

paper in a high-caliber research journal. For each aim, describe the protocol including details about subject selection, inclusion and exclusion criteria, randomization (if appropriate), location of subject activities, duration, and any other implementation details that reviewers will want to know. Clearly describe all data that will be collected as outcome measures and describe how this information will be obtained by naming instruments and methods. Describe who will do the data collection and provide the when, where, and how often details. For each aim, discuss how the data will be analyzed by naming specific statistical tests and methods of analysis. Please—do not "wing it" when writing the statistical analysis component of the Methods section. If you are not a bonafide statistician and not completely confident in your skills (which covers the vast majority of people who write grants), recruit a statistican to your team and work closely with this individual when developing all phases of the Methods section, and especially the description of the analytical strategy.

After providing a complete gameplan for each aim, the remaining text in the Methods section should be devoted to three additional questions that reviewers will want answered: (1) how will your research team interpret (make sense) of the results that are obtained—that is, what is the process for making decisions about the data and what it means? (2) What are some of the limitations in your study design or potential pitfalls (problems) that may occur as you implement the protocol, and what do you plan to do if these problems emerge?; and (3) What is your timeline or workplan—what is the sequence and duration of the various activities that need to occur to complete the project? Your workplan should be displayed graphically as illustrated in Figure 16–12.

Write a full paragraph that walks reviewers through the project timeline; do not simply insert a table displaying your work plan without accompanying explanatory text. The discussion of limitations and potential pitfalls should be thorough; it's better for you to identify potential problems and discuss coping strategies than to have reviewers discover them and criticize you for not being alert to certain potential glitches in the protocol. Experienced reviewers are aware that no protocol can be perfect and that successful project management requires ongoing coping and tweaking. However, reviewers expect a candid discussion of concerns to demonstrate that you have considered all aspects of the study and have anticipated predictable pitfalls. In your discussion of limitations, be sure to identify potential sources of data contamination (for example, cross-talk among subjects in different study groups) and discuss how you will try to minimize this contamination.

The wrap-up paragraph in the Methods section should be very similar to the wrap-up paragraph in the background and significance component of your appli-

Project Activities	Pre-	Year - 1						Year - 2					
		Apr-May	Jun-Jul	Aug-Sep	Oct-Nov	Dec-Jan	Feb-Mar	Apr-May	Jun-Jul	Aug-Sep	Oct-Nov	Dec-Jan	Feb-Mar
Project Organization	▓	▓											
MD Training			▓										
Nurse Training			▓										
Staff Training													
Project Organization													
Data Collection Procedure	▓	▓											
EC Enrollment				▓	▓	▓							
EC Implementation				▓	▓								
Baseline Data				▓									
Outcome Data							▓	▓					
Data Analysis								▓		▓			
Write and Submit									▓	▓		▓	▓

FIG. 16–12. Example of a table displaying a project work plan.

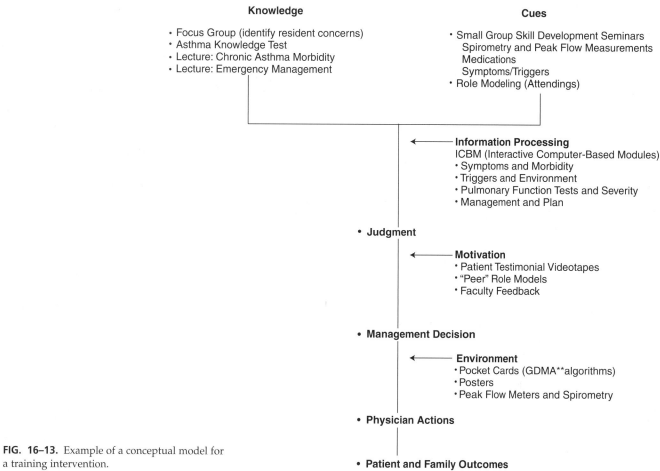

Educational Model for Physicians' Curriculum

Knowledge
- Focus Group (identify resident concerns)
- Asthma Knowledge Test
- Lecture: Chronic Asthma Morbidity
- Lecture: Emergency Management

Cues
- Small Group Skill Development Seminars
  Spirometry and Peak Flow Measurements
  Medications
  Symptoms/Triggers
- Role Modeling (Attendings)

Information Processing
ICBM (Interactive Computer-Based Modules)
- Symptoms and Morbidity
- Triggers and Environment
- Pulmonary Function Tests and Severity
- Management and Plan

• **Judgment**

Motivation
- Patient Testimonial Videotapes
- "Peer" Role Models
- Faculty Feedback

• **Management Decision**

Environment
- Pocket Cards (GDMA**algorithms)
- Posters
- Peak Flow Meters and Spirometry

• **Physician Actions**

• **Patient and Family Outcomes**

FIG. 16–13. Example of a conceptual model for a training intervention.

cation. Your goal in this paragraph is to remind the reviewer why this project is needed and emphasize what is unique about the strategy you will employ to study this research question.

CONCEPTUAL MODELS

Figure 16-13 is an example of a graphic display of a conceptual model for a grant that proposes to implement a training intervention. Why would you want to create a graphic representation like this and devote a paragraph of text to describing it? There are a number of reasons for including a model in the overview component of your Methods section. The first three reasons listed below help reviewers do their job and the last three items primarily help investigators.

- Provide a rationale or framework for the structure of your study; that is, why do you propose to conduct the project this way? In many grants that I critique, the underlying assumptions and reasoning that influenced the structuring of the project are never explained.

- Help reviewers understand the background "context" for the project that influence the implementation of the project or the results that may be obtained.

- Help reviewers understand the underlying assumptions or theories for the intervention that is proposed. For example, if the project involves efforts to change provider behaviors or provide patient education, what is the investigator's basis for selecting a particular strategy?

- Provide a classification or analysis system to categorize subject behaviors and actions.

- Provide a mechanism to interpret or explain the outcomes.

- Help explain or understand variability among subjects or treatments; that is, provide a framework to help answer the question, Why did we get these results?

BULLETPROOFING

The Methods section is a target-rich environment for reviewers who are eager to criticize. An important strategy for successful grantsmanship is to bulletproof your proposal as much as feasible before it is submitted. After you have typed what you hope is the final word in your Methods section, go back to the first paragraph and make a list of everything that reviewers could possibly criticize as you re-read your plan. Then write a one-sentence "defense" (rationale) for each of these potential criticisms. As needed, insert these bulletproofing sentences into the text to justify or defend the methods you have chosen. Reviewers often go south on proposals because they do not understand the reasoning or logic behind the investigators' decisions, not because they disagree with the methodology selected. In my experience, this bulletproofing review will also identify areas that are not well explained or employ questionable methods and these areas simply need to be changed to enhance the proposal. Experienced reviewers will expect you to explain why you did not select an alternative approach in situations where options exist. An important part of bulletproofing is to strategically insert sentences that justify why you propose to use method A versus method B or method C.

Bulletproofing also involves providing reviewers with sufficient density of detail that they can evaluate key decision points. Reviewers will expect thorough explanations of all aspects of methodology where there are decision points; for example, decisions about how often to collect data and what instruments or equipment to use. Reviewers will want to evaluate the research team's decisions in the following six areas, and therefore the narrative description of these areas should be reviewed carefully to make sure you have provided adequate information:

- Sequence, duration, frequency, and redundancy of data collection (measurements)
- Critical details for technical procedures such as exposure times, temperature, concentrations, equipment, and instruments
- Subject sampling (recruitment strategies, inclusion and exclusion criteria, number of subjects, randomization process, strategies for dealing with subject attrition)
- Statistical tests and analyses
- Data management—collection, entry, editing, storage, retrieval, access, and security
- Sequencing of project activities throughout the proposed funding period.

Subject sampling is an easy target for reviewers to attack. In particular, you will need to convince reviewers that you have adequate numbers of subjects to conduct the proposed statistical analyses. In particular, most individuals who review research grants submitted to state and federal agencies and also for the major private foundations have been well educated about the concept of "power analysis" and will keenly look for a description of the statistical methods that were used to establish the sample size requirements needed to detect statistically significant differences among study groups.[11]

One final note about support letters before leaving the Methods section. A support letter is a notice of intention to *perform a service in support of a project*. Make sure to provide support letters from all individuals who are not part of your core team but who will perform critical tasks, services, and consultations during the course of the project. For example, support letters should be obtained from administrators of clinical or laboratory facilities that you will use to implement project tasks, from supervisors of support staff, for example, research associates or laboratory technicians, who will have responsibilities in your protocol, and from consultants who will serve as advisors or perform specified tasks such as conducting training or serving as an external evaluator. Many support letters are vaguely written and are essentially cheerleading letters (e.g., "great idea, hope you get funded, glad to help if you do") that provide little meaningful information about the role and tasks to be played by the individual who wrote the letter. To avoid cheerleading letters, a more proactive strategy is to write the letter yourself and send it to the individual who will perform the service if the project is funded. Send these letters as drafts and encourage the recipients to make any revisions that are indicated, print the letter on their institutions' letterhead, sign it, and return to you. My experience is that consultants and other project support personnel rarely make changes and usually are glad that you removed a task from their "to do" list. Figure 16–14 is an example of the format for a support letter.

I recommend a three-paragraph letter. The first paragraph should read like the first "attack the gap" paragraph of the background and significance section—it should identify the problem to be addressed by this proposal, describe a key outcome, and pledge support for the project. I try to use the phrase "This project addresses a significant gap in our knowledge of (fill in the blank)" and work the word "innovative" into the text of the first paragraph. The second paragraph stipulates the specific tasks to be performed, when they will occur, and the duration or frequency of these tasks; it also indicates the nature of the compensation for these services. The writer should also alert reviewers to pertinent task-related experience in the second paragraph as demonstrated in Figure 16–14. The third paragraph is

January 6, 1999

Jane R. Green, PhD
Associate Professor
Department of Respiratory Care
The University of Wyoming Health Science Center
Laramie, Wyoming

Dear Dr. Green,

I am pleased to write this letter in support of the Multidisciplinary Project in Health Promotion and confirm my willingness to contribute to the project as described in the second paragraph. This project addresses a significant gap in our knowledge of how best to prepare health care professionals for public service: does interdisciplinary training create health professionals who are more capable and willing to work in cross-disciplinary teams? Implementation of an integrated curricular experience for students in clinical laboratory science, respiratory care, occupational therapy and physician assistant studies will make interdisciplinary primary care more than an abstract concept in the minds of the students. The evaluation plan for the project will allow us to assess impact of this approach as these individuals begin their professional careers. For these reasons, I look forward to supporting this innovative project.

PARAGRAPH 1: IDENTIFY GAP; DESCRIBE KEY OUTCOME; PLEDGE SUPPORT

Per our previous discussion, I will be pleased to contribute to this project by: (1) conducting 16 hours of seminars annually for students on patient education strategies in years 1, 2 and 3, (2) conducting an annual retreat for the steering committee and core faculty in years 1, 2 and 3 of the project and, (3) serving on the project steering committee which will meet monthly. I understand that this grant will assume 10% of my base salary for all three years in exchange for these services. I have served as the educational consultant on interdisciplinary patient and provider education grants in the areas of asthma, altered pain perception, diabetes mellitus, oral health for HIV+ patients, renal failure, rheumatoid arthritis, and substance abuse.

PARAGRAPH 2: SPECIFY TASKS & COMPENSATION; DESCRIBE EXPEREINCE

This pilot project will help faculty evaluate the implementation logistics, attitudes toward cross-disciplinary training and effect on early career job selection which will substantially increase our knowledge of interdisciplinary education strategies.

PARAGRAPH 3: DESCRIBE BENEFITS

Sincerely,

Michael Blue, PhD
Educational Specialist

CC: Fred Brown, Ph.D.
        Director, Division of Professional Development

FIG. 16–14. Example of a support letter using the three paragraph template.

essentially written for the reviewers' benefit to remind them about the critical nature of the gap, or problem, and the likely benefits of this project.

Make sure to obtain letters from individuals who will actually perform the designated services and from administrators who actually have control over facilities, personnel, and equipment. If you will serve as the principal investigator/project manager, your immediate supervisor should also contribute a support letter that generally follows the format outlined above, but in the middle paragraph pledges to allow you the "protected" time (e.g., 30 percent time for 2 years) for the project activities indicated in the proposal and in the budget

request. As we will discuss in the following section on budget issues, one of the biggest reviewer red flags is concern that the PI will not have enough protected time to accomplish project tasks and manage the project.

In conclusion, the Methods section of the grant application is the final component of the research plan, which for NIH and many other organizations that emulate the PHS 398 application format consists of the specific aims page (may be called project objectives), background and significance, preliminary studies, and the research methodology. Box 16–6 summarizes questions that reviewers want answered in each component of the research plan and indicates key writing strategies.

BOX 16-6

Summary of Questions to be Answered and Writing Strategies for Components of the Research Plan Based on PHS 398 Format Used by NIH

A. Specific Aims: What do you intend to do? (1 page)
1. Start with one paragraph summary of the overall study; purpose, methods, expected outcomes
2. Depending on study design, state the research questions to be answered OR the hypotheses to be tested
3. State 3–4 specific aims that describe what are you going to do to produce data that will answer the research question or test the hypothesis

B. Background & Significance: Why is this work important? (2–3 pages)
1. Convince reviewers of project need and value:
   - Define the knowledge gap you will address in this project (Attack The Gap)
   - Build a convincing case for why this gap is important to study
   - Describe a compelling benefit: What will a better understanding of this knowledge gap allow us to do in the future?
2. Summarize theory and research outcomes leading to the present proposal
3. Discuss the work of other investigators even-handedly, acknowledging important contributions that paved the way for your proposed investigation, and clearly identifying limitations in the knowledge base that represent unknowns or which have not been explored adequately

C. Preliminary Studies: What has already been done by your research team? (6–8 pages)
1. Describe projects your team has completed that are directly related to this study and which set the stage (e.g., are logical preliminary steps) for this current proposal.
   - Describe your published findings. Do not just append copies of articles.
   - Graphically display key preliminary data, but also explain these data in the narrative.

D. Research Design and Methods: How are you going to do the work? (up to 15 pages)
1. Begin the methods section with a project overview. Help the reviewer understand your overall approach by explaining the research questions and the design of your study.
2. Provide a table that graphically displays the overall study design.
3. If appropriate, describe and visualize the conceptual model that communicates the underlying logic of how you organized the research study
4. Use the specific aims as the organizing structure for the remainder of the method section; organize information about each aim as displayed below

Aim	Interventions	Data to be Collected	Instruments	Statistical Analysis
Type full text of each aim	Describe protocol for each aim	Describe types of data to be collected	Name methods & instruments to collect data	Name statistical tests

RED FLAGS—METHODS SECTION
(NO = RED FLAG!)

- Does the methods section begin with a "big picture" overview and conclude with a "pull it all together" wrap-up paragraph?   YES   NO
- Is a model proposed to serve as the framework (logic) for the project?   YES   NO
- Is the overall study design displayed in a table?   YES   NO
- Are aims, methods, data collection, and analysis linked together?   YES   NO
- Are key decision points explained and justified with adequate detail?   YES   NO

- Is a timeline presented and discussed? Does it appear to be realistic?   YES   NO
- Are alternative study designs discussed?   YES   NO
- Are potential limitations and sources of data contamination acknowledged and coping strategies proposed?   YES   NO

Writing the Budget Justification

The art and science of writing budget requests is a grantsmanship skill of its own; a detailed exploration of the many facets of budget planning is beyond the scope of this chapter. Research activity is intertwined with governmental and institutional regulations that influence distribution of awards within institutions. At many health science centers, the manuals explaining the rules and regulations that govern the allocation of direct (the money you get) and indirect (i.e., the money your institution gets for overhead, now known as F&A, or Facilities and Administrative Costs) are hundreds of pages long. The fine-grain details of what budget items are allowable, or not, and under what conditions for state and federal grants are seemingly endless. Many of the textbooks on grant writing and grantsmanship listed at the end of the chapter provide in-depth discussion of financial and project management issues including do and don't examples. Reif-Lehrer[7] has useful recommendations for budgeting strategies as do Carlson, Collins and Tremore, and Smith in the general resource list. This section is designed to alert you to a group of universal principles that apply to the budgets of all grants whether the source of funding is a small local philanthropic foundation, a state agency, a major nonprofit organization, or the NIH, and to demonstrate a template that can be used to write clear, compelling, and convincing justifications for personnel on your project.

The planning and level of detail evident in your budget and the supporting narrative justification communicates much to reviewers about how you are likely to manage the project. Here are seven suggestions. (1) "Size" your budget request appropriately. As discussed earlier in the chapter, do your homework and determine the range of financial awards, average award, and typical project duration for the funding agency that you plan to approach. If the organization's typical award is $50,000 for 2 years, don't request $180,000 for 3 years. This guideline particularly applies to foundations, but in reality most of the federal agencies also have publicized award ranges for various types of grants or the size of the grant is predetermined as in the case of RFAs. (2) For a research grant, create your overall budget by assembling the individual budgets needed to accomplish each specific aim. Everything you will need to accomplish the aim should be accounted for in the budget request: staff members' salaries, equipment purchase, lease and repair, facility rentals, maintenance and warranties, consumable supplies, communication costs, data management costs, transportation costs, stipends for patients, and on and on. (3) Follow the budget directions for the funding agency precisely. If in doubt, place phone calls to determine answers rather than guessing. (4) Justify everything. Do not assume that any expense item will be obvious to reviewers. (5) Do not create a bargain (low bid) budget in the hopes that a funding agency will award you financial support because "you are giving them a lot for a little." Experienced reviewers and grants program managers will be skeptical of the low-bid approach because they know that a common reason for project failure is trying to do too much for too little. (6) Have everything checked well in advance of the deadline submission date by your institutions' grants management office if you have such an organization at your institution and/or by the accounting manager in your department. (7) Create two budgets. Budget A is your "wish list" support request that is submitted with the application. Budget A reflects your best estimate of the financial resources needed to conduct the project in an ideal situation. B is your "we can live with this" budget. Budget B designates items that are negotiable and items that are essential. Some degree of budget negotiations occur after the award notification is received and investigators fare better during budget "whacking" if they know in advance what they are willing to eliminate without compromising project viability. Investigators can be caught off guard when they receive an unexpected phone call from a grants program manager who says: *Good news— XYZ Foundation has approved your project for funding; congratulations! .... But ... we would like to reduce your budget by 15 percent so we can fund one more deserving project.*

Here are a few tips for standard budget items:

Personnel: At the level of NIH, major foundations, and state agencies, designating less than 30 percent time for the principal investigator will raise concern that the PI will be overextended with other responsibilities and not have adequate time to attend to the day-to-day details of the project. For major projects with substantial budgets, funding agencies may expect PI to devote at least fifty percent of their time to directing the project, particularly if the investigator is relatively inexperienced.

Equipment and supplies: Avoid requests for deluxe models of equipment (i.e., requesting funds for a Mercedes SUV when a Ford Explorer will probably be adequate). Justifications for deluxe items truly need to be clear, compelling, and convincing. Don't guess; obtain bids from vendors that indicate exact prices and quote these bids in your budget justifications. Don't frontload your budget request by requesting equipment and supplies (and personnel too) in year one that won't be needed until year three. Frontloading leads reviewers to suspect that this equipment may be used for purposes other than activities associated with the grant.

Travel: At the state and federal level, do not exceed the allowable per trip expenditures and the total number of trips per fiscal year that are stated in budget directions. These guidelines change from time to time, so—don't guess or assume. Carefully justify all travel requests and in general, be parsimonious in requesting travel, especially for personnel who are not key contributors.

Renovation of facilities: In general—don't bother requesting funds for remodeling or construction of physical space.

Consultants: Clearly justify each consultant's role, tasks to be performed, time commitment, and compensation. Do not list several "big name" consultants in your budget who have ill-defined roles or vague tasks. Reviewers at all levels are sensitive to the padding strategy, which is enhancing the apparent star power of your research team by listing several "RFPs" (i.e., really famous people) as either coinvestigators or consultants but who have token involvement in the project.

Co-investigators: The same guidelines apply for coinvestigators as for consultants. Each coinvestigator should be a participant because of a clear need for that individual's expertise and experience. However, coinvestigators who are listed on the budget page as nonsalaried contributors make me nervous. What control or accountability will exist in this situation? The time commitment for a coinvestigator needs to be commensurate with that person's assigned tasks. An individual listed at 10 percent time for the project (i.e., 4 hours per week) but who is responsible for several major project activities is not likely to be successful in accomplishing these tasks unless sacrifices are made in other areas of responsibility that may not be appreciated by other administrators in the organization.

Writing Justifications for Project Personnel

At some point during the critique of grant applications, all reviewers will ask themselves this question: Does the team assembled for this project have the individual and collective expertise and experience to be successful? For me, this question is often critical if I am "on the fence" about the overall merits of the proposal. One way to win over wavering reviewers or to "seal the deal" if a reviewer is looking for one final reason to give a good rating to an application is to write informative and convincing justifications for key project personnel. As mentioned earlier, grant writers often fail to communicate the strengths of the team members when preparing the narrative justification that accompanies the budget request. The template below provides a guide for writing personnel justifications that gives reviewers the information they need to understand an individual's role on the grant and his/her qualifications and experience. Using this template is another way to help reviewers do their job which in this case is to assess the capacity of the project team for the proposed work. Figure 16–15 is an example of a personnel justification that was prepared using this template. As demonstrated in this example, at least half the text should be devoted to key tasks, supervision responsibilities, pertinent training, and prior work experiences.

- List name, degree, current title (e.g., Sandra Black, PhD; Associate Professor, Bioinformatics).
- Identify department, school, university.
- Indicate the percentage of time that will be devoted to the proposed project.
- Identify job title on this project (e.g., Director—Data Management).
- Describe key tasks this person will perform.
- Identify any supervision responsibilities that this person will have on the grant.
- Describe pertinent training and prior work experiences.

One note of caution when describing personnel in grant applications. It can be confusing and annoying to reviewers if the grant writer fails to use exactly the same job titles for project staff when their roles and assignments are described at various points in the proposal. I recently read an application where a single person was variously described as the clinical nurse specialist, research nurse, research coordinator, nursing research manager, and project coordinator. In fact, all of their references were to a single individual who was listed as

---

Archie Dennis, PhD, MPH is a Senior Associate in the Center for Health Professions Education at the UAHSC and is an associate professor at the University of Arizona School of Educational Policy and Research. He will devote 10% of his time as co-investigator and physician education coordinator. He will play a major role in the development and evaluation of the physician education component, including the computer-based asthma knowledge pre/post-tests and ICBMs, and also assist with the patient education component, assuming major responsibility for design and production of the videotapes. Dr. Dennis will supervise the 50% time educational media specialist who will do software programming for the computer-based tests and patient management simulations in the physician education intervention. Dr. Dennis earned his PhD from Yankton State University in 1971. He has been a medical education specialist at the University of Washington Medical School (1971–76), the University of Tennessee Medical School (1976–85) and at UAHSC since 1986 and has served as a consultant to more than 100 universities. He has directed bilingual patient education programs for the American Dietetic Association, the American Heart Association and the Tennessee Kidney Foundation.

FIG. 16–15. Example of a personnel justification.

the project manager (yet another title) on the budget page. Prior to writing the proposal, it's a good idea to make a list of all the players in the project and designate one clear title for each person that is used every time that individual's role is mentioned.

There are billions of dollars available to support your projects; your job as a grant writer is to communicate the story of your project with clear, compelling, and convincing language. If you do this, you will help reviewers do their job and ultimately, with persistence, I am confident your grant writing efforts will be successful. Remember, there are two ways to make sure you do not get a grant funded: one, never submit the grant, and two, don't resubmit the grant if at first you are not successful. **GOOD LUCK!**

Resources on Writing Grant Applications

Web Resource on Proposal Writing

The Foundation Center's Proposal Writing Short Course.
http://fdncenter.org/learn/shortcourse/prop1.html
Examples of completed grant proposals from the Foundation Center.
http://fdncenter.org/learn/faqs/html/propsample.html

Books

Barbato J, Furlich D. Writing for a Good Cause: The Complete Guide to Crafting Proposals and Other Persuasive Pieces for Nonprofits. New York: Simon & Schuster, 2000.

Bauer D. The Teacher's Guide to Winning Grants. San Francisco: Jossey-Bass, 1999.

Brewer E. Finding Funding: Grantwriting and Project Management from Start to Finish. Thousand Oaks, CA: Corwin Press, 1995

Brown L, Brown M. Demystifying Grant Seeking: What You Really Need To Do To Get Grants. San Francisco: Jossey-Bass, 2001.

Browning B. Grant Writing for Dummies. New York: Hungry Minds, 2001.

Carlson M. Winning Grants Step by Step: The Complete Workbook for Planning, Developing, and Writing Successful Proposals, 2nd ed. San Francisco: Jossey-Bass, 2002.

Collins S (ed). The Foundation Center's Guide to Winning Proposals. New York: Foundation Center, 2003.

Fey D. The Complete Book of Fund-Raising Writing. Rosemont, NJ: Morris-Lee, 1995

Gitlin L. Successful Grant Writing: Strategies for Health and Human Service Professionals. New York: Springer, 1996.

Karsh E, Fox A. The Only Grant-Writing Book You'll Ever Need. New York: Carrol & Graf, 2003.

Knowles C. First-Time Grantwriter's Guide to Success. Thousand Oaks, CA: Corwin Press, 2002

New C, Quick J. Grantseeker's Toolkit: A Comprehensive Guide to Finding Funding New York: John Wiley. 1998.

Ramsey L, Hale PD. Winning Federal Grants: A Guide to the Government's Grant-Making Process. Alexandria, VA: Capitol, 1994.

Tremore J, Smith N. The Everything Grant Writing Book. Avon, MA: Adams, 2003.

References

1. Orientation Handbook for Members of Scientific Review Groups. National Institutes of Health, 1992.
2. Miner LE, Miner JT. Proposal Planning and Writing. Westport, CT: Greenwood Press, 2003.
3. Reif-Lehrer L. *Grant Application Writer's Handbook,* 2nd ed. Boston: Jones and Bartlett, 1995.
4. Cuca JM, McLoughlin WJ. Why clinical research grant applications fare poorly in review and how to recover. Cancer Investigation 1987;5(1):55–58.
5. Schwartz SM, Friedman ME. A Guide to NIH Grant Programs. New York: Oxford University Press, 1992.
6. Rush AJ, Gullion CM, Prein RF. A curbstone consult to applicants for National Institute of Mental Health grant support. Psychopharmacology Bulletin 1996;32(3):311–320.
7. Reif-Lehrer L. Grant Application Writer's Handbook, 4th ed. National Book Network. 2004.
8. Bauer D. The "How To" Grants Manual: Successful Grantseeking Techniques for Obtaining Public and Private Grants, 4th ed. Phoenix: Oryx Press, 1999.
9. Ogden TE, Goldberg IA. *Research Proposals—A Guide to Success,* 2nd ed. New York: Raven Press, 1995.
10. Read P. Foundation Fundamentals: A Guide for Grantseekers, 3rd ed. New York: The Foundation Center, 1994.
11. Sackett DL. Evidence Based Medicine. How to Practice and Teach EBM, 2nd ed. Edinburgh: Churchill Livingstone, 2000.
12. Lipsey MW. Design Sensitivity: Statistical Power for Experimental Design. Newbury Park, CA: Sage, 1990.

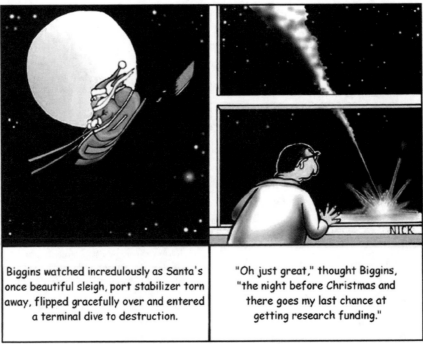

Reprinted by permission of Nick D. Kim.

Appendix

Paper Format

Theses and dissertations have a generally accepted format that is different from the format that most journals want their submissions to follow. A thesis or dissertation is an original piece of work that contributes to our fund of knowledge. Theses and dissertations are formal academic written presentations of a scientific endeavor. They are the hallmarks and capstones of a prescribed academic curriculum. Typically in the United States, a thesis is a part of research-based master's degree education. A dissertation is the culmination of a research-based doctoral degree education. The philosophical difference between a master's and a doctoral education is the expectation that doctoral education should result in a work that is more complex and innovative in its contribution to our knowledge.

Although there is some variability in format and requirements among colleges and universities, the format presented below, probably, would be acceptable by most. Every graduate school will have a preferred format for theses and dissertations. Requirements for the format will be published in the institution's student materials. Likewise, there is usually a preferred style manual, and often it is the required style manual. Guidelines may be available online and, in some instances, a template may be available for downloading. Style manuals may also offer formats for theses and dissertations.

A General Outline for a Thesis or Dissertation

1. Title Page or Front Page
   a. Title, Author
   b. School, Institution
   c. Required wording
   d. May include signature lines for committee or be followed by signature page
2. Dedication or Acknowledgments (or both), but not required or necessary
   a. Dedication—honor someone special to the author
   b. Acknowledgments—Recognition of people who have provided support or input. By tradition, thesis/dissertation committee members and the major advisor are acknowledged for their contributions.
3. Table of Contents
   a. Should include beginning page number for all chapters, sections, and subchapters or subsections.
   b. Should include pages with a list of tables and a list of figures.
      i. These items should be a table of contents for tables and figures
4. Abstract
   a. A brief summary or description of the work. Guidelines are available in the literature, but many institutions will have their own.
   b. In some formats, the abstract may be located elsewhere in the work, rather than at the beginning. Again, check local requirements.

Typically there are five chapters in the work (but there is variability) with multiple subsections. Below is an example from the author's experience.

5. Chapter 1: Introduction
   a. The problem or statement of the problem
   b. Need for the study
   c. Purpose of the study
   d. Research hypotheses, null hypotheses, or research questions
   e. Limitations of the study
   f. Definition of terms
6. Chapter 2: Review of Related Literature (or Literature Review)
   a. A review of what is known about the problem studied
      i. Should be as complete as possible.
      ii. Reference heavy
7. Chapter 3: Methods and Procedures (or Methodology)
   a. Introduction
   b. Design of the study
   c. Population or sample of the study
   d. Experimental procedures or instruments
   e. Process of statistical and data analysis
   f. Limitations of the methodology

8. Chapter 4: Results
   a. Presentation of the data
9. Chapter 5: Discussion
   a. Summary, conclusions, interpretations
   b. Implications
   c. Recommendations
   d. Closing
10. References
    a. Follow specified guidelines or format in required style manual.
11. Appendices
    a. Used to provide materials germane to the investigation
       I. survey instruments, letters, and so forth.

A General Outline for a Manuscript to Be Submitted for Publication (See Chapter 13)

Every journal has guidelines for manuscripts. Be familiar with and follow these guidelines explicitly. Typically, theses and dissertations are too long for most journals, so that format is rarely acceptable. As a general rule, a journal wants a manuscript to be concise and to the point. Some journals may have limits on the length of manuscripts or, at least, recommended length. The exact format for a paper depends on the type of paper being submitted; original research, clinical review, case study, and so forth. A general outline follows.

1. Title Page
   a. Title of manuscript
   b. Author(s)
   c. Titles and Affiliations
   d. Address(es)
   e. Contact person
2. Abstract
   a. There may be a prescribed format.
3. Introduction
   a. Statement of problem(s)
   b. Review of literature
4. Methodology
5. Results (may not be needed for some types of papers)
6. Discussion, Summary, Conclusion (may be the major component)
7. References

In some types of papers, methodology and results may be a single section. Every journal will have requirements for tables, figures, and photographs.

Glossary

absolute value   The value of a number regardless of its sign.

abstract   The summary of a study in clear and concise terms. Usually limited to 100 to 300 words.

abstract thinking   Thinking oriented toward the development of an idea without application to, or association with, a particular instance, independent of time and space. Abstract thinkers tend to look for meaning, patterns, relationships, and philosophical implications.

accessible population   Portion of the target population or group to which the researcher has reasonable access.

accidental sampling   A method of sampling in which subjects are included in the study because they happen to be in the right place at the right time. One method of obtaining subjects for a study is to enter all available subjects coming into a room until the desired sample size is reached (also known as convenience sampling).

accuracy   The extent to which a scale correctly represents the amount or classification of a variable.

across-method triangulation   Combining research methods or strategies from two or more research traditions in the same study.

adverse effect   An undesirable and unintended, although not necessarily unexpected, result of therapy or other intervention.

alpha (α)   Level of significance or cutoff point used to determine whether the samples being tested are members of the same population or of different populations. Alpha is commonly set at .05, .01, or .001.

analysis of covariance (ANCOVA)   A method of removing pretreatment variations (as measured by the control variable) from the post-treatment means (criterion variable) before testing the significance of the post-treatment differences among the groups. Analysis of covariance provides a basis for ruling out pretreatment differences when the interest is in testing post-treatment differences.

analysis of variance (ANOVA)   A statistical method that tests the difference between two or more means when studying groups. Independent variables are nominal (categorical) and dependent variables are interval values. Asks whether the squared variation of the case scores around their treatment means (within)

is greater than the squared variation of the means themselves around the grand mean (between). These two totals are expressed as a ratio. Comparison of variances reflects different sources of variability (i.e., within vs. between).

analysis of variance, one-way (See ANOVA)   Only one independent variable is manipulated.

anonymity   Condition in which subjects' identities cannot be linked to their individual responses.

a posteriori   By observation of facts or results (literally, "after").

applied research   Research designed to answer practical questions.

a priori   By reasoning from self-evident facts (literally, "before").

area probability sample   A form of multistage cluster sample in which geographical areas, such as census blocks or tracts, serve as the first-stage sampling unit. Units selected in the first stage of sampling (e.g., all the households on a selected block) are listed, and such lists would be subsampled.

assent   Agreement by an individual not competent to give legally valid informed consent (e.g., a child) to participate in research.

assignment   Method of placing of subjects in study groups that can be random, matched, stratified, and so forth.

associated keywords   A set of words used as identifiers of the topic area.

associative relationship   A connection among variables or concepts that exist together in the real world so that when one variable changes, the other variable also changes.

assumptions   Statements taken for granted or considered true, even though they have not been scientifically tested.

attributes   Characteristics of persons or things (e.g., age, eye color).

attrition   The loss of participants during the course of a study. Attrition can introduce bias by changing the composition of the sample initially drawn, particularly if more subjects are lost from one group than another.

autonomy   Personal capacity to consider alternatives, make choices, and act without undue influence or interference of others.

average   An ambiguous term generally suggesting typical or normal. The mean, median, and mode are specific examples of mathematical averages.

baseline measure   The measurement of the dependent variable before the introduction of an experimental intervention.

basic research   Discovery research that seeks to add knowledge or to support or refute theories.

beneficence   The principle that one should do good and, above all, do no harm.

benefit–risk ratio   The proportion of potential benefits compared to potential risks of an intervention, weighed to determine whether it is ethical.

beta (β) coefficient   Standardized regression coefficient that allows comparison of relative importance of variables in regression analysis.

bias   That quality of a measurement device that tends to result in a misrepresentation of what is being measured in a particular direction. For example, the questionnaire item, "Don't you agree that your physician is doing a good job?" is biased because it encourages favorable responses.

bibliography   A list of source materials or references that are used or consulted in the preparation of a work. The references of the bibliography are usually cited in the text.

binary or binomial variable   A variable with only two attributes (e.g., sex, with the attributes male and female). Also called a dichotomous variable.

bivariate analysis   The analysis of two variables simultaneously to determine the empirical relationship between them. The construction of a simple percentage table or the computation of a simple correlation coefficient would be examples.

bivariate correlation   Analysis technique that measures the extent of the linear relationship between two variables.

boolean logic   Refers to the logical relationship among search terms. It consists of three logical operators; OR, AND, NOT.

box-and-whisker plot   Exploratory data analysis technique to visualize some of the major characteristics of complex data. Sometimes used to display spread, symmetry, and outliers at the same time in a graph.

bracketing   Qualitative research technique of suspending or laying aside what is known about an experience being studied.

canonical correlation   Extension of multiple regression with more than one dependent variable.

case study design   Intensive exploration of a single unit of study, such as a person, family, group, community, or institution.

causal relationship   Relationship between two variables in which one variable (independent variable) is thought to cause or determine the presence of the other variable (dependent variable). Three criteria must be satisfied: (1) the cause precedes the effect in time, (2) the two variables are empirically correlated with one another, and (3) the observed correlation between the two variables cannot be explained away as being the result of the influence of some third variable that causes both of them.

cell   The box created by the intersection of column and row in a table or matrix. The cell is where the number or information is inserted.

census   An enumeration of the characteristics of some population. A census collects data from all members of the population, in contrast to a survey, which is limited to a sample.

central limit theorem   A theorem stating that even when statistics, such as means, come from a population with a skewed (asymmetrical) distribution, the sampling distribution developed from multiple means obtained from that skewed population tends to fit the pattern of the normal curve.

central tendency   A statistical index of a typical set of scores that comes from the center of the distribution of scores. The three most common indices of central tendency are the mean, median, and mode.

chi square (X^2)   A test to assess whether observed frequencies of nominal data differ from expected frequencies. A nonsignificant value indicates the classes are independent. A significant value indicates an association. Range is zero to infinity.

chronology   A type of unstructured and sequential observation that provides a detailed description of a person's or population's behavior.

citation   The reference to an authority or author of a document.

clinical trial   A prospective study comparing an intervention to a control involving human subjects.

cluster sample   A multistage sample in which natural groups (clusters) are sampled initially, with the members of each selected group being subsampled afterward. For example, select a sample of clinics, and then draw a sample of patients from each.

code book   A document used in data processing and analysis that tells the location of different data items in a data file and the meanings of the codes used to represent different attributes of variables. Often a notebook, this document lists all methods used so someone else could duplicate the work.

coding The process of transforming qualitative data into numerical symbols. Often done for computer input prior to analysis.

coercion To compel someone by threat of harm or excessive reward to do something they would not ordinarily undertake (e.g., obtaining participants for dangerous research projects by offering large sums of money).

cohort study A study in which some specific group is studied over time, although data may be collected from different members in each set of observations (e.g., a study of the clinical practice of physician assistants who graduated in 1976, in which questionnaires were sent every 5 years).

comparative descriptive design Used to describe differences in variables in two or more groups in a natural setting.

comparison group Commonly known as the "control group," a group not receiving a treatment, reward, or intervention.

compatibility The degree to which the innovation is perceived to be consistent with current values, past experience, and priority of needs.

complete observer The passive researcher with no direct social interaction in the setting.

complete participation When the researcher becomes a member of the group and conceals the researcher role.

concept A term that abstractly describes and names an object or phenomenon, thus providing it with a separate identity or meaning.

conceptual definition A definition that provides a variable or concept with a theoretical meaning and is established through concept analysis.

conceptual framework A set of highly abstract, related constructs that broadly explains phenomena of interest, expresses assumptions, and reflects a philosophical stance.

conclusions Opinion or interpretation of the results or meaning of a study.

confidence interval The range of values within which a population parameter is estimated to lie.

confidence level The estimated probability that a population parameter lies within a given confidence interval.

confidentiality Management of data in research so subjects' identities are not linked with their responses. This differs from anonymity, in which the subjects' identities are not known.

confounding variable An uncontrolled variable that may compete with a manipulated variable for interpretive priority. Makes a clear interpretation of the results of a study difficult or impossible.

consent form A form used to document a subject's agreement to participate in a study.

constant comparison Iterative method of content analysis where each category is searched through the entire data set and all instances are compared until no new categories can be identified.

construct (pronounced with emphasis on first syllable) An image, idea, or theory that has some general meaning not directly observable.

construct validity The degree to which a measure relates to other variables as expected within a system of theoretical relationships. In other words, construct validity is based on the logical relationship among variables (e.g., patients who report they are satisfied with their physician assistant are more likely to comply with treatment).

content analysis Systematic examination of text (field notes) by identifying and grouping themes and coding, classifying and developing categories.

content validity The extent to which the method of measurement includes all the major elements relevant to the construct being measured.

contingency tables Cross-tabulation tables that allow visual comparison of summary data output related to two variables within a sample.

control Rules imposed by the researcher to decrease the possibility of error and increase the probability that the study's findings are an accurate reflection of reality.

control group A group of subjects to whom no experimental stimulus, treatment, or intervention is administered and who should resemble the experimental group in all other respects (also known as comparison group).

convenience sampling Simply entering available subjects into the study until the desired sample size is reached (also known as accidental sampling).

copy editor The person who makes corrections on a manuscript to achieve consistency in style, word usage, and spelling, following the appropriate publication guidelines.

correlation Consistent relationship between two variables such that one variable can be predicted from knowledge of the other. With a positive correlation, both variables increase together; that is a positive value increase. Positive does not mean good, beneficial, advantageous, or better. With a negative correlation, one increases when the other decreases or one variable is high and the other is low. Negative does not mean bad, adverse, worse, or least.

correlation analysis   Statistical procedure conducted to determine the direction (positive or negative) and magnitude (strength) of the relationship between two variables.

correlation coefficient (*r*)   A statistic that shows the degree of relationship between two or more variables.

correlation matrix   A table showing the correlation coefficients of sets of variables.

correlational research   Systematic investigation of relationships between two or more variables to explain the nature of relationships in the world and not to examine cause and effect.

cost–benefit analysis   Economic technique that examines costs and benefits of alternative ways of using resources to determine which way produces the greatest net benefit, assessed in monetary terms.

cost-effectiveness analysis   Type of outcomes research that compares costs and benefits of different ways of accomplishing a clinical goal (e.g., diagnosing a condition, treating an illness, or providing a service). The goal is to identify the strategy that achieves the desired result for the least cost.

covariate analysis   See analysis of covariance.

covert data collection   Collection of research data without the subjects being aware that data are being collected.

critical analysis of studies   Minute examination of the merits, faults, meaning, and significance of studies.

crossover design   Experimental design in which more than one type of treatment is administered to each subject; the treatments are provided sequentially, rather than concurrently, and comparisons are made of the effects of the different treatments on the same subject.

cross-sectional study   A study that is based on observations representing a single point in time. Contrasted with a longitudinal study, which is based on two or more observations over time.

cross-tabulation   A determination of the number of cases occurring when simultaneous consideration is given to the values of two or more variables, such as sex (male/female) cross-tabulated with smoking status (smoker/nonsmoker). The results are presented in a table format according to the values of the variables.

data   The reports of observations of variables.

data coding sheet   A form for organizing and recording data for rapid entry into a computer.

data collection   Precise, systematic gathering of information relevant to the research purpose or the specific objectives, questions, or hypotheses of a study.

data entry   The process of entering data (usually in coded form) onto an input medium for computer analysis.

data triangulation   Collection of data from multiple sources in the same study.

deception   Misinforming subjects for research purposes.

decision theory   Theory that is inductive in nature and is based on assumptions associated with the theoretical normal curve. The theory is applied when testing for differences among groups with the expectation that all of the groups are members of the same population.

deduction   The logical model in which specific expectations of hypotheses are developed on the basis of general principles.

deductive research   Moving from prior hypotheses to observation or empirical research; other than discovery research.

degrees of freedom (df)   Number of values that can vary independently, usually one less than the total number of values or variables.

Delphi technique   A method of measuring the judgments of a group of experts for assessing priorities or making forecasts.

demographic variables   Characteristics or attributes of the subjects that are collected to describe the sample.

dependent variable   A phenomenon that is affected by the researcher's manipulation of an independent variable.

description   The precise measurement and reporting of the characteristics of a population or phenomenon under study.

descriptive correlational design   Used to describe variables and examine relationships that exist in a situation.

descriptive method   A research plan undertaken to define the characteristics, relationships, or both, of variables, based on systematic observation of these variables.

descriptive statistics   Calculated values that represent certain overall characteristics of a body of data.

design   Blueprint for conducting a study that maximizes control over factors that could interfere with the validity of the findings.

diary Written record of a subject's observations and feelings, which is collected by the researcher for analysis.

dichotomous variable A variable that places subjects into two groups (e.g., male/female).

directional hypothesis A hypothesis that states the specific nature of the interaction or relationship between two or more variables.

discriminant analysis A form of regression analysis used to place a variable in a category.

dispersion The distribution of values around some central value, such as an average. The range is a simple example of a measure of dispersion.

disproportionate stratified sampling A sampling strategy in which the researcher samples different proportions of subjects from different strata in the population to endure adequate representation of subjects from strata that are comparatively smaller.

distribution A collection of measurements usually viewed in terms of the frequency with which observations are assigned to each category or point on a measurement scale.

double-blind experiment An experiment in which neither the subjects nor those who administer the treatment know who is in the experimental group or control group.

ecological fallacy Erroneously drawing conclusions about individuals based solely on the observation of groups.

editor The person in charge of a research publication, who decides which articles are to be published, manages the overall production of the publication, and heads the editorial staff.

effect size A statistical expression of the magnitude of the difference between two variables, or the magnitude of the difference between two groups, with regard to some attribute of interest.

Eigen value The variance explained by each factor, a product of factor analysis. Each factor has a possible total of 1.0, so Eigen values cannot exceed the number of factors. The Eigen value shows the relative importance of each factor by the amount of covariance of variables associated with the underlying (unobserved) common factor (which tends to be the most important factor).

emic view A term used in anthropology meaning "inside view" as opposed to etic view meaning "outside view."

empirical generalizations Statements that have been repeatedly tested through research and have not been disproved.

empiricism The philosophical doctrine that all knowledge is derived from sense experience.

epistemology The science of knowing; a branch of philosophy that investigates the origin, nature, methods, and limits of human knowledge.

equivalence Type of reliability testing that involves comparing two versions of the same instrument or two observers measuring the same event.

ethical inquiry Intellectual analysis of ethical problems related to obligation, rights, duty, right and wrong, conscience, choice, intention, and responsibility to obtain desirable, rational ends.

ethical principles Principles of respect for persons, beneficence, and justice relevant to the conduct of research.

ethics The values or guidelines that should govern decisions in research or medicine. The social obligation the researcher has to his or her subjects.

ethnographic research A qualitative research methodology for investigating cultures. This method involves collecting, describing, and analyzing the data to develop a theory of cultural behavior.

etic view A term used in anthropology meaning "outside view" as opposed to emic view meaning "inside view."

evaluation research Has as its objective the description and evaluation of some existing social policy or program (oriented toward program research). Differs from applied and basic research.

exclusion criteria Sampling requirements identified by the researcher that eliminate or exclude an element or subject from being in a sample.

expedited review Review of proposed research by the IRB chair or a designated voting member or group of voting members rather than by the entire IRB. Federal rules permit expedited review for certain kinds of research involving no more than minimal risk and for minor changes in approved research.

experimental group The subjects who are exposed to an experimental treatment or intervention.

experimental method A research plan undertaken to test relationships among variables based on systematic observation of variables that are manipulated by the researcher.

experimenter effects A source of bias in experimental research in which subjects react to personal attributes of the experimenter or pick up cues about what the experimenter is seeking and modify their behavior accordingly.

exploratory factor analysis A method of analysis in which the variance of the first factor is completed and removed from influence before analysis is begun on a second factor. It is performed when the researcher has few previous expectations about the factor structure.

external validity   The degree to which the results of a study generalize to the population. The process of testing the validity of a measure, such as an index or scale, is conducted by examining its relationship to other, presumed indicators of the same variable.

extraneous variables   Variables which exist in all studies that the investigator cannot control and is not studying. They can affect the measurement of study variables and the relationships among these variables.

F   Designation letter for the value derived from an "*F* test."

F **ratio**   A statistical value used in analysis of variance and other statistical methods.

F **table**   A table of values that represent the percentage points of the "*F*" distribution.

F **test**   A test for comparing two or more means: the ratio of variance between groups divided by the variance within groups (error). As the number of observations in each sample (*n*) increases, the critical value of *F* increases; smaller differences between the variances of the samples become significant because variations tend to level out as the proportion of the population sampled increases.

factor   The independent variable in single-variable studies. Most commonly used to describe groups of related independent variables within a larger group of variables.

factor analysis   A complex computerized method for determining the general dimensions or factors that exist within a set of concrete observations.

fatigue effect   When a subject becomes tired or bored with a study.

feasibility study   A study of whether a research project can or should be carried out, as determined by examining the time and money commitment; the researcher's expertise; the availability of subjects, facilities, and equipment; the cooperation of others; and ethical considerations.

field notes   Term used for records of observation, interview transcription, document sources.

field research   A form of research that consists of observations made in nature (the field) that are often not easily reduced to numbers.

findings   The translated and interpreted results of a study.

focus group interview   An interview in which the respondents are a group of individuals with some trait in common who are assembled to answer questions on a given topic in order to generate data.

forced choice   Response set using a scale that has an even number of choices, such as four or six, so that respondents cannot choose an uncertain or neutral response.

frequency distribution   A description of the number of times the various attributes of a variable are observed in a sample.

frequency polygon   Graphic display of a frequency distribution, in which dots connected by a line indicate the number of times a score value occurs in a set of data.

generalizability   The quality of a research finding that justifies the inference that it represents something more than the specific observations on which it was based. Sometimes this involves the generalization of findings from a sample to a population. Other times, it is a matter of concepts: If you are able to discover why patients consume alcohol, can you generalize that discovery to other substance abuses?

gestalt   A psychological theory that the objects of mind are really clusters of linked ideas that cannot be split up into parts. A system of phenomena having properties that cannot be derived solely from the components of that system.

grounded theory   Hypothesizing inductively from data, notably using subjects' own categories, concepts, and so forth.

Guttman scale   A type of composite measure used to summarize several discrete observations and to represent some more general variable.

Hawthorne effect   A term coined in reference to a series of productivity studies at the Hawthorne plant of the Western Electric Company in Chicago. The researchers discovered that their presence affected the behavior of the workers being studied. The term now refers to any impact of research on the subject of study.

heterogeneous   Having a wide variety of characteristics; the use of heterogeneous subjects reduces the risk of bias in studies not using random sampling.

history effect   The effect of an event unrelated to the planned study that occurs during the time of the study and could influence the responses of subjects.

homoscedasticity   Descriptive term for the combination of two assumptions: homogeneity of variance and normally distributed dependent variables.

hypothesis   A provisional theory set forth to explain some class of phenomena, either accepted as a guide to future investigation (working hypothesis) or assumed for the sake of argument and testing. A statement to be tested in a study. An expectation about the nature of things derived from a theory. A statement about the relationships.

hypothesis testing   The determination of whether the expectations that a hypothesis represents are, indeed, found to exist in the real world.

human subjects   Living individuals whose physiologic or behavioral characteristics or responses are studied in a research project.

inclusion criteria   Sampling requirements identified by the researcher that must be present for the element or subject to be included in the sample.

independent variable   A phenomenon that is manipulated by the researcher and is predicted to have an effect on another phenomenon. A variable whose values are not problematical in an analysis but are taken as simply given. An independent variable is presumed to cause or determine a dependent variable.

in-depth interview   Face-to-face conversations used to explore details of topic.

index   An observation or measure that indicates the presence of a phenomenon, relationship, or characteristic. May also be the baseline (i.e., starting point) for a series of observations or measurements of the same variable.

indicator   A thing or person that indicates and, therefore, can serve as a proxy for a concept.

indirect measurement   Measurement of indicators or attributes of an abstract concept rather than of the abstraction itself.

induction   The logical model in which general principles are developed from specific observations.

inductive research   Any form of reasoning in which the conclusion, although supported by the premises, does not follow them necessarily. Research as discovery is used to develop or generate hypotheses. Inductive research is used to move from observation to development of hypotheses.

inferential statistics   Statistical methods that make it possible to draw tentative conclusions about a population based on observations of a sample selected from that population and furthermore make a probability statement about those conclusions to aid in their evaluation; inferential methods include sampling theory, hypothesis testing, and parameter estimation.

informed consent   The process used to inform subjects of the risks, benefits, and goals of research studies. It usually involves a printed information section and a signature page attesting to understanding those risks and benefits and consent to participate. Consent and the consent form may also outline the subject's expected obligations to the study.

institutional review   A process of examining study proposals for ethical concerns by a committee representing an institution.

institutional review board (IRB)   A specially constituted review body established or designated by an entity to protect the welfare of human subjects recruited to participate in biomedical or behavioral research.

intercept   The value of y when x equals zero in a regression statistic.

internal validity   The extent to which the individual items constituting a composite measure are correlated with the measure itself. This provides one test of the wisdom of including all the items in the composite measure. Threats to internal validity include history, maturation, testing, instrumentation, selection, loss of subjects, causal time-order, compensation, demoralization, and diffusion or imitation of treatments.

interrater reliability   The degree of consistency between two raters who are independently assigning ratings to a variable or attribute being investigated.

interrupted time series design   A study design involving the collection of data at different points in time, as contrasted with a cross-sectional study. Also known as longitudinal study.

interval scale   Interval scale is arbitrarily assigned and at equal intervals but has no zero point.

interview   Structured or unstructured verbal communication between a researcher and a subject, during which information is obtained for a study.

judgmental sample   Purposive sample; a type of nonprobability sample in which the researcher selects the units to be observed on the basis of his or her own judgment about which ones will be the most useful or representative.

key terms   See associated key terms.

kurtosis   A quality of the distribution of a set of data dealing with whether or how much the data "pile up" around some central point; the quality of "peakedness" or "flatness" of the graphic representation of a statistical distribution.

level of significance   In the context of tests of statistical significance, the degree of likelihood that an observed, empirical relationship could be attributable to sampling error. For example, a relationship is significant at the .05 level if the likelihood of its being only a function of sampling error is no greater than 5 out of 100.

Likert scale   A type of ordinal measurement in survey questionnaires. A verbal frequency scale, Likert items uses the response categories: strongly agree, agree, disagree, and strongly disagree.

limits of confidence   A term used in constructing confidence-interval estimates of parameter values to specify our confidence that the interval includes the parameter value; using procedures for constructing a

95 percent confidence interval, for instance, we would enclose the true parameter value within its limits on 95 percent of such attempts; the higher the level of confidence, the wider the interval.

linear regression   A method of predicting the relationship of one independent variable and one dependent variable.

linear relationship   A relationship between two variables such that a straight line can be fitted satisfactorily to the points on the scatter plot; the scatter of points clusters elliptically around a straight line rather than a curve.

literature review   A review of previous relevant literature that serves as the basis or beginning point for a research endeavor.

longitudinal study   A study design involving the collection of data at different points in time.

Mann-Whitney U test   A nonparametric hypothesis-testing procedure used to decide whether two given independent samples could have arisen by chance from identically distributed populations; a test for comparing two populations based on independent random samples from each.

matrix   A two-dimensional organization; each dimension is composed of several positions or alternatives; any particular "score" is a combination of the two dimensions.

mean (M or $\bar{x}$)   The sum of the scores in a distribution of a population or collection of things divided by the number of scores. In common usage, the average.

measurement   A scheme for the assignment of numbers or symbols to specify different characteristics of a variable. Characteristics include validity, accuracy, precision, and reliability.

measurement error   A deviation from accurate or correct measurement. Random error is as likely to occur in one direction as the other around the mean. Bias is systematic error that tends to occur regularly in one direction, owing to faulty procedure or measurement technique.

measures of central tendency   Statistical procedures (mean, median, mode) for determining the center of a distribution of scores or a typical value.

median   The midpoint or midscore in a distribution. The middle number in a sequence of numbers.

meta-analysis   The statistical integration of the results of several independent studies.

methodological triangulation   The use of two or more research methods or procedures in a study.

minimal risk   A risk is minimal where the probability and magnitude of harm or discomfort anticipated in the proposed research are not greater, in and of themselves, than those ordinarily encountered in daily life or during the performance of routine physical or psychological examinations or tests.

mode   The most frequent score in a distribution.

mortality   Subjects who are lost to a study or drop out from the study or a group. It does not necessarily mean the death of the subject.

multiple linear regression   Multiple regressions incorporate more than one independent variable into an equation. This procedure almost inevitably more fully explains the dependent variable because few phenomena have a simple cause, and it removes the effect of distorting influences from the other independent variables.

multistage sampling   A process generally used with cluster sampling in which levels (stages) of sampling occur. For example, you want to study particular traits of patients admitted to hospitals in your city who are hypertensive, regardless of the admitting diagnosis. You would have to sample all the hospitals for hypertensive patients, then sample those patients, then study the traits.

multivariate analysis   The analysis of the simultaneous relationships among several variables. Examining simultaneously the effects of age, sex, and social class of patients seen by different providers would be an example of multivariate analysis. Specific techniques include factor analysis, multiple correlation, multiple regression, and path analysis, among others.

multivariate analysis of variance (MANOVA)   Extension of the basic analysis-of-variance design to include more than one independent variable. Also known as multiple-factor analysis of variance.

narrative review   When the reviewer reads and thinks about a collection of relevant studies and then writes some narrative account of whether the hypothesis under consideration seems to be supported by the evidence.

natural setting   Field settings or uncontrolled, real-life situations examined in research.

needs assessment   Questions concerned with discovering the nature and extent of a particular social problem to determine the most appropriate type of response.

neopositivism   Empirical scientific method of research that deals with observable facts that must be objectively verifiable via natural scientific method.

nominal scale   Designation of subclasses by assigning numbers or symbols that represent unique characteristics. The weakest level of measurement because it denotes the least information about observations (e.g., eye color: blue = 1; brown = 2).

nondirectional hypothesis   A hypothesis stating that a relationship exists but not predicting the exact nature of the relationship.

nonparametric statistics   Tests that do not directly incorporate estimates pertaining to population characteristics. Examples are chi-square, log-linear models, Wilcoxon matched-pairs signed ranks tests. Nonparametrics tests are used with ordinal data.

nonprobability sampling   A sample selected in some fashion other than those suggested by probability theory.

nonsampling error   Imperfections of data quality that result from factors other than sampling error, such as misunderstanding of questions by respondents, erroneous recording by interviewers and coders, or keypunch errors.

nontherapeutic research   Research conducted to generate knowledge for a discipline that does not benefit those in the study; it may benefit future patients.

normal distribution curve   The characteristic values and frequencies of a variable based on empirical observations that are predicted to follow a predicted graphic curve.

null hypothesis   A statement that statistical differences or relationships have occurred for no reason other than the laws of chance operating in an unrestricted manner. The null hypothesis is sometimes stated instead of or in addition to the hypothesis. It is a form of the hypothesis stated in a negative manner.

objectivity   A characteristic of the scientific method; the condition in which to the greatest extent possible the researcher's values and biases do not interfere with the study of the problem.

observation   Systematic watching of behavior and discussion in naturally occurring settings.

one-tailed test   A directional hypothesis test that incorporates a rejection region in only one tail of the probability curve used for a given statistic. In setting up a directional hypothesis, the researcher must be confident beforehand that there is no reason to expect differences in an opposite direction. Used only when there is a good reason to make a directional prediction.

operational definition   The concrete and specific definition of something in terms of the operations by which observations are to be categorized; definitions of variables

ordinal scale   The assignment of numbers or symbols to identify ordered relations of some characteristic, the order having unspecified intervals. Ordinal scales do

not represent the magnitude of differences, only order or ranking.

orthogonality   Statistical independence of two or more variables.

orthonormality   A situation in which all variables are normally distributed.

outcomes research   A type of research developed to examine the end results of patient care; the strategies used are a departure from traditional scientific endeavors and incorporate evaluation research, epidemiology, and economic theory perspectives. In nonpatient care settings, the focus is on objective measurement of change.

outliers   Extreme scores, which can change the mean and violate homogeneity of variance.

p **value**   The probability value level used to accept or reject a study value as significant or nonsignificant. For instance, $p < .05$, $p < .01$. Thus, if researchers report that a difference was "significant at the $p < .05$ level," they are simply saying that the probability that the outcome was due to chance is less than 5 percent.

paired sample (matched sample)   Two matched samples or groups that are studied before and after the same intervention. Also used to describe a single group that undergoes the same measurement before and after some intervention.

paradigm   A way of looking at a natural phenomenon that encompasses a set of philosophical assumptions and that guides one's approach to inquiry.

parameter   A characteristic of a population or sample.

parametric test   Statistical test that requires interval data and the assumption of a normally distributed population.

participant observation   Systematic watching of behavior and discussion in which the researcher also participates as a role in the setting in addition to observing what is taking place.

path analysis   A form of multivariate analysis in which the causal relationships among variables are presented in graphic form.

Pearson's *r* or Pearson's product-moment correlation coefficient   Parametric test used to determine the relationship between variables.

phenomenon   (singular; plural is phenomena) Any object or event, the characteristics of which can be observed.

pilot study   A smaller version of a proposed study conducted to develop or refine the methodology, such as the treatment, instrument, or data collection process.

placebo   A chemically inert substance given in the guise of medicine for its psychologically suggestive effect; used in controlled clinical trials to determine whether improvement and side effects may reflect imagination or anticipation rather than actual power of a drug.

population   The total number of members (or persons) in a defined study group or area. Any class of phenomena arbitrarily defined on the basis of its unique and observable characteristics. A set of people or events from which a sample is taken.

population distribution   The frequency with which all units or observations in a population would be assigned or expected in each category or point on a measurement scale.

population mean   The estimate of the mean of the population based on the mean of the sample and normal distribution.

poster session   Visual presentation of studies at a professional gathering, using pictures, tables, and illustrations on a display board.

power   The probability that a statistical test will detect a significant difference that exists.

power analysis   Analysis used to determine the risk of a Type II error, so the study can be modified to decrease the risk if necessary.

practice effect   Improvement of subject performance because of increased familiarity with the experimental protocol.

precision   The exactness of the measure used in an observation or description of an attribute.

prediction   The ability to estimate the probability of a specific outcome in a given situation.

predictive validity   The degree to which an instrument can predict some criterion observed at a future time.

principal investigator   In a research grant, the individual who has primary responsibility for administering the grant and interacting with the funding agency.

privacy   Control over the extent, timing, and circumstances of sharing oneself (physically, behaviorally, or intellectually) with others.

probability sample   The general term for a sample selected in accordance with probability theory, typically involving some random-selection mechanism. Specific types of probability samples include area probability sample, simple random sample, and systematic sample.

proofs   In publishing, the "hard copy" of the typesetter's work. Proofs may resemble the finished pages of the publication or may be "galley proofs"—plain, one-column text to be reviewed and corrected (usually by the proofreader and editor) before the pages are laid out.

proposal   Written plan identifying the major elements of a research study, such as the problem, purpose, and framework, and outlining the methods to conduct the study. A formal way to communicate ideas about a proposed study to receive approval to conduct the study and to seek funding.

proposition   An abstract statement that further clarifies the relationship between two concepts.

protocol   The formal design or plan of an experiment or research activity; specifically, the plan submitted to an IRB for review and to an agency for research support. The protocol includes a description of the research design or methodology to be employed, the eligibility requirements for prospective subjects and controls, the treatment regimen(s), and the proposed methods of analysis that will be performed on the collected data.

purposive sample   A type of nonprobability sample in which the units to be observed are selected on the basis of one's own judgment about which ones will be the most useful or representative. Same as judgment sample.

qualitative analysis   The nonnumerical examination and interpretation of observations for the purpose of describing and explaining the phenomena that those observations reflect.

quantitative research   The use of applied mathematics to assist in the research process.

quasi-experimental designs   Research designs used when the researcher has little interest in establishing cause-and-effect relationships but is more concerned about measuring constructs and collecting data from a representative sample of individuals. The internal validity of these designs is threatened, and causal inferences about the effect of independent variables on dependent variables are difficult to make.

quota sample   A type of nonprobability sample in which units are selected into the sample on the basis of prespecified characteristics, so that the total sample has the same distribution of characteristics as are assumed to exist in the population being studied.

R^2   Coefficient of determination. Indicates the percent variance of y accounted for by x_1 and x_2 in combination.

random sample   A collection of phenomena so selected that each phenomenon in the population has an equal chance of being selected.

range   The highest score in a distribution minus the lowest score.

ratio scale   The assignment of numbers to identify ordered relations of some characteristic, the order having been arbitrarily assigned and at equal intervals, but with an absolute zero point. The ratio scale specifies values and differences that are applicable to arithmetic operations and to statements about phenomena. Age is a ratio measure (scale).

references   The specific items or units used as information resources for a study or written report. References can be texts, journal articles, individuals, and so forth. They are generally noted in the body of a report and listed in the bibliography.

regression analysis   The analysis of the relationship of sets of scores for two variables.

regression coefficient   The amount of increase of one variable with each unit of increase in another.

rejection region (significance level)   A level of probability set by the researcher as grounds for the rejection of the null hypothesis. If a calculated value of probability falls within the rejection region, the researcher interprets the difference or relationship as statistically significant.

relative risk (RR)   A ratio that represents the probability of developing an outcome within a specific period when a risk factor is present, divided by the probability of developing the outcome in the same period if the risk factor is not present.

reliability   The external and internal consistency of a measurement. In the abstract, whether a particular technique, applied repeatedly to the same object, would yield the same result each time.

representativeness   That quality of a sample having the same distribution of characteristics as the population from which it was selected. By implication, descriptions and explanations derived from an analysis of the sample may be assumed to represent similar ones in the population. Representativeness is enhanced by probability sampling and provides for generalizability and the use of inferential statistics.

research design   The plan, protocol, format, and parameters of the research project.

research hypothesis   A statement expressing differences or relationships among phenomena, the acceptance or non-acceptance of which implies the existence of a null hypothesis that is susceptible to a probability estimate.

research methods   The methods used in systematic inquiry into a subject in order to discover or revise facts, theories, and so on. Examples include experiments, survey research, field research, content analysis, replication, historical research, comparative research, and evaluation research.

research proposal   Written proposal that provides a preview of why a study will be undertaken and how it will be conducted. It is a useful device for planning

and is required in most circumstances when research is being conducted.

research question   A formal statement of the purpose of the investigation stated as a question

respect for persons   An ethical principle requiring that individual autonomy be respected and that persons with diminished autonomy be protected.

response formats   Types of replies allowed by questions (e.g., open-ended versus close-ended).

response rate   The number of persons participating in a survey divided by the number selected in the sample, in the form of a percentage; the percentage of questionnaires sent out that are returned.

risk   The probability of harm or injury (physical, psychological, social, or economic) occurring as a result of participation in a research study. Both the probability and magnitude of possible harm may vary from minimal to significant. Federal regulations define only "minimal risk."

robust   Remaining useful even when its assumptions are violated (said of a statistic).

sample   A collection of phenomena selected to represent some well-defined population.

sample distribution   The frequency with which observations in a sample are assigned to each category or point on a measurement scale.

sampling bias   Inherent bias in a sample. Sources: nonrandom, systematic sampling; incomplete or inaccurate sampling frame; nonresponse. Sampling bias causes systematic error not compensated for by increasing the size of the sample.

sampling error   An estimate of how statistics may be expected to deviate from parameters when sampling randomly from a given population.

sampling frame   The list of units or criteria composing a population from which a sample is selected. If the sample is to be representative of the population, it is essential that the sampling frame include all (or nearly all) members of the population.

sampling ratio   The proportion of elements in the population that are selected to be in a sample.

sampling size   The number of subjects, usually designated as "n," in each category, group, and so forth used in the research study.

sampling statistics   Calculated values that represent how sample characteristics are likely to vary from population characteristics.

scale   A specific scheme for assigning numbers or symbols to designate characteristics of a variable. Nominal, ordinal, interval, and ratio are examples of scales. Scales can be single-item or multiple-item measures.

scatterplot   A two-dimensional dot plot that places data in an *x* and *y* grid.

scientific method   A process of discovery by systematic investigation.

secondary analysis   A form of research in which the data collected and processed by one researcher are analyzed—often for a different purpose—by another. This is especially appropriate in the case of survey data.

semantic differential scale   A specialized type of Likert-like scale that measures the meaning of an object to an individual using a scale.

significance   The level of calculated probability that was sufficiently low as to serve as grounds for rejection of the null hypothesis.

single-factor analysis of variance   A statistical model used for testing the significance of difference among two or more means when these means reflect the consequences of different levels of a single independent variable. See analysis of variance (ANOVA).

skewed   Term used to describe unusual or odd distributions.

snowball sample   A nonprobability sampling method often employed in epidemiology research. Each person interviewed may be asked to suggest additional people for interviewing. Used to track down the source of a communicable disease.

specification   Explanatory and clarifying comments about the handling of difficult or confusing situations that may occur with regard to specific questions in a questionnaire.

spurious relationship   A relationship that gives a false impression because it is without a base in theory or common sense.

standard deviation (SD)   The square root of the mean of the squared deviation scores about the mean of a distribution; more simply, the square root of the variance. SD gives a basis for estimating the probability of how frequently certain scores can be expected to occur in a sample.

standard error of the mean   The standard deviation of a distribution of sample means; describes the likely deviations of sample means about the population mean.

standardized score   A value that results from methods of converting values from different distributions into scores that can be compared.

static-group comparison   Studies based on experimental and control groups but using no pretests.

statistic   A characteristic of a sample. Statistics provides the mathematical models for reasoning, providing a framework for reasoning from data so that generalized statements about the data can be made. Types include descriptive and sampling statistics.

statistical inference   The process of estimating parameters from statistics.

statistical power   The degree of a test's sensitivity.

statistical significance level   The level of probability that an association between two (or more) variables could have been produced by chance. Expressed as a "*p* value" and referred to as the level of significance. Arbitrarily set by the investigators, but commonly at the .05 or .01 level.

statistical test   A test that addresses the question, "Could the observed relationship between *x* and *y* have occurred by chance?" Statistical tests state the relationship between variables by some specified degree.

stratification   The sorting of the units composing a population into homogeneous groups (strata) before sampling.

survey techniques   Research methods to collect data from populations. These include face-to-face interviews, survey questionnaires (by mail or in person), telephone interviewing, and group interviewing.

systematic sample   A type of probability sample in which every *k*th unit in a list is selected for inclusion in the sample: for example, every 25th patient visiting a clinic.

t-table   A statistical table of percentage points of the "*t*" distribution. Used with statistical analyses that produce a "*t*" value.

t-test (Student's t-test)   Test of the difference between two population means, based on the observed difference between two sample means and their distribution.

theory   Statement that integrates a large number of simple laws and their associated variables, contributing to scientific knowledge and generating new testable hypotheses.

triangulation   Use of three or more different research methods in combination; often used as a check for validity.

two-tailed test   A nondirectional hypothesis test that incorporates rejection regions in both tails of the probability curve used for a given statistic. Also known as nondirectionality tests.

type I error   Rejecting a null hypothesis when it should have been retained.

type II error   Retaining a null hypothesis when it should have been rejected.

units of analysis   The what or whom being studied, such as individual people.

univariate analysis   The examination of the distribution of cases on only one variable at a time. Usually reported in the form of frequency distributions, central tendencies (averages), and dispersions (ranges and standard deviations).

validity   The degree to which a scale is in fact consistently measuring the variable that it was designed to measure.

variable   An observable characteristic of an object or event that can be described according to some well-defined classification or measurement scheme; an observable phenomenon.

variable, dichotomous   (also binary, dummy) A variable with only two values.

variance   The mean of the squared deviation scores about the mean of a distribution.

voluntary   Free of coercion, duress, or undue inducement. Used in the research context to refer to a subject's decision to participate (or to continue to participate) in a research activity.

weighted mean   A procedure for combining the means of groups of different sizes.

Wilcoxon test   A nonparametric test for use with related samples.

Wilks lambda (λ)   A commonly used test for group mean equality in multivariate tests.

***x*-axis**   The horizontal axis on a graph, also called the abscissa.

***x*-variable**   Variable plotted on the horizontal axis, usually the independent variable

***y*-axis**   The vertical axis on a graph, also called the ordinate.

***y*-variable**   Variable plotted on the vertical axis, usually the dependent variable.

***z*-score (lowercase *z*)**   A commonly used standard score that gives a measure of relative location in the distribution where the mean is 0.

***z*-score (uppercase Z)**   A standard score, based on manipulation of the *z*-score, where the mean of the distribution is 50 and the standard deviation is 10 to provide a whole number score that allows comparison.

Note: Page numbers followed by f refer to figures; page numbers followed by t refer to tables; page numbers followed by b refer to boxes.